For the Least of My Brethren

Dear Christina

you were such an important part of St. Michael's Hospital. You will be missed, however, you should know that you will never be forgotten. Your professional, kind, caring approach in all that you did in your daily work will inspire others to do their best each day. You were my right hand for 11 wonderful years. I learned from you and will value our friendship forever.

Best wishes for good health and happiness in your retirement.

In Love,
Ello.

For the Least of My Brethren

A Centenary History of St Michael's Hospital

Irene McDonald, c.s.j.

Toronto and Oxford
Dundurn Press
1992

Editing: Curtis Fahey
Design and Production: Ron & Ron Design Photography
Printing and Binding: Gagné Printing Ltd., Louiseville, Quebec, Canada

The writing of this manuscript and the publication of this book were made possible by support from several sources. The publisher wishes to acknowledge the generous assistance and ongoing support of **The Canada Council, The Book Publishing Industry Development Program** of the **Department of Communications, The Ontario Arts Council,** and **The Ontario Publishing Centre** of the **Ministry of Culture and Communications.**

Care has been taken to trace the ownership of copyright material used in the text (including the illustrations). The author and publisher welcome any information enabling them to rectify any reference or credit in subsequent editions.

J. Kirk Howard, Publisher

Canadian Cataloguing in Publication Data

McDonald, Irene, 1922–
      For the least of my brethren: a centenary history of St. Michael's Hospital

1. St. Michael's Hospital (Toronto, Ont.) – History.
2. Hospitals – Ontario – Toronto – History.
3. Catholic hospitals – Ontario – Toronto – History.   I. Title.

ISBN 1-55002-181-8   (bound)   ISBN   1-55002-182-6   (pbk.)

RA983.T672S32   1992   362.1'1'09713541   C92-095376-X

Dundurn Press Limited
2181 Queen Street East
Suite 301
Toronto, Canada
M4E 1E5

Dundurn Distribution
73 Lime Walk
Headington, Oxford
England
OX3 7AD

To all the women and men whose part in the building of St Michael's Hospital is recorded here, and to those countless others whose indispensable contribution has not been fully recognized, I gratefully dedicate this book.

Contents

Glossary of Abbreviations

ACU	Acute Care Unit
AO	Archives of Ontario
ARCAT	Archives of the Roman Catholic Archdiocese of Toronto
ASMH	Archives of St Michael's Hospital
ASSJ	Archives of the Sisters of St Joseph
CCHA	Canadian Council on Hospital Accreditation
CCU	Coronary Care Unit
CIU	Clinical Investigation Unit
CTA	City of Toronto Archives
CV	Cardiovascular
DHC	District Health Council
FACC	Fellow of American College of Cardiologists
FACS	Fellow of the American College of Surgeons
FCOG	Fellow of the College of Obstetricians and Gynaecologists
FRCP	Fellow of the Royal College of Physicians
FRCS	Fellow of the Royal College of Surgeons
HCMT	Hospital Council of Metropolitan Toronto
ICU	Intensive Care Unit
LMCC	Licentiate Medical Council of Canada
LRCP	Licentiate Royal College of Physicians
MAB	Medical Advisory Board
MAC	Medical Advisory Committee
MB	Bachelor of Medicine
MB,BS	Bachelor of Medicine, Bachelor of Surgery (UK)
MB,ChB	Bachelor of Medicine, Bachelor of Surgery (Latin)
MCPSO	Member of the College of Physicians and Surgeons of Ontario
MRCS	Member of Royal College of Surgeons
MRI	Magnetic Resonance Imaging
OHA	Ontario Hospital Association
OHIP	Ontario Hospital Insurance Plan
OHSC	Ontario Hospital Services Commission
OHRDP	Ontario Hospital Redevelopment Plan
OMA	Ontario Medical Association
OMCW	Ontario Medical College for Women
SCC	Senior Coordinating Committee (of the OHSC)
SJHS	St Joseph Health System
UTA	University of Toronto Archives
UTHA	University Teaching Hospitals Association
WCB	Workers' Compensation Board

Acknowledgments

My first acknowledgment must be to the Sisters of St Joseph of Toronto, especially to Sister Imelda Cahill, general superior at the time the decision was made to begin this work, and to her successor, Sister Mary Beth Montcalm, who has continued to support the project. I am honoured to have been entrusted with the task of preparing a history of St Michael's Hospital for my congregation.

I am indebted to Sister Christine Gaudet and to Jeffrey Lozon, the former and current presidents of St Michael's, who put at my disposal the hospital records and a place to work on them. I am particularly indebted to Sister Camilla Young, whose superb organization of the hospital's archives has greatly facilitated my search, and to her successor, Marina Engelsakis, whose competent, ready assistance has been of great value. The help of Sandy Collins, Alex McDonald, and John Fagan of the hospital's department of medical photography is gratefully acknowledged.

I have been greatly assisted by the staffs of the Archives of Ontario, the City of Toronto Archives, and the University of Toronto Archives. Other archivists deserving of my deepest thanks are Sister Mary Jane Trimble of the Archives of the Sisters of St Joseph and Sister Frieda Watson, archivist for the Roman Catholic Archdiocese of Toronto, and her staff. Without exception, the archivists at all these institutions are true professionals. In addition to her advice with regard to archival documents, Sister Frieda rendered invaluable service by reading and offering criticism of the manuscript along the way. Her comments both encouraged and prodded the author, while improving the product.

I am grateful to the sisters with whom I live; they have lived through my preoccupation with this work and have shared my excitement over it. I am especially grateful to Sister Rita DeLuca, who typed the first draft.

To Sister Mary Thomas Ford, who cheerfully typed and retyped numerous drafts, and to my editor, Curtis Fahey, who painstakingly did what editors do, I owe a huge debt of gratitude. Both sacrificed personal time to meet my time constraints.

9

Lastly, my greatest debt is owed to all those who recorded the happenings down the years and kept them against the day when they could all be pieced together to produce a history of St Michael's Hospital. The credit for furnishing the material is theirs; the responsibility for any flaws in interpreting and presenting that material rests solely with the author.

Preface

For the Least of My Brethren is a history of the first one hundred years of St Michael's Hospital. It is a record of steps taken, difficulties encountered and, occasionally, mistakes made in the achievement of the hospital's mission – full and responsible partnership with government and society at large in the provision of health care to the people of Toronto and of Ontario.

While the bare facts of St Michael's history can be identified in the official documents of the times, the documents alone cannot adequately convey the vision and courage, the energy and resourcefulness, the compassion and commitment of the leading figures in that history, nor of the countless others who supported them. This book is an attempt to put names and faces on the people behind the documents.

The records tell a story of a changing health-care scene, and of how this story shaped St Michael's over the century. There is the pioneer handful of sisters, unprepared for health care, who grew in numbers and professional qualifications sufficient to provide the hands-on leadership for this first Catholic hospital in Toronto and first Catholic school of nursing in Canada – a leadership that has tapered off only in the past very few years. There is the medical staff – beginning with one young man, just out of medical school and fired with enthusiasm, and evolving through one hundred years into a fully rounded staff, among whom are several with solid international reputations in research and practice.

There is the story of bills to be paid and of those who searched for the money to pay them, especially the board members all down the years, and there is the story of increasing government intervention – beginning with the grudging admission of St Michael's in 1895 to the league of hospitals that might apply for the forty-cent-a-day grant from the city of Toronto, and ending with a provincially sponsored health plan which in 1992 may pay as much as $1000 a day for an inpatient's care. Between these two dates, for more than half a century St Michael's was largely supported by the donated services of the sisters, and even later their salaries were channelled to fund the capital costs of the new technologies and the facilities to house them.

There is the record of St Michael's involvement in medical education through the years – from the withering query of an 1899 city councillor, "Are medical students *really* going to St. Michael's?," to the 1980s and 1990s when this hospital became a popular choice for internship and post-graduate training for medical students from across Canada. There is the proud eighty-year record of St Michael's involvement in nursing education, both basic and post-graduate, the parameters of which were radically changed with the shift into the community colleges in the years following 1974; St Michael's other on-site educational programs followed a similar path.

After groping its way to a first affiliation agreement with the University of Toronto, St Michael's went on to become and remain a respected senior partner within the university's health sciences complex, despite the long shadow cast from the first by its older hospital partner (Toronto General) and later by its better-endowed partners.

The movement in patient care has been a spiral upwards from a one-room emergency, a simple outpatients clinic, and a few dozen beds to a sprawling 900-bed facility – and downwards and outwards to an emphasis on ambulatory and day care as well as tertiary care. Through it all, St Michael's one constant has been its sick poor; those familiar with this hospital may suggest that that's where St Michael's heart still is in 1992.

Sister Irene McDonald, C.S.J.
Toronto, Ontario, September 1992

1
A Start Is Made

The story of great and enduring human enterprises is, in large part, the story of great people who have endured – men and women whose lives have been deeply interwoven with the history of their times, vigorously continuous with what went before and what would come after. These people grasped the challenges and the opportunities contained in their moment of time and, in so doing, moved their particular enterprise above and beyond what they had inherited to a new level of life and, in the case of hospitals, of service. The history of St Michael's Hospital is about such people and their times, and about the contribution they made toward shaping St Michael's over the last century. The St Michael's that exists today, on its one hundredth anniversary, is testimony to their efforts.

The beginnings, growth to maturity, and character of St Michael's Hospital can be understood only within the context of the surrounding culture – political, social, economic, and religious – which has pressed and prompted, hampered, or even hurt the hospital at every stage of its development since its founding in 1892. Indeed, a history of St Michael's must also take into account the fifty dynamic years that preceded the hospital's founding, years that had a profound effect on the shape of the city of Toronto and on its institutions.

But the challenge to health and to the health-care providers of Toronto goes back even a further fifty years: Lieutenant-Governor John Graves Simcoe chose to found the new town of York in 1793 on what was then a mosquito-ridden swamp, a choice that for decades would be a factor in the annual outbreaks of typhoid, diphtheria, and scarlet fever, with their toll of human misery. One of these outbreaks would be the catalyst for the founding of St Michael's Hospital.

A Community in Formation, 1793-1847[1]

The steady trickle of British immigrants to the new town of York between 1793 and the War of 1812 came largely from the British upper and middle classes. These people came to fill military, civil,

13

and professional posts, and brought with them a particular set of beliefs, attitudes, and social skills. As a result, for two to three decades the town of York remained conservative and thoroughly British in its social makeup and outlook, and Anglican in its religious adherence. The influx of settlers from the United States between the American revolution and the War of 1812 did little to alter the basically British character of the town.

After the War of 1812-14 there began another wave of immigration, this time from a Great Britain in the throes of rapid industrialization. A measure of the strain inherent in absorbing the newcomers, and also of the charity of the citizens of York, was the foundation in 1817 of the Society for the Relief of Strangers, an organization that for years would be the principal agency concerned with assisting distressed immigrants, the sick, and the abandoned. Later, in the summer of 1832, the town was faced with its most serious social crisis to date – the arrival of eleven thousand immigrants, many poor and sick with cholera, from impoverished Ireland. One can only imagine the extent to which such an influx changed the balance and the established order of the young town, fairly comfortable and secure in its homogeneity but primitive and inexperienced in its capacity to extend social services.

Social services were strained most particularly in the summer, when cholera was at its worst; in the summer of 1834 it claimed five hundred fatalities, out of a population of less than 14,000. York Hospital (the future Toronto General Hospital) was given over completely to the care of the victims, and cholera sheds were set up on the hospital grounds. A Board of Health, whose powers appear to have been more apparent than real, was created to deal with the epidemic. Accounts of the sanitary conditions of the time do not paint a pretty picture – food and water supplies contaminated from garbage piled in the streets, pigs roaming at will through the town, and privy waste overflowing in backyards or dumped into the harbour.

But life went on, and even vigorously. In 1834 the town was incorporated as the first city in Upper Canada and its name was changed from York to Toronto. The only hospital at the time was the General Hospital; it was badly in need of new facilities, which would not come until 1855. Still, the new city boasted a good harbour, plank roads, a gas-lit main street, and waterworks throughout. Upper Canada College had been founded in 1830, publicly endowed and entrusted with the mission of preparing future leaders for society. King's College, which included a faculty of medicine, opened its doors in 1844. Within the dynamic ten to fifteen years following the city's incorporation, there evolved a strong and assertive business class with extensive wholesale, banking, and insurance operations. All things considered, Toronto was on a modest upward swing.

The religious and ethnic composition of the town also changed rapidly after the War of 1812. Irish Catholics started construction of St Paul's Church in 1822; simultaneously the conservative, pro-British, and vehemently anti-Catholic Orange Order made its emergence, and, in the words of historian J.M.S. Careless, "the long Orange Walk through Toronto history" had begun.[2] There came to York/Toronto, as well, English non-conformists, Scottish Presbyterians, and Irish Methodists. The stable, established order of an English-Anglican gentry was soon faced with an expanded middle-class and a burgeoning lower class, and the social nature of the city was further destabilized with the influx of Irish Catholics fleeing the potato famine of 1846-47.[3] Uneducated, untrained, and impoverished, they inevitably settled into the lowest level of Toronto society, the first of its urban poor.

Thirty thousand "famine Irish" flooded into Toronto in the summer of 1847. Typhus had broken out on the ships carrying them to the New World, with the result that many died on the voyage and countless little children arrived motherless or fatherless or both. Worse still, disease came with the immigrants. Again the General Hospital responded magnificently, erecting and equipping sheds on the hospital grounds for the care of the new arrivals. The hospital superintendent, Dr George Grasett, himself fell victim to typhus, as did the first Catholic bishop of the diocese of Toronto, Michael Power, as well as other Torontonians who overcame their fear to come to the aid of the stricken immigrants. The city possessed little in the way of public welfare and, understandably, the Board of Health was overwhelmed and quite unable to cope with the extent of the wrenching human tragedy – "whole families lying under the shelter of fences and trees ... within the very heart of town ... begging for food."[4] All of this within a city that, a few years before, was enjoying a confident and prosperous youth.

Charbonnel's Legacy, 1850-92

It was to this troubled scene that Armand-François-Marie de Charbonnel came as Roman Catholic bishop in 1850. Well-born and well-connected, Bishop Charbonnel lost no time in using his connections for the sake of his new flock. He was familiar with the Sisters of St Joseph and their works in his native France.[5] Now his call went out to them at their first North American foundation, established in St Louis, Missouri, in 1836; in 1851 four sisters of St Joseph came, two from St Louis and two from Philadelphia – a week's journey by boat and stagecoach from the latter city. They took charge of an already established orphanage at 100 Nelson (now Jarvis) Street. A year later, the energetic bishop brought the Basilian Fathers, under whom he had done his classical studies in France, to help with the preparation of priests. Charbonnel immediately served notice on the powerful Egerton Ryerson, chief superintendent of education in Canada West (Ontario), that Roman Catholics "must have, and we will have full management of our schools."[6] The School Bill of 1853 established the dual educational system that gave the Catholics of Canada West a separate financial structure for their schools and their own boards of trustees.[7]

Although he spoke English with some difficulty, Bishop Charbonnel was a catalyst for change on a wide scale. One of the most notable achievements of his episcopate was a comprehensive Catholic welfare system which he gradually put in place through the efforts of the Sisters of St Joseph, Catholic laywomen, and the St Vincent de Paul Society – the last modelled on an organization that Charbonnel had known in France. The scope of the bishop's social-welfare activities was nothing short of spectacular: not just the usual food, clothing, and shelter, but a savings bank, a fuel cooperative, distribution of tools to workmen, and an employment agency.[8]

Historian Murray Nicolson records that by the end of the century the destitute and downtrodden Irish had achieved some measure of independence and sense of self-worth, an accomplishment owing in large part to the efforts of the French bishop and the religious orders, French in origin, which he imported and whose personnel became, within a few years, Irish and working class.[9] The silver lining was beginning to shine through the cloud for the Irish of Toronto; beside it there glowered, however, a Protestant crusade that lasted for almost eighty years. The crusade was originally triggered by the influx of so many diseased, dirty, poor (and sometimes drunk and disorderly) Irish into what had been until then an upper and middle-class town; it was perpetuated by the anti-Catholic, anti-Irish crusade waged by the press, especially George Brown's *Globe*, and by the Orange Order, whose outrages even Brown condemned.[10]

The Sisters of St Joseph were deeply engaged throughout these turbulent forty years between their arrival in Toronto and the founding of St Michael's Hospital. They quickly (1852) moved beyond the care of orphans into the schools and, with the Loretto Sisters, who had arrived four years ahead of them, and the Christian Brothers, were partners in a Catholic school system which by 1892 had thirteen schools and 4500 pupils.[11]

Notre Dame des Anges,
Precursor of St Michael's Hospital

The sisters moved their headquarters in 1854 from the original foundation on Nelson Street between Richmond and Lombard streets, to Power Street where they opened a boarding and day school for girls. From there in 1871, the congregation having experienced a spurt of rapid growth, the headquarters were moved to St Alban Street (now Wellesley Street). The Nelson Street orphanage was converted to an industrial school for girls, known as Notre Dame des Anges.[12] The word "industrial" is misleading; the house was intended as a comfortable boarding place for girls coming to the city to attend normal school, learn a trade, or seek employment.

Some interesting bits of information about Notre Dame des Anges:[13] in 1873 the rate for board was $2.50 per week; a canonical visitation in January 1880 lists a superior and seven sisters living there, as well as "25 inmates, of whom 3 are Protestant." An 1884 record of the school (in which it is referred to as the Notre Dame Industrial Home) suggests that it served as a kind of employment agency – "servants provided with situation: 87." Nonetheless, it was a difficult place to finance, the same record showing "arrears for board, $432.00" and unpaid wood and grocery bills. An undated handwritten list of women at Notre Dame des Anges, probably about this time, names persons kept while "out of situations" and unable to pay board; the occupations of the women were listed as seamstress, machinist, general servant, immigrant (thirty-two were listed), and orphan (fourteen listed).

In 1885 the Notre Dame des Anges operations were moved to 32 Bond Street. Nine years earlier, what appears to have been a circular from Archbishop John Joseph Lynch to the Catholic people of Toronto stated: "We have purchased the Baptist Church on Bond St., near our Cathedral, for Catholic purposes – a children's church, a lecture hall, reading rooms for various religious confraternities … The Church proper can seat a thousand persons … We have considered the mode of collecting the sum required [to pay for it] … that each Catholic of the city contribute the wages, earnings, or income of one day in this year."[14] Attached to the above document are several printed blank forms for subscription, printed in the name of the St John Baptist Catholic Institute and receipted with Archbishop Lynch's stamped signature.

In connection with this purchase, there is preserved an old mortgage document which indicated that the Regular Baptist church, through its trustees, had bought the lot for £1,000 on 27 June 1855. The Toronto census of 1871 shows 1900 Baptists in a population of 56,000; the same census lists 20,600 Anglicans, 11,800 Roman Catholics, 9,600 Methodists, and 8,900 Presbyterians.[15]

There is no record of what renovations Archbishop Lynch had made to the property for church use, or of what specific renovations were later made to accommodate Notre Dame des Anges. There is evidence that one $10,000 loan and others totalling $6,575 were arranged by the sisters in payment for the building.[16] There remains an 1887 document, on the letterhead of Notre Dame des Anges, 32 Bond Street, which bears a sketch of the edifice – a sturdy three-storey building with a two-storey attachment, shielded by a high fence. The document illustrates a remarkable change in the clientele from those listed in 1880: eleven private boarders, two medical students, three artists, two conservatory of music students, six normal school students (the normal school was within walking distance, off Yonge, at Gould Street), 5 business college students, eight bookkeepers and clerks, fourteen machinists and dressmakers, four milliners, four apprentices, six domestic servants, and four "kept free" – sixty-nine residents in all. The majority do not seem to fit the industrial school classification; this may indicate a change in philosophy of the house, yet as late as 1891 it was receiving an annual grant of $200 from the city in its capacity as an industrial school for girls.[17]

The Isolation Hospital

On 26 November 1891 a special meeting of the sisters' General Council (the senior administrative body of the congregation) was called to consider a proposition set before it by the Board of Health through Dr Norman Allen, medical superintendent of the Diphtheria Hospital, who had already pleaded his case both with the sisters and with the archbishop. Allen asked that "three Sisters be sent to the Isolation Hospital – one to act as Matron, having the entire charge. Two trained nurses are already on duty and a third to be called in." The request added that "whatever was decided upon for the Sisters' remuneration the Board of Health would consent to settle unhesitatingly."[18]

The open-ended nature of the proposal indicates that the board and its health officer were in desperate circumstances. The council immediately called for volunteers; from among these they appointed Sister Juliana as directress or matron, as well as Sister de Sales and Sister St Felix, a novice.[19] [Speaking at the graduation exercises of St Michael's Hospital School of Nursing in 1903, Allen recalled that the sisters were the *only* volunteers who went to the relief of the afflicted.] It was agreed that the Board of Health would be asked to pay $5 per week for each sister – that is, one-half of what the trained nurses would be getting.

It was to the old Isolation Hospital in Riverdale Park (earlier known as the Old House of Refuge, which was concerned with the reformation of prostitutes[20]) that the sisters went in 1891; the construction of the new Isolation Hospital, which would later become Riverdale Hospital, did not begin until 1892. Construction of the new hospital was in response to an order from the High Court "prohibiting the further use of the building on Broadview Ave., north of the jail, as an Infectious Disease Hospital."[21] In other words, the building was in such a state as to be condemned for use; a further idea of the state it was in can be inferred from the record that only two offers, one for $120 and one for $160, were received when it was finally put up for sale, offers which the city fathers rejected, voting to give the facility instead to the city engineer to pull down and to allow him to take the material for whatever use he could make of it.[22]

The sisters entered the Isolation Hospital at the height of the epidemic; 1,917 cases of diphtheria were treated at the hospital during the months they were there, out of a total of 2,691 during all of 1891 and 1892.[23] Care of these victims was not for the faint-hearted; as late as November 1893, of the 326 diphtheria patients admitted that year to the Isolation Hospital, 63 had died.[24] Late that same year the new Behring antitoxin serum was used –with success – to treat a patient in the Isolation Hospital, and the future became considerably brighter.

During the time the sisters were at the Isolation Hospital Dr Allen was lobbying the General Council to have them assume charge of the new isolation hospital under construction, while the council was actively considering sites for establishing a hospital of its own.[25] The beleaguered Dr Allen was successful in warding off several attempts to withdraw the sisters, but in November 1892, with the epidemic beginning to show signs of subsiding, the last of the sisters left the Isolation Hospital and were rewarded with two weeks in Barrie and St Catharines "for a necessary change of air."[26] By this time, the council had sent two other sisters, Columba and Attracta, to the Hôtel-Dieu Hospital in Montreal "to gain some knowledge of nursing."[27]

The Founding of St Michael's Hospital

While the sisters' experience at the Isolation Hospital appears to have been one of the deciding factors in a series of events that was moving them towards involvement in health care, the drama of that experience must not be allowed to obscure other factors which powerfully influenced their decision. Certainly the desirability of having their own hospital must have crossed their minds during the early years when so many of their young sisters and their students became ill and/or died, and the need for improvisation of temporary infirmary facilities recurred again and again. The annals contain no record of sisters having been admitted to the General Hospital when ill; on the contrary, there is an entry of a sister having had a breast tumour removed, under ether anaesthetic, at the convent.

Too, the desirability, and even the need, for the sisters to open a hospital for the people of Toronto, especially the sick poor, had become increasingly evident. In October 1869, after the Toronto General Hospital had been closed for a full year for lack of funds, Bishop Lynch proposed to that hospital's board that the Sisters of Charity take over the domestic management of the institution, a move which, he suggested, would save the hospital hundreds of dollars annually.[28] While it is not known for certain that he was referring to the Sisters of St Joseph, it is highly probable that he was, for they were often referred to as Sisters of Charity, even in semi-official records.[29]

That Bishop Lynch was serious is evident from the energy with which he followed up his original proposal over a period of five years, several times requesting meetings with the General's trustees, submitting a second proposal, and publishing the latter in the newspapers complete with an embarrassing reminder to the trustees that "by refusing the extended offer you pronounce upon the life or death of many of your fellow citizens." So concerned was Lynch about the sick poor that he even offered to clear out a section of the House of Providence (an institution founded by Bishop Charbonnel in 1856 for the relief of the poor and destitute, operated and staffed by the Sisters of St Joseph) for their care, setting up a "supplementary hospital" to the General.

In politely declining the bishop's offer of the sisters' services, the trustees pointed out that, although they themselves would be open to the idea, the citizens of Toronto would "assume the Sisters would use their opportunities of inculcating the precepts and doctrine of their Church."[30] To decline the offer must have been a difficult decision for the trustees, who, in the absence of systematic government support for charitable institutions, were struggling desperately to meet expenses.

The above forms a backdrop for a decision that began to take shape in October 1890. As the General Council considered the future of the debt-ridden Notre Dame des Anges, one of the councillors proposed that it should become a hospital. No further mention is made of the proposal until a year later when the council considered the offer of a Mr B.B. Hughes to sell his property to the congregation, for use as a hospital, for the sum of $65,000. It was at that same council meeting that the original plea of Dr Norman Allen for sisters to help at the Isolation Hospital was considered and acceded to.

This brings us to the question of Dr Allen's influence in the sisters' eventual decision to open a hospital. In sketches of St Michael's, one finds the suggestion that it was founded in response to requests from Dr Allen. The author has found nothing in the congregation records to substantiate this claim. In fact, a hospital had been proposed thirteen months before he ever surfaces in the congregation records, and a site was already being actively sought at the time he first appears. (Dr Walter McKeown, a future surgeon at St Michael's, brought him to the episcopal palace and to the convent to plead his case for the sisters' help, first with the archbishop, and then with the council.) The B.B. Hughes offer of a hospital site continued to be the subject of council discussion throughout the sisters' involvement at the Isolation Hospital.[31]

On 1 May 1892 the council decided that Notre Dame would be the site of its first hospital in Toronto; thereafter events moved with incredible speed, for two months later, on 1 July 1892, the hospital opened its doors to its first patients.

The original capacity (twenty-six beds) was increased the next year to seventy-three beds when a further area of the building was given over to hospital use. How the name was decided upon is not recorded; council minutes dated 17 August 1892 – six weeks after the hospital's opening – contain a reference to St Mls. Hospital (*sic*), the first reference by name to the new facility. Its proximity to St Michael's Cathedral, together with the fact that the Toronto archdiocese is under the patronage of St Michael the Archangel, probably suggested the name. Indeed, the hospital was well supplied with patrons, for the wards were not numbered but were given saints' names – twenty in all – St Anne's, St Agnes's, and so on, and of course, St Joseph's and St Patrick's.[32]

While there is no detailed record of what renovations were necessary to convert the building to hospital use, ledger entries of July and September 1892 show expenditures of $500 and $200 as "payments on elevator" as well as expenditures for bedsteads and mattresses.[33] A later entry, for the year ending 30 June 1893, notes: "House alterations for Hospital Purposes, $2,307.47," and a further $1,106 for mattresses, bedding, and other furniture. In June 1893 the first telephone entry is shown ($22.50), and twice-yearly thereafter for several years. For a time the north wing was set aside for male patients, and the sisters' living quarters were in the main building, among the patients. This arrangement was a subject of debate in General Council, and finally the male patients were moved to the main building and the sisters took over the more private accommodations in the north wing (the only recorded defeat of Mother de Chantal, soon to be introduced, in debate!).[34]

St Michael's was one of only three hospitals mentioned in the 1893-94 calendar of the University of Toronto's faculty of medicine. The entry read: "[St Michael's Hospital] contains 80 beds, and during the nine months of its existence about 560 patients have been admitted. The following members of the Faculty are members of the staff of St Michael's Hospital: Prof. I.H. Cameron, Prof. J.E. Graham, Prof. A. McPhedran, Prof. W. Oldright, J. Amyot."[35]

The details are sparse with regard to how the medical staff was recruited. The council minutes merely record: "The names of several doctors were taken down, who are to be on the staff. A meeting of these physicians to take place at the Hospital, when they will decide what is best to be done in dividing the staff."[36] That the medical staff be self-governing would thus appear to have been accepted from the first. But within weeks the brakes were put on over-confident young surgeons:

> The question as to the propriety of young doctors ... undertaking critical operations without notifying senior or consulting physicians – as has been done on one or two occasions lately – was discussed. It was considered advisable that the Superior should have an understanding with the Medical Staff about this matter, and have some definite rule for the house doctor, so that serious cases should have the full benefit of the Hospital staff.[37]

This decision shows a remarkable insight, on the part of medically unsophisticated women, into the proper use of the medical hierarchy for the benefit and protection of the patient and of the young doctor – and ultimately, of themselves and of the hospital. The concern expressed then, within six weeks of opening the hospital, would continue to concern administrators all down the years.

Finally, a few words are in order concerning a man who figures prominently in this chapter – Dr Norman Allen. An 1885 graduate in medicine from Toronto's Trinity University, Allen had then done post-graduate work in England where he obtained his MRCS (England). Upon his return to Canada, not yet thirty years of age, he became Toronto's second medical officer of health in April 1891 – just in time for the diphtheria epidemic. Two years later Allen was dismissed because of "extravagant and unbusiness-like use" of Board of Health moneys.[38] It is difficult to assess the validity of this charge for the board was, itself, chronically the victim of a city hall that was tight-fisted where public health matters were concerned.[39]

Though trained in surgery, Allen then joined the staff of St Michael's as a specialist in dermatology. Here again he appears to have been a controversial figure (but not for the same reasons).[40] In 1922 Allen was apparently recovering nicely from gall-bladder surgery, performed at St Michael's by Dr George Wilson, when he developed tetanus and died. A coroner's inquest followed (similar deaths had been reported elsewhere in Ontario about the same time), at which it was determined that the source of infection was catgut improperly sterilized by the manufacturer.[41]

Allen's family established a permanent memorial in the form of a prize for the highest standing in surgery to a member of each graduating class of nurses. He himself bequeathed $1000 to Sister de Sales (one of the original sisters at the Isolation Hospital) as a token of his esteem for her as a devoted nurse.

2

Hostile Forces at Work

When St Michael's Hospital opened in 1892, Toronto had a population of 144,000 of whom 65 percent were Canadian born and 30 percent were British-born.[1] So, in spite of a smattering of German, Italian, and Slavic immigrants, the workforce was generally English-speaking.

Torontonians were earnest in their observance of Sunday rest and worship as well as in their service to their church and community. Education was officially compulsory and, in addition to the free public schooling that now extended to the secondary level, there were state-aided Catholic separate schools. In terms of medical care, there were already four general hospitals – the 400-bed General and the smaller St John's, Grace, and Homeopathic Hospitals – as well as the recently established Children's Hospital.

Major public buildings, which would endure, were in place: the Legislative Buildings in Queen's Park, Union Station, and the Post Office. What is now the "old" City Hall was then under construction. The streets were still cedar-paved but asphalting was not far in the future. Although horse-drawn streetcars were beginning to be replaced by electric ones, fire engines were still horse-drawn. For private transportation, wealthy citizens sported handsome carriages and spirited horses. Gas lighting was being introduced into the city at this time.

Toronto was well supplied with newspapers – among them, the *Globe*, the *Evening Telegram*, and the newest (1892), the *Star*. St Michael's had two department stores near at hand, on the corner of Queen and Yonge streets – Simpson's (with two telephones for orders) and Eaton's (with elevators). Both were less than twenty years old.

Closer still to the hospital, Metropolitan Church (Methodist) and St Michael's Cathedral presided grandly over Bond Street to the east, and the last home of the fiery little rebel, William Lyon Mackenzie, was up Bond to the north. Under construction to the northwest was dour Massey Hall, whose management would surprise and delight generations of St Michael's nursing students by sending over from time to time a handful of tickets to the symphony. And St Michael's had other, less imposing neighbours whose names are not recorded. These would gradually be replaced by a hospital that refused to stop expanding.

The Opening Shot

A threat to the growth, if not the very survival, of the young hospital came within a year of its founding. On 2 June 1893 the *Globe* reported that Alderman J. Orlando Orr, who was also a doctor associated with the General, had introduced a resolution concerning Toronto's hospitals at a meeting of the city council executive. The following account of this meeting appeared in the newspapers:

> The items of $7,000 for sundry homes and hospitals, city patients on mayor's order, and $20,000 Toronto General Hospital city patients on mayor's order, took some time to consider. Alderman Orr moved that the sums be amalgamated, and that the medical health officer be empowered to state the hospital to which he might send city patients. He found fault with the manner in which the Toronto General Hospital, the only hospital that admitted medical students, was being treated. The result of sending patients, where expenses were paid for by the corporation, to sectarian and private hospitals was that the student population of the city was being decreased. The General was a non-sectarian hospital, and all corporation patients should be sent there. (Hear, hear). Some of the hospitals where city patients had been sent during the past year had no qualified medical resident, and as a matter of fact, the physicians were leaving St. Michael's Hospital because they could get no properly trained nurses for their patients. He knew that in that same hospital the city had been paying 40 cents per day for the upkeep of persons who were well enough to act as nurses and assist in cooking.
> It was decided to cut the whole estimate down from $27,000 to $20,000 and a resolution was passed to the effect that the city should contribute nothing except to the General Hospital, which was non-sectarian.

These charges brought an immediate and spirited rebuttal from Dr Robert Dwyer, medical superintendent of St Michael's Hospital, in a letter to the editor of the *Globe*, also dated 2 June 1893:

> In Friday's issue of your paper certain statements were made by Ald. Orr concerning St. Michael's Hospital. These statements were made during a committee meeting of the City Council, and are as follows:

1. That I am not a qualified physician.
2. The nursing is defective.
3. That no advantages are given to students.
4. That patients are kept after being cured and given work to do, such as cooking, etc.
5. That patients are not properly attended.

To all of the charges I give an absolute denial as follows:

1. I am a graduate of Toronto University, and a licensed practitioner, and I am and have been the resident medical superintendent of St. Michael's, dating from its inception.
2. We have a competent staff of nurses, while of their faithfulness and efficiency the staff and I are the best judges, and they are fully up to standard.
3. The students of the Women's Medical College have had clinics all winter, and the same liberty has been given to Toronto University – a privilege which has been taken advantage of, as will be seen by the curriculum.
4. Patients are not given work to do when convalescent any more than at the General Hospital, where one of the printed rules is that convalescent patients must assist the nurses.

The fifth charge may be characterized as grossly untrue.

Dr. Orr further states that Dr. Sheard (M.O.H.) substantiated the above statements. From my knowledge of Dr. Sheard, I will take the liberty of doubting this.

> R.J. Dwyer, M.D., M.C.P.S.O.,
> Medical Superintendent,
> St. Michael's Hospital, June 2, 1893.

Dwyer's point-by-point response to Orr's charges was echoed and elaborated upon by St Michael's medical staff:

Owing to statements made concerning St. Michael's Hospital by Dr. Orr, as reported by the public press, a meeting of the Staff was called on Thursday afternoon, 8th June, and it was unanimously resolved:

1st. That the resident physician is a thoroughly qualified and efficient superintendent.
2nd. That the nursing has been satisfactory, and the nurses have been [illegible] and attentive.
3rd. That the Hospital has been used extensively for clinical instruction by the Faculty and Students of the Women's Medical College and that the Students of the University of Toronto have had the same privileges.

4th. That the management and equipment are excellent.

5th. That patients have been admitted and treated without regard to creed.

6th. That a downtown Emergency Hospital is desirable for the reception of severe accident cases.

7th. Moreover, that since Dr. Orr's statements have influenced the public as well as the City Council prejudicially to the interests of the Hospital, we desire to contradict them, and express the hope that St. Michael's Hospital will continue to receive the same aid from the City Council that it had in the past.

C.R. Cuthbertson, M.D.; M. Wallace, M.D.;
T.F. McMahon, M.D.; Walter McKeown; R.B. Nevitt;
J.A. Amyot; Edmund E. King; I.H. Cameron; C. McKenna; A. McPhedran; A.H. Garratt; D. Campbell Meyers; John Caven, M.D.; Wm. Oldright.

Some of the above were already men of repute in the medical fraternity. Drs Cameron, McPhedran, and Caven were on staff at the General; Dr Cameron is listed in the university medical faculty calendar of 1894-95 as professor of clinical surgery, Dr McPhedran as associate professor of medicine and clinical medicine, and Dr Caven as professor of pathology. Dr Oldright was professor of hygiene and later became associate professor of clinical surgery. Dr Amyot was assistant surgeon at St Michael's and demonstrator in pathology at the university and later became associate professor of pathology and bacteriology. Several of the signatories were active at the time in the Toronto Medical Society, Dr Oldright being elected president and Dr McMahon vice-president in 1895.[2] Both were active in presenting cases and in discussion, as was Dr Nevitt. Others were on their way up in the profession.[3]

Dr R.B. Nevitt, dean of the Ontario Medical College for Women,[4] had already filled in a few more of the blanks in a letter to the *Mail* on 3 June 1893:

> When the hospital was opened for the admission of patients, foreseeing the advantages which might accrue to the students, I made application to be allowed to use the clinical opportunities on behalf of the students. The request was granted .... At the present moment there are eight or ten lectures given weekly to the attending classes of students. In addition I, with other members of the active staff, have frequently brought individual students to see the work done in the hospital. Alderman Orr's arguments then fall to the ground, and medical students will not be drawn to other cities where more clinical lectures are given, unless St. Michael's is "crippled" by unfriendly efforts.

It appears that Dr Nevitt had done some investigation on his own, for his letter continues: "I am assured by the hospital authorities that no fraud has been contemplated, attempted, or accomplished. The books of the institution are open for inspection."

A further letter to the *Mail*, signed merely "One of the Staff, St. Michael's Hospital," addressed the quality of the institution's medical staff and challenged the basis for the withdrawal of the grant:

St Michael's has resident within its walls two University graduates, one of whom also occupies the position of lecturer at one of our Medical Colleges .... Apart from the Sisters of St. Joseph, St. Michael's Hospital has a large staff of properly trained nurses, the head nurse, Miss Harrison, being a graduate of Brooklyn Hospital, and a lady who stands at the very head of her profession.

The medical and surgical staffs number among their members many of the most eminent physicians and surgeons of the city. If any charge of mismanagement or wrong can be brought against this ... institution by all means let it be probed to the bottom, but do not let it be said that this hospital shall be unjustly assailed for no other reason than that it has the name of being a Roman Catholic institution.

Despite these claims, one cannot but wonder about the quality of the nursing that would have been available at the fledgling St Michael's. Harrison may have been the only fully trained nurse on staff; two of the sisters had had a few months' experience in Montreal, but none of the others had any formal preparation for nursing and the first nursing students would not graduate for another year. Contrast this situation with that of the General, whose school of nursing, opened in 1881, was by 1894 the largest in the country, with some of the young graduates staying on staff at the hospital at the handsome salary of $12 a month, plus uniform.

While St Michael's was the only "other" hospital singled out as being inappropriately subsidized, the motion in city council would, in effect, have cut off funds to St John's Hospital as well, a small institution operated since 1885 by the Anglican Sisterhood of St John the Divine.[5] At the time of the debate, patients applying for a "city poor order" had the option of going to St Michael's, St John's, or the General, with the usual allowance from the civic treasury of forty cents per day to the hospital of the patient's choice.

Advised that a delegation from the hospital was about to appear before city council with a request that the resolution be rescinded, the editor of the *Globe* was swift to take a position:

Council decided to withdraw this practice on the broad principle that the General Hospital is a public, non-sectarian institution ....

the principle is a right one, and should be adhered to ... it does not require much thought to see where an extension of the present principle will lead us ....

Nothing will more readily break down the sectarianism so rampant among the people of Canada than the maintenance of common public institutions such as the General Hospital, on the governing board of which Catholic and Protestant ... may sit side by side, and in the wards of which Catholic and Protestant clergy may minister to their adherents.[6]

And a letter published in the *Mail* asked: "Is not the Toronto General Hospital, under the capable management of Dr. Charles O'Reilly, sufficient for the needs of the city? If not, then let sufficient grant be given it ... but by all means let Toronto avoid an innumerable set of hospitals under different ecclesiastics."

The newspaper accounts, clearly indicating the interest in the issue, ranged from humorous to nasty. Under a heading "Alderman Orr's Bad Break," one paper referred to Orr's blunder in mistaking Mother de Chantal as superintendent and to his charge that she ruled like an "absolute monarch." (Mother de Chantal was superior of the hospital at the time.) Another newspaper charged the council with being "in fear of the Lodge," a charge not without grounds, for as Murray Nicolson has noted: "As an organization, the Orange Order held Victorian Toronto in its grasp .... Through its membership it controlled the militia, the police, civic employment, city hall, ward politics, and the work place." [7]

Monsignor Treacy, the first priest to serve as chaplain at St Michael's, wrote in 1940 : "A Catholic hospital in Toronto forty-seven years ago was an island surrounded by a considerable expanse of Boyne water, and it needed tact, influence and diplomacy to forestall private and public opposition."[8] The gravity of the situation shows through in yet another headline: "Still In The Swim: St. Michael's Hospital Will Not Die Without A Struggle."

The "struggle" was powerfully engaged when a veritable Who's Who of Catholic laymen went "to wait upon" the mayor and the executive council to protest against Alderman Orr's statements and the proposed withdrawal of civic patients from St Michael's. These included, among others, Hugh Ryan, the railroad magnate; Frank Smith, a senator since 1871 and member of five federal Conservative governments who was to be knighted within the year; and J.J. Foy, counsel to the archbishop of Toronto and later MPP and attorney-general of Ontario.

The principal point which these men impressed upon city council was that, though the hospital was managed by the Roman Catholic Sisters of

St Joseph, it was completely non-sectarian. Against this, the aldermen argued that they favoured sending the city patients to the General, where medical students could have the advantage of examining their cases; the students who attended the medical schools each year depended upon the city-order patients for their clinics and other studies. The patients, they said, naturally disliked being the subject of lectures, and frequently there was a tendency to prefer St Michael's where greater privacy was to be obtained. The deputation withdrew, to await an answer.

Finally, in a strongly worded circular to his clergy, Archbishop John Walsh issued the church's response to the council's proposed action. (Though he did not refer to the incident, Walsh could not but remember that his carriage had been stoned when he arrived in Toronto four years earlier to occupy his see, and that the Bond Street Convent had also been stoned that same day.) The archbishop deplored this "wretched intolerance and religious bigotry" and reminded Catholics that they must "protect, help, and uphold St. Michael's Hospital .... We must enable it to keep its doors open for the sick poor, whether Catholic or Protestant." Further, "We require of the clergy to announce from their pulpits on Sunday next our express desire that all our sick poor shall henceforward go to St. Michael's Hospital for medical treatment, and we expect of our clergy that they will faithfully carry out our desire in this respect."[9] The archbishop showed that he was not unaware of the political overtones of the situation when he added a postscript: "It is but fair to state that His Worship the Mayor and several Aldermen did their duty nobly by St. Michael's Hospital, and the fact will not be forgotten by our people."

So the medical staff, Catholic laymen,[10] the archbishop, and former patients[11] rallied staunchly in defence of St Michael's, not yet a year old. What of the sisters? Both Dr Nevitt's and the archbishop's statements suggested that discussion with them had taken place, but no direct response from the sisters (even in their General Council minutes) is recorded, nor from Mother de Chantal whose name by now many Torontonians would have come to know through the newspapers. And where did the Toronto General stand in the debate? William Howland, ex-chairman of its board, supported by Mayor Robert John Fleming (also a board member), stated that the Toronto General was not in sympathy with the movement to withdraw grants from other hospitals and reduce the facilities for treatment of the sick in Toronto. Dr Charles O'Reilly, the medical superintendent, said that each hospital should "stand on its own merits."

The foregoing debate over the allocation of public funds to St Michael's Hospital so early in its history highlighted a number of questions, quite apart from the question of religious bigotry. First of all, is a charitable institution "sectarian" by reason of its ownership and management, and should it therefore be considered ineligible for public funds? Further, does the state, by supporting religious-sponsored institutions, inhibit the solid growth and development of similar public institutions? On these points, it is of interest that the practice of continuing the grant to the House of Providence, also sponsored by the Sisters of St Joseph, was not questioned. Was it because the size of the grant – two cents per patient per day – was negligible, or was it because the House of Providence posed no threat to those involved in medical education? Or was it because to question this grant was politically risky? Also, did the support of city-order patients in a number of hospitals really have an adverse effect on medical education in Toronto? Dr Orr had stated that "if the policy of crippling Toronto General Hospital were persisted in the medical students would go away to Montreal where they could get more clinics." In mid-1893 the General had 400 beds, while St Michael's had somewhere between twenty-six and seventy-five – hardly a significant threat.

Did there exist, or was there foreseen, a unique, partnership between the General and the University which must be carefully and consciously protected and cultivated? Dr Orr had insisted that "the presence of *a* large and perfectly appointed hospital was a necessary adjunct to the magnificent State-aided university," and Cosbie, the General's historian, records that from 1887 onwards there was close collaboration between the two institutions, with the university's trustees and the hospital's board jointly deciding upon the site and design of the new Toronto General, still in the planning stage at the time of the current controversy.[12]

Finally, can the quality of patient care be sustained with a lay (non-medical) administrator? The archbishop had nicely delineated the roles in question when he wrote: "This lady [Madame de Chantal] is the responsible Superintendent of the institution as far as its general and economic management is concerned, but she has nothing whatever to do with the medical treatment of the patients; and the institution has a qualified resident physician, who is medical superintendent."

The Debate Continues

Finally, in April 1894, after returning again and again to the debate, and after at least one near-defeat of Dr Orr's motion, Toronto council cut St Michael's off the list of institutions to which city patients might be sent and for whom the forty cents per diem per patient might be claimed. The withdrawal of the grant was to become effective on 1 July 1894.

As it turned out, this setback was only temporary. Chief among the developments that led to a reversal of city policy in this regard was the tremendous boost – in capacity, in potential, in institutional pride and confidence, and in public support – given to St Michael's by the addition of a new surgical wing and operating room. The hospital's cause was also assisted by the archbishop, who lobbied powerfully for the institution, and by Dr Dwyer, who was quick to correct publicly some misleading statistics presented to city council by the medical officer of health.

Archbishop Walsh's circular letter of 1892 had been, in general, pastoral and conciliatory in tone, dwelling not so much on the action of council as on the need to ensure that the poor would continue to be received and cared for at St Michael's. In contrast, on the occasion of the laying of the new wing's cornerstone on 13 May 1894, Walsh launched a direct offensive. First he countered attacks on St Michael's "sectarianism" with some comparative statistics:

> The institution [is] under Church control, yet, out of twenty physicians connected with it, fifteen are Protestant. In its first twenty-two months, St. Michael's had 321 Protestant patients .... Protestant ministers [are] perfectly free to visit the members of their church who might need their ministrations .... All the managers save one of the General Hospital are Protestant, all members of its medical staff are Protestant, all its trained nurses are Protestant .... [He then compared Grace Hospital and Sick Children's to St Michael's in the same way.]
>
> In the face of these indisputable and undisputed facts, the majority of the City fathers favour the aforesaid hospitals on the ground that they are non-sectarian, and discriminate against St. Michael's on the pretence that it is sectarian .... It were more honest, more manly ... had they come out squarely, and openly avowed that their shafts were aimed at St. Michael's for the simple reason that it is a Catholic institution as regards its management.
>
> Be it remembered that we ask no favour. We demand only our rights as regards this matter .... We claim that our sick poor be allowed to be sent to St. Michael's Hospital, and that the same amount shall be paid for their hospital treatment ... as would be paid for them if sent to other hospitals. We ask no more, and we will not be satisfied with less.

The gauntlet had been thrown down, and powerful emotions surfaced in response. One editorial expressed fear that this was but the thin edge of the wedge:

> If Archbishop Walsh wins in the fight ... and succeeds in securing a permanent place for St. Michael's Hospital on the civic charity list, it will only be a question of time until there will be a demand here,

too, for the creation of a second institution, under sectarian auspices, for the treatment of contagious diseases [a reference to a
struggle currently underway in Ottawa] …. Now is the time to take
a firm stand in the matter …. Instruction should be given to recognize only the General Hospital.

Evident also was an element of nasty suspicion: a trustee of the General Hospital wrote: "No denomination shall seize on public funds to propa-
gate their religion under the guise of caring for the sick or poor."[13] Finally,
there was the not-so-veiled threat: "If he protests so vigorously, the very
large amount that Protestants now ascribe to Catholic charities is very apt
to be withheld in the future, for no ecclesiastic can be permitted to adopt
his tone of voice when addressing the people of this city."

A year later the medical officer of health touted, and was briefly commended for, the "saving" to the city of $3,000 which his department had
been able to effect by rigorous screening of whom he "allowed to live at
the public institution at the City's expense." Dr Dwyer pounced upon the
figures, publicly charging that the very amount saved by the city had, in
fact, been spent by St Michael's, which had continued to receive the city's
sick poor free of charge.

Whatever the reason – the archbishop's challenge, the near-comple-
tion of the superior new facilities at St Michael's, or the dogged analysis
and exposition of the facts by its young medical superintendent – city
council had a change of heart.[14] From 1 August 1895 St Michael's was
restored to its place among the institutions to which city-order patients
might be admitted at public expense.[15]

Was the forty cents per city patient per day worth the struggle? Most
assuredly it was, for the hospital's financial statement for the twelve
months previous shows that payment for such patients constituted fully
38 percent of the total revenue, exclusive of loans [See Appendix B]. But
apart from the money, the struggle secured the hospital's right to be, a
right that would not be challenged again so publicly, nor with such raw
antipathy, for many years.

Mother De Chantal

To round out this account, we will now take a closer look at some of the
figures who played important roles in St Michael's formative years. One
of these was the first superior of the hospital, Mother de Chantal McKay.

This impressive woman was born Mary Isabella Cole in 1827 in Tipperary, Ireland. The date of her immigration to Upper Canada is not
known, nor is it known whether or not she was already a widow when
she came. The young widow entered the Sisters of St Joseph in 1855 and

three years later, at just thirty-one years of age, was appointed superior of the House of Providence which had been opened a year earlier on Power Street. To support their work there, the sisters had to solicit alms from door to door. They took in washing, the water for which had to be carried up from King Street, a task often begun at two or three o'clock in the morning. It is unlikely that Mother de Chantal dispensed herself from a share in this heavy manual work.

Her term of superiorship was the beginning of a lifelong series of leadership positions to which Mother de Chantal was appointed or elected: superior and founder of an orphan asylum in London (1868) and of an industrial school for girls (1871); member of her congregation's General Council in 1872 and again in 1887 and 1890; general superior – the highest office in the congregation – (1875); superior of the House of Providence again (1878); and superior of Notre Dame des Anges (1890). In the last post she directed the conversion of this industrial school for girls into St Michael's Hospital while serving concurrently on the General Council.

The records of the Sisters of St Joseph show Mother de Chantal at the forefront of every new community development and in every community crisis: selected by the archbishop as one of two sisters to whom he entrusted the instruction of the female inmates of the Don jail (1870); converting Sunnyside orphanage into a temporary infirmary for the many students stricken with scarlet fever at the sisters' private school for girls (1883); one of the three sisters present when doctors undertook surgery on a sister in the convent, under ether (1880); and one of the two sisters present when Archbishop Lynch breathed his last (1888).

Mother de Chantal was deeply involved in major renovation programs – at Notre Dame des Anges (1892) and at the Cobourg convent (1883). She was involved in real estate transactions – the acquisition of sites for the Sunnyside orphanage (1875) and Notre Dame des Anges (1878); and she arranged for a communal plot in St Michael's Cemetery (1877) for the congregation's dead.

She was a person to whom gifts were often given as "firsts" – a gas lamp in 1873, only days after the first gas lighting was arranged for the convent on St Alban Street; a horse from an admirer in 1876. And she herself gave handsome gifts – for the benefit of the sisters' health she provided, not medicines, but season's tickets on the *Chicora*, a steamer running to Niagara and Lewiston. Sisters turned out *en masse* each year to celebrate her feast day.

There is strong evidence that the suggestion to found a hospital was Mother de Chantal's idea,[16] an idea she felt so strongly about that she went on foot to beg for funds among the wealthy of Toronto (See Appendix A).

Accustomed as she was to positions of authority for more than thirty years, it is quite possible that she projected in her person an authority and decisiveness that spelled "absolute monarch" to men unaccustomed to seeing women at the helm of public enterprises. Described in the congregation's records as a "woman of exceeding beauty and majestic proportions" (the latter, perhaps, not seen as a compliment by women of the late twentieth century), Mother de Chantal emerges as a person who had touched life at some of its deepest levels. As such, she could and would muster the strength to guide the young hospital through the storm of public controversy and personal attack that accompanied the withdrawal of the grant. We shall meet other Mother de Chantals in the ensuing 100 years at St Michael's.[17]

Dr Robert J. Dwyer

We have been able to infer, from her background and her character, the probable influence of Mother de Chantal in bringing to birth St Michael's Hospital. But the person who, more than any other, dominated the scene at St Michael's for the ensuing thirty years was the slight and seemingly indefatigable Dr Robert Dwyer.

Dwyer was born in Napanee, Ontario, in 1867,[18] a descendant of immigrants from Tipperary, and he graduated in medicine from the University of Toronto in 1892 – the year St Michael's was established. It is not known how he came to be associated with the hospital immediately upon graduation, but one can conjecture that it was through Mother de Chantal; probably the Tipperary people looked up, and looked after, one another. Or he may have boarded at the old Notre Dame as a medical student, even though the original intent for that place was to offer living accommodations to women. The 1887 records of Notre Dame lists two medical students among the residents.

An eager student, Dwyer was elected to the Toronto Medical Society in October 1892 and as early as the following January was making presentations at the society's meetings, exhibiting pathological specimens (a ruptured heart, a stomach with an ulcer which had perforated the liver, and so on), and taking a very active part in discussion of the cases presented.[19]

Dwyer married Teresa Lumage of St Louis in St Patrick's Cathedral, New York, in 1898 and two years later became the father of a little girl who died at only ten months of age, soon after he had left for study in Europe (London, Berlin, Vienna). In 1903 Dwyer resumed his duties as physician at St Michael's and was given, as well, an appointment in the faculty of medicine at the University of Toronto. The faculty calendar lists him as one of only eight faculty members, out of a faculty of eighty-eight, to hold the advanced medical degree of MRCP. (At that time, there were not more than five holders of the MRCP degree in Canada, and thirteen in the whole American continent.[20])

The esteem in which Dwyer was held within his profession is evident in an article in the *Canadian Journal of Medicine and Surgery* of April 1920, following his death of heart disease in January of that year:

> Canada has lost one of her foremost physicians in the person of R.J. Dwyer. "Bob" was an unique student. He was not enamoured of lectures and books .... He did, however, [make] a special study of pathology, by post-mortem work, as no other man of his time.[21]
>
> On graduation he became first house surgeon and later medical superintendent at St. Michael's Hospital where ... he perfected his acquaintance with disease at the bedside – becoming one of the best clinical physicians in America. Dwyer went to London and the continent, and in due course obtained his M.R.C.P – a degree which few Canadians hold.
>
> The deceased was a great teacher ... not only by reason of his gift of imparting knowledge, but for his ability to communicate his penetrative diagnostic acumen.
>
> [Dr. Dwyer's associates] trusted him and believed in him implicitly. In illustration – the deceased once requested one of the orderlies, an aged Hibernian, to go up to a ward and help to remove to the morgue the remains of a patient who had died .... [The orderly] was "three sheets in the wind" and made his way to the wrong bed. At his touch, what he took to be the corpse raised up on his elbow and remonstrated at the interference, whereupon the faithful, inebriated orderly exclaimed: "Lie down; you're dead; you're dead; for Dochtor Dhwyer says you're dead."[22]

When the sisters opened the doors of St Michael's Hospital they still had everything to learn about hospital work. Dwyer joined the hospital in its infancy; there can be little doubt that this man, with his professional skill and vision, his energetic work habits, his culture, his lived faith, and his personal charm, was in large part responsible for setting the infant firmly on its feet, and starting it on its long walk to senior status within the teaching hospitals of Toronto and of Canada.

Hugh Ryan

One last person deserving of a few words is Hugh Ryan, who was responsible for providing St Michael's with its new wing.

The former church-boarding house, no matter how creative the remodelling effort, was probably not a very impressive St Michael's Hospital. Some may have thought it would never amount to much, an opinion that might well have been in the minds of the city fathers who had openly declared their preference for supporting one really good hospital in Toronto. As a hospital board member throughout the events of 1893-94, Hugh Ryan would have been aware of this perception. Through his construction business he had been made aware, too, of the importance of emergency facilities for injured workmen near the heart of the city.[23] A man of faith, he was also doubtless moved to give something back to his community for all that he had been given.

The Hugh Ryan wing – the building a gift of Mr Ryan, the furnishings a gift of his wife, Margaret – was opened on Thanksgiving Day, 1895.[24] The only condition Ryan made part of the deed was that the hospital be kept open night and day to receive anyone in need of its services, without consideration for creed, colour, or nationality. Intended for the exclusive use of surgical cases, the three-storey building of Credit valley stone topped with red pressed bricks had an operating theatre one and one-half storeys high, with a gallery to accommodate fifty students. Clearly the hospital intended to be involved in medical education.

Steam-heated, with gas and incandescent lights throughout, the new wing boasted a feature quite remarkable for the times – in the ten-bed wards, the space allotted to each bed was provided with hot- and cold-air registers so that varying degrees of temperature might be maintained for differing spaces and needs of patients. An enthusiastic press spoke glowingly of the new wing as a model of sanitation, lighting, and ventilation.[25]

The public wards faced Bond Street and boasted an adjoining convalescent room on each of the three floors, filled with easy chairs, a bookcase, and writing table. But it was for the private and semi-private rooms, which faced south, opening onto a sunny verandah, that Mrs Ryan must have really given her imagination (and her pocket book) free rein – brass bedsteads, oak bedroom sets, engravings on the walls, a service of china and silver, and soft rugs on the hardwood floors.

On the north side on each floor were the sisters' and the housekeepers' rooms, as well as the kitchens, freeing up the whole of the original building to become the medical wing. The new and the old wings were joined by corridors to a centre building, also new and set farther back from the street, which housed the emergency ward, administrative offices, and apartments for the resident surgeon. The main entrance to the hospital was now through the door of this building, over which was the inscription "He hath borne our infirmities."

The bed capacity was thus brought to 110 – eleven public wards, twelve semi-private, and twelve private rooms. The new rooms were numbered with Roman numerals, I to XX. "Inspected that day by nearly all the public and professional men of the city," as recorded by the press, the transformed facility must have made it clear to all that St Michael's was here to stay and was to be taken seriously.

Hugh Ryan, the bewhiskered donor of this handsome gift, of such symbolic as well as practical importance in putting the hospital on a firm footing, was called in his day "a model millionaire." He had come to Canada from County Limerick, Ireland, and worked his way up in the railroad construction business, until he was finally in charge of building a thousand miles of railroad as well as the Sault Ste Marie Canal. It was said of him that, among the thousands of men he employed, he never had a strike, not because he was generous, but because he was just. He was a lifelong student of his Catholic faith and Catholic discipline, and his advice was sought by the highest authorities in the church.

Ryan's former home in Rosedale, where he died in 1899, became (and remains in 1990) the impressive main building of Branksome Hall, a private girls' school.[26] Margaret Ryan died in Egypt during a visit to that country in February 1904.

3

Bustle and Bonding

W ith a superior new wing, rising public esteem, a volume of patients second only to that of the General, and an established school of nursing (soon to be described), St Michael's was well positioned to grow with a growing city. By 1896 Toronto had, in addition to twenty private hospitals, eight hospitals where free treatment could be obtained, with a capacity for 1,039 patients.[1] During the last few years of the nineteenth century and up until the First World War, Toronto experienced a period of vigorous growth. Supported by a steady flow of immigrants, especially from the British Isles, enterprises of every kind (building, industrial, financial) thrived, especially along King Street and the waterfront.

The number of non-Anglo-Saxon immigrants to Toronto increased markedly during those years, reaching 30,000 by 1911. Many were poor and unskilled, of Italian, Austrian-Hungarian, and Russian birth, including Jews. Up to 10,000 of these crowded into St John's Ward west of Yonge and above Queen streets, not far from St Michael's. As they struggled with the complexities of life in their new world of promise, they strove at the same time to maintain their ethnic identities, thereby adding to the city a richness that would not, until much later, be recognized and celebrated. It was but a short step from ship-side to construction-site, and jobs were plentiful; by the time the war broke out many had exchanged their status as "foreigner" to that of moderately well-to-do and influential citizen.

The residential pattern of the city changed during these years, influenced by the growth of a streetcar system that was converted from horse-drawn to electric-powered in 1894. Then began the shift of the middle-class residential districts and the upper-class estates to the outskirts of the city, while the lower socio-economic neighbourhoods ringed the inner business and industrial core. Slum conditions there were, to be sure – with high winter unemployment, alcohol abuse, and so on – but there were no tenements, for most workers managed to have their individual family homes, no matter how poor they were. The plight of the single immigrant man, however, was a harsh one; the influx of immigrants to Toronto in the years here described severely overtaxed the available housing, and single men were forced to settle for sordid, crowded boarding-houses in a section of the city not far from St Michael's – a situation that eventually became the focus of a major public-health initiative.[2]

There were significant changes in women's lives during these years, with increased opportunities for employment in offices, stores, and factories. Admission to the professions, however, did not come easily for women. To slip a high-buttoned shoe through the doors of Osgoode Hall was among the early struggles and finally, in 1889, the first Canadian woman gained admission to the courts of law; she was Clara Brett Martin, after whom the new (1989) Offices of the Attorney General on Bay Street are named.

By 1898 women had gained a modest foothold among students at the University of Toronto – except in medicine, from which they were excluded until 1906. However, from 1883 to 1906 they had their own Ontario Medical College for Women and at least one woman faculty member – Ann Augusta Stowe, daughter of Emily Howard Stowe, the first Canadian woman authorized to practise medicine. As already indicated, women medical students were received at St Michael's from the time of its opening.

In 1895 St Michael's accepted its first woman doctor for internship; she was Pearl Smith, believed to be the first woman to intern in a Canadian hospital. Smith was preparing to join her Baptist-missionary fiancé, the Reverend Jesse Chute (also a medical doctor), in India, where they served for forty years.[3] Their son, Dr A.L. Chute, became dean of medicine at the University of Toronto, serving from 1966 to 1972.

In 1901, after four years of refusals, the Toronto General Hospital accepted its first woman resident physician, Dr Helen MacMurchy. Evidently she passed muster, for in 1902 the trustees resolved to appoint a female intern each year. MacMurchy had applied as well at St Michael's, as did two other women doctors, but St Michael's would not have its second woman intern (Dr Mary Callaghan McCarthy) until 1904-05.[4]

In 1911 the Sisters of St Joseph opened a residential college for women – St Joseph's College, affiliated with the University of Toronto through St Michael's College. One of the original five women students records that they were "very unwelcome" at that previously all-male bastion.[5]

The number of sisters grew with the growth of the city, from the four pioneers who came to Toronto in 1851 to a congregation of 248 in 1904,[6] of whom sixteen were stationed at St Michael's Hospital.

Until 1920 the majority in the congregation was Irish, either Irish-born or first-generation Irish-Canadian.[7] By 1913 the sisters had ten foundations in the Archdiocese of Toronto and one, St Joseph's Hospital, in Comox on

Vancouver Island. Several urgent invitations to open hospitals had been refused – Oshawa (1902), Cobalt (1906), Port Perry (1911) – on the grounds that there were too few sisters for new hospital undertakings.

Meanwhile, the congregation's elementary and secondary schools flourished, their students comparing more than favourably with those from other schools within the educational system of Ontario. By 1911 sister-teachers were receiving $300 per annum from the school boards and the congregation was making every effort to ensure they obtained the necessary qualifications in the academic subjects as well as in music and art. At least five were well on in their university work by war's start.[8]

At St Michael's the archbishop was apparently no longer involved directly – as he had been initially – in the appointment of sisters to key positions. However, his influence in the affairs of the congregation was felt very immediately on more than one occasion. Meeting with the General Council in 1899, the newly arrived Archbishop Denis O'Connor issued a flurry of directives which were, to say the least, not guaranteed to encourage any professional aspirations the sisters may have had: the superior of the hospital was subject to the medical superintendent; the work of nursing should be confined entirely to the nurses – the duty of the sisters was to see to the domestic affairs of the house and look after the nurses; the sisters were responsible to the nurses' parents for their health and conduct; the medical superintendent should have the power to receive and reject subjects for the training school, and to define the numbers of nurses required; the sisters were not to be present at surgical operations, except those of a simple nature.

The fidelity with which these directives were carried out appears uneven; probably some accommodation was arrived at between the busy Dr Dwyer and the superior and sisters which satisfied the consciences of all concerned. It is clear that the sisters had charge of the medical and surgical wards from the first. However, from earliest days, a lay woman appears on the staff payroll as operating-room nurse. For three years following the resignation of Julia O'Connor in 1916 there was no operating-room nurse listed on the payroll; this may have been the time when one of the sisters, of whom there were thirty on staff, first took charge of the operating room.[9]

The incumbent archbishops served successively as presidents of the advisory board of the hospital, with the board members taking turns chairing the meetings until, finally, in 1940 J.J. Fitzgibbons became the first lay member to serve for a term. Often it is unclear whether the superior's communications with the archbishop were in his capacity as president of the board or as ecclesiastical superior. In 1905 Archbishop O'Connor decreed that all councillors should reside at the motherhouse, a directive that necessitated replacing Sister Demetria MacGregor (a councillor, and superior/administrator at St Michael's) by Sister Irene Conroy.

In the city, religious tolerance was increasing. Being Catholic was no longer equated with being poor. Striving, perhaps, to demonstrate their broadmindedness, public figures sometimes referred to St Michael's catholicity rather than to its Catholic sponsorship.[10] As well, government had legislated convent property to be free from taxation. These were gains of no mean significance but, on the lighter side, there remained one concession the sisters had to make: in 1904 the huge bell atop the convent tower, which for decades had roused the sisters at 5 a.m., had to be replaced by an in-house electric bell, since the former disturbed the neighbours roundabout, including the premier of Ontario.[11]

In the public-health field, the incidence of typhoid fever, which persisted stubbornly throughout the first decade of the century, was dramatically curbed in 1912. In large part, this was because of the installation of a water-filtration plant at Toronto Island and a sewage-disposal plant at Scarborough Bluffs, together with the introduction of water chlorination (1909) and the use of anti-typhoid vaccine (1912). Tuberculosis, however, remained a threat of sinister proportions, accounting for 14 percent of all deaths, in all ages and all social conditions, as late as 1904.[12]

So the city where St Michael's Hospital was gradually taking root was a city bursting with vitality and change, increasingly open to the future. As for the hospital itself, one must remember that it began as the simplest of organizations – a sister acting as superior/administrator was in charge of the general and non-medical affairs; a medical superintendent was responsible for medical matters; six sisters were responsible to one or other of these two, depending on the situation; and five nursing students were directed by a teacher – in a building that initially housed twenty-six patients. These were the fourteen staff members we know about; presumably there were an additional one or more male staff members to handle the furnaces and the cleaning and to help with the male patients, and some further staff to help in the kitchen and laundry.[13]

This cosy little arrangement did not last for long. The health-care requirements of a growing city called early and repeatedly for expansion of St Michael's physical plant. Expanded facilities and operations introduced more complexity and, consequently, the need for more formal organization, both in general administration and in medical affairs, including the introduction of an advisory board. Let us attempt to capture the feel of those days.

The Early Sisters

There is little doubt that the first sisters left the imprint of their characters, their personalities, and their sense of mission upon the young hospital. They formed the stable core group – some remaining upwards of twenty or thirty years at the hospital – around which others (doctors, nurses, patients) would come and go. As a consequence, the pattern was early established in the hospital community of holding in balance what may appear to be opposites: strict self-discipline combined with tolerance toward the needy poor; thrift combined with a ready dispensation of charity; trust in divine providence combined with hard work and the full use of human and political resources; hiddenness and simplicity in personal and community life combined with readiness to tap the power residing in church, government, and private philanthropy – all for God, whom the sisters saw and served in the sick. These qualities were destined inevitably to rub off, to a greater and lesser degree, on those who formed the hospital community.[14]

The first change among the original seven sisters came in the summer of 1893 when Mother de Chantal was replaced by Sister Assumption Keenan. (Mother de Chantal's term as superior, begun at Notre Dame des Anges, expired in 1893, and the constitutions of the congregation required that she be relieved of the office.) Born at Kingston, Ontario, Mother Assumption was in her mid-fifties when she assumed this position, having spent thirty-six years in religious life. She had most recently been superior of St Nicholas Home, an institution located on Toronto's Lombard Street accommodating fifty working boys. Having apparently recognized early that she was quite unprepared for hospital administration, Mother Assumption set off in July 1895 to tour hospitals in the United States to see how things were handled there.

Responsible for everything except the medical management of patients, the superior had an array of functions, many of which would become eventually whole departments in themselves. She was spokesperson for the hospital to the General Council, which concerned itself with personnel appointments and capital funding, including loans and land acquisitions. Room rates and nurses' allowances were subject to council approval, and council was the final arbiter in disciplinary matters.[15] The superior appears to have provided for the keeping of accounts, including a record of gifts. (In a newspaper entry of 31 December 1894 the sisters named and thanked a host of donors for gifts of money ranging from $5 to $100, as well as for turkeys, oranges, biscuits – the Christie Brown Company gave a barrel of biscuits year after year at Christmas – flowers, candy, and even sheeting and pillow ticking.) The superior appears to have been the contact person with the various denominational clergymen who visited the hospital from the beginning, and was also a strong presence in the young school of nursing established, as we shall see momentarily, simultaneously with the hospital's opening in 1892.

During Mother Assumption's nine-year term of office (1893-1902) much of the property surrounding the hospital was secured for its use, owing primarily to her foresight and economy. Her biographer speaks of the "untold difficulties Mother Assumption successfully contended with, in the upbuilding of the institution." From the perspective of the 1990s, one of the difficulties must have been the sheer loneliness of her position and the absence of peer support, given the almost-cloistered condition of the sisters relative to the hospital superintendents of the day.

Sister Juliana Morrow, who had assumed the position of matron at the Isolation Hospital in 1889, transferred to St Michael's as assistant superior when the hospital opened in 1892. She died of cancer two years later. Sister Juliana was an aunt of Fred Morrow, whose generous bequest helped to make possible the relocation of the motherhouse from downtown Toronto to Morrow Park, Willowdale, in 1960.

Sister M. Attracta Hynes, a veteran of the congregation's elementary schools and of the Isolation Hospital, received some few months nurse's training in Montreal. After two years further training in St Michael's first (1894) class of nurses, she graduated at forty-six years of age. She spent the remaining thirty years of her life at St Michael's "putting her good judgement and practical mind to service in many different departments with unique success."[16] Sister St Felix Heeney, another of the Isolation Hospital pioneers, was also one of the founding members of St Michael's. She graduated with the second graduating class of nurses, and spent more than twenty years caring for patients and instructing nursing students on the medical wing.

Sister Julia Curry, an immigrant from County Tipperary, Ireland, was already stationed at Notre Dame des Anges when it was converted to a hospital. She stayed on as procuratrix (buyer) until a few months before her death, almost thirty-five years later. Described as "an old-fashioned saint," Sister Julia appears to have been a good business woman, too. Provincial inspectors repeatedly commented on the high quality of the food she purchased, and of the records and inventory she kept. As early as 1903 she had moved into contract buying, and by 1918 nearly all food, medical, and surgical supplies were furnished by contract.

The best-known and most widely remembered of the pioneers was Sister Francis de Sales Ryan – hereafter referred to as Sister de Sales – an immigrant from Kilkenny County, Ireland. Prepared initially as a teacher,

Sister de Sales went as a volunteer to the Isolation Hospital and then to St Michael's. She was thirty-eight years old when she graduated as a nurse in 1895; she spent the next forty years at St Michael's, in charge of the surgical floor for most of that time. It was said of her that she "possessed a personality that was unique – a curious blend of the religious and the human – and most attractive." Among the countless tributes after Sister de Sales's death, none expresses better the apostolic side of her character than that contained in a letter to the superior general by one of the doctors; to him she was "the most consistent expression of Our Lord Jesus Christ that I have ever encountered in this world; my own charity has been deepened and my spirit strengthened in the long period through which it was my privilege to work with her." When Sister de Sales died in 1932 her niece, Sister Margaret Phelan, was already superior of St Michael's and would return a second time, after holding the highest office in the congregation.[17]

Admittedly, accounts of the early sisters by those who knew them were not uniformly flattering. A nurse recalls that Sister de Sales once summoned her out of bed at 11:00 a.m., after a hard tour on night duty and a successful struggle to get to sleep against the competing carillons from Metropolitan Church, for the sole purpose of tidying up a ward kitchen left in less-than-perfect order. She recalled as well, however, Sister de Sales's uncanny ability to interpret clinical symptoms and to make a diagnosis as quickly and as accurately as many a physician.[18] In this connection, Sister de Sales may be considered representative of dozens of future nurses, both religious and lay, who would live out their whole nursing careers at St Michael's and, through intelligent use of their clinical contacts, develop remarkable assessment skills and superior care and comfort measures.

The First Patients

On 1 July 1892 the first three patients were admitted – two women and one man – the latter a twenty-seven year-old priest with tuberculosis who was discharged six weeks later "much improved." Twenty-four patients were admitted the first month, twelve women and twelve men, eight of the twenty-four giving their birthplace as Ireland and four as England. The average age, if we exclude the one ninety-one-year-old woman with rheumatism, was thirty-four years; in September of that year the average age of those admitted was thirty-one years. Admitting diagnoses in the first month ranged over a wide spectrum: among them, two typhoid, two rheumatism, two epididymitis, one spinal curvature, one syphilis, one gonorrhea, one hysteria – the latter a domestic, with no relatives in North America. (In scanning the admission register of the first five years one is struck by the prevalence of tuberculosis and venereal disease in all their stages and complications; also typhoid, and to lesser extent Bright's disease. Beside these, one notes the infrequency of stroke and heart disease, and even of cancer.) The admitting doctors were C. McKenna, Robert Dwyer, R.B. Nevitt, M. Wallace, J.J. Cassidy, Walter McKeown, T.F. McMahon, J.F.W. Ross, and I.H. Cameron; the latter two, as we shall see, were men active at the university and at the General. All of these doctors appear regularly in the admission register of the initial five years.[19]

The first death was on 17 August 1892 – a thirty-three-year-old man with bronchopneumonia. Six months later there appears the sparse and stark record of two female domestics, aged twenty and twenty-two years old, admitted from out of town on 28 January 1893 with diagnosis of pyosalpinx (a form of severe pelvic inflammation), both of whom died within three months – fifty years too early for the marvels of sulphanil-amide and penicillin.[20]

After the Hugh Ryan wing was built in 1895, the doctors were kept busy in the well-equipped operating theatre and emergency ward; indeed, there were strong recommendations for St Michael's to become exclusively an emergency hospital, withdrawing its claim to a share of public ward in-patients. The newspapers reported in colourful detail all the accident cases brought to the emergency ward, ranging from frequent streetcar accidents to construction falls, fights, fires, and even attempted suicides (often by poisoning). In September 1897, during a disastrous fire on Yonge Street between Adelaide and King, the horses drawing the fire engines panicked when a steam whistle blew, and plunged into the crowd. As a result, two firemen, four other adults, and an eight-year-old boy were brought to St Michael's emergency ward with fractured skulls, compound fractures of legs and arms, and internal injuries – no small challenge to a new hospital. The little boy died, but the six adults recovered, their progress faithfully reported by the newspapers over a two-month period.

Early Legislation

Legislation covering the care of the sick evolved slowly in Ontario. The Act of Incorporation granted to the Sisters of St Joseph in 1855, four years after their arrival in Toronto, acknowledged the "benefits which must arise" from the congregation's intent to relieve "the poor, the sick, and other necessitous" and authorized the congregation to purchase and hold property for this purpose.[21] The act was altered and more clearly defined in 1898, empowering the corporation to "erect, construct, equip, and maintain and operate buildings and other erections for the proper carrying on of its education, hospital, and other charitable works ...."[22] Under the act, authority was vested in the mother superior and council to establish such regulations as were deemed necessary or useful for the proper management of the corporation and its operations, undertakings, and works, and all property was vested in the corporation. This latter clause established the pre-eminence of the superior general and council in the government of the hospital; the hospital was subsumed within the Act of Incorporation of the congregation rather than being separately incorporated.

While the statutory power to hold property for the conduct of the hospital operations and to manage same was thus conferred on the congregation, there remained the question of funding. The first financial statement (Appendix B) indicates that provincial funds would begin to flow in 1893. From this it may be inferred that the hospital had applied for such under the Charity Aid Act, 1874.[23] At the time it was enacted this act had named certain institutions to be immediately eligible for public funds, and stipulated that others might be added after inspection by, and recommendation from, an inspector appointed under the Prison and Asylum Inspection Act, 1868.[24] Under these arrangements, thirty-two hospitals in Ontario were receiving public funds in 1893.[25]

Under the Charity Aid Act those institutions receiving provincial grants were required to accept provincial inspection. If the inspector found the institution deficient in what was required to fulfil its stated objects, government aid might be cancelled until the inspector recommended that it be resumed. (See Appendix C.)

The inspectors – two "fit and proper persons" were appointed for all the province's public asylums, hospitals, jails, and reformatories in 1883 – did much to improve management procedures (for example, by requiring that by-laws be established by each hospital and submitted to the legislature for approval), the safety and comfort of buildings, dietary and sanitary provisions, and statistical and accounting practices.

Under the Charity Aid Act, Schedule A institutions, which included the general hospitals, were eligible for a basic grant of twenty cents a day for each day of actual maintenance and treatment of indigent patients, in addition to a possible extra ten cents a day contingent upon the institution receiving aid from sources other than the province. This original provision of a possible thirty cents per patient per day decreased over the first ten years of St Michael's operation to eighteen cents as the number of hospitals sharing the appropriation increased.[26]

The Early Board

The first mention of St Michael's board is contained in an overview of the hospital carried in the newspapers when the Hugh Ryan wing was opened. It was an advisory board, composed of eight members: president, Archbishop Walsh; 1st vice-president, Hugh Ryan; 2nd vice-president, Frank Smith; committee – Mayor Warring Kennedy, Thomas Long, Matthew O'Connor, and W.T. Murray; secretary, Hugh T. Kelly.

Archbishop John Walsh, Hugh Ryan, and Frank Smith have already been introduced. Matthew O'Connor was a prominent building contractor, active in the separate school board. Hugh T. Kelly, from the partnership of Foy and Kelly, barristers located at Bay and Adelaide streets will appear at greater length presently. Thomas Long, an immigrant from County Limerick, Ireland, had served for eight years in the Ontario legislature, was a founder and president of the Collingwood Shipbuilding Company, and in the latter capacity pioneered the opening of communications with Lake Superior ports. He became a generous benefactor of the congregation and of the hospital, contributing half of the cost of the congregation's first automobile in 1917, and $10,000 to each of three institutions – St Michael's, House of Providence, and Sacred Heart Orphanage – in 1919.[27] William Thomas Murray, another immigrant from County Limerick, had been prepared for the dry goods business in Paris and London, and was by 1895 president of the large dry goods firm (W.A. Murray Company Limited) founded by his father. Warring Kennedy, who served as mayor in 1894-5, was probably appointed on the recommendation of an early inspector who urged that each hospital have substantial municipal-government representation.[28]

In what amounted to his inaugural address as president of the board, on the occasion of the formal opening of the Hugh Ryan wing, Archbishop Walsh laid out three elements of the philosophy of the hospital.[29] St Michael's was not, he said, established in a spirit of antagonism to any similar institution, but rather to fill a perceived need, and no rivalry must be allowed between it and other hospitals, save the rivalry of doing good; secondly, St Michael's would be open to the sick of every race and creed, and all would be treated with the same skill and devotion; thirdly, the religious convictions of the patients would be scrupulously respected, and the clergymen of every denomination would be perfectly free to minister to the spiritual wants of those who might require their services.

While the responsibilities of the board in these years are not recorded, it was involved primarily in the appointment and promotion of medical staff. As well, the board spoke for the hospital in the public arena and, when necessary, lobbied vigorously on the hospital's behalf.[30] It was also active in a public-relations capacity on formal occasions – for example, when the archbishop invited, and hosted with the sisters, a visit of Governor-General and Lady Aberdeen to the hospital in December 1897. One board member, Hugh Ryan, testified before city council to his "daily attendance" at the hospital and to his "intimate knowledge of the best hospitals in Europe, the U.S., and Canada." Ryan was, truly, the first of many dedicated and knowledgeable men (and later, women) who would serve on the board of St Michael's Hospital.[31]

The beginnings of a formal link with the medical schools are evident in the agendas for board meetings in 1901 and 1904. About the same time the board was, in addition, beginning to consider finances and building plans.[32]

The School of Nursing

As noted earlier, provincially appointed inspectors were required by law to make regular inspections of those hospitals receiving public grants and to report their findings to the government. Nursing, as a major component of a hospital's operation, thus fell within the inspectors' general mandate. Inspectors had special commendation for those hospitals that provided nurses' training and thereby aided the development of the nursing profession in Ontario.[33]

Simultaneous with the formal opening of the hospital in 1892, St Michael's opened its school of nursing, the first in Canada under Catholic auspices[34] and the third school of nursing in Toronto – coming after Toronto General's (1881) and Sick Children's (1886). Miss Harrison (the records do not contain her first name), a graduate of Bellevue Hospital, New York City, was in charge of the school. Little is known of Harrison or of how she was recruited.[35] Something of her philosophy and methods may be deduced, however, from her training at Bellevue, one of the first three American schools of nursing, all established in 1873. Florence Nightingale's correspondence with Bellevue Hospital's board has been called the "charter for American schools of nursing," with Bellevue singled out in a special way as bearer of the Nightingale principles of nurse training with their strong emphasis on character formation.[36]

The first St Michael's graduation exercises were held in December 1894 – after two years of training – for seven nurses, including Sisters Columba and Attracta who had had some preliminary experience at Hôtel-Dieu, Montreal, and earlier at the Isolation Hospital.

School of nursing records indicate that five of the second graduating class completed their preparation in 1895, and five in 1896. This appears to have been the time of transition from the original two-year program to a three-year one, an impression corroborated by a statement from a graduate of 1895; graduates of 1897 and thereafter had a three-year period of training.[37] Since the school records show a graduating class each year, the situation was established early that a corps of advanced students was on

51

hand to provide skilled nursing care while intermediates and beginners were learning and practising the fundamentals – an apprentice system that future nurse-educators would gradually replace by what they judged to be a more academically sound preparation. Early ledger entries give evidence of the efforts made to provide for nurses' instruction: an entry of February 1893 of $43 for "charts and Mannikin," and an entry of April 1897 of $21.36 for "Medical Books (Nurses)."

Classes were small, possibly limited by available housing, until after the Margaret Ryan residence was opened in 1898. From their names, it would appear that the students were predominantly of Irish or English ancestry, with a steady trickle of French and some Scottish. The immigration, other than British and French, that preceded the First World War was for many years only sporadically represented in St Michael's school of nursing. The first graduate of Italian parentage, Matilda Simoni (1912), was quickly recruited by the Toronto Board of Education for its newly begun "School Nurse Programme." According to annals contained in the hospital archives – unsigned, but presumed to be the work of Sister de Sales – within three years of its opening, applications to the school numbered 120, only thirty-six of whom were judged to have the necessary qualifications. What the qualifications were is not specified, but the annalist goes on to record that the number was further reduced by the hard realities of the probationary month. A first-hand account of the life and times of the nursing student of a century ago is given by Elizabeth O'Leary, a graduate of the first class:

> I started my training as a nurse at St Michael's in the autumn of 1892, about four months after the hospital opened its doors. The course was then two years and, as a rule, we were on duty twelve hours a day. However, you must remember that there were not many trained nurses available anywhere in those days, and we thought nothing of staying on duty till ten or eleven o'clock at night, or getting up in the middle of the night to watch sick patients or relieve a nurse who had taken ill.
>
> Reverend Mother M. de Chantal was the Superior of the hospital, and Miss Harrison, a graduate of Bellevue Hospital, was the first Directress of Nurses, followed later by Miss Margaret Kelman. The Sisters in charge of the wards and floors were Sister M. Francis de Sales (Surgical Ward), Sister M. Anne, Sister Rosalie, Sister M. St Felix (Medical Ward), and Sister Columba, in the Pharmacy. Lessons were given in Anatomy and Medicine by our beloved Chief Physician, Dr. John Roche, and others.[38] Practical

work was taught by Miss Harrison and the Sisters. Our residence consisted of two large rooms on the main floor of the hospital, one used as a sitting-room and the other as a dormitory. There were no ward maids or dietitians, but I remember the delicious food prepared by the Sister in charge of the kitchen. It tempted many a sick patient's appetite. We made our own dressings and bandages, and sterilizing was done on a stove, but later we had what was then a very modern sterilizer. Aseptic technique was as important then as it is now. We had not heard of oxygen tents or intravenous infusions, but we were taught how to make a sick person comfortable and to treat him with kindness.[39]

An account of 1895 provides further information about nurse preparation at St Michael's: "There were lectures, recitations, demonstrations, and instructions in practical nursing in the wards. The doctors lectured the nursing students in Anatomy and Physiology; Practical Nursing; Obstetrics; Antiseptic Surgery and Bandaging; Dressing and Treatment of Wounds, Dislocations, and Fractures; Ventilation; and Materia Medica and Toxicology." A year later the course of study was expanded to include "the recognition of symptoms, and an accurate understanding of the means used by the doctor to overcome particular diseases." The advantages to the school of having "the University professors lecture to the nurses" were a source of pride. Likewise, the opportunity nurses had to participate in the care of the numerous patients treated in the busy emergency ward was seen to be a distinct advantage in their preparation.

The valedictorian at the February 1897 graduation exercises paid tribute to her head nurse, Alice Doyle, who "had made theory keep pace with practice."[40] The same young graduate outlined elements of the school's philosophy:

The whole tendency of our training has been to discipline us into strong, self-reliant, self-contained women …. as we have studied to become capable nurses, we have striven to acquire that control of our minds and hearts, our wills and our desires, necessary to ensure a proper use of that authority which the relationship of nurse to patient embraces …. We have learned to value the strict obedience, the accurate and intelligent carrying out of directions. Every detail of life here is serving to build up the character of the ideal nurse; and the ideal nurse – what is she but the ideal woman, with some practical knowledge of nursing?

Remarks such as these indicate that, in the brief space of four years, there had been a shift away from merely "doing" nursing to some under-standing of the basis for the doing. Also of interest is the reference to "the-ory," which would only much later be emphasized in nursing. Finally, the sociological context of nursing practice appears to have been glimpsed by the 1897 graduate.

Whether by chance or by design, nursing was beginning to be seen as a respectable, and respected, career for gentlewomen, and nurse leaders were using the trend for the advancement of the profession and its image. With respect to the applicants in June 1897, the annals of the school referred to "ladies born and bred [as] many of them are," and at about the same time the superintendent of the Toronto General (a woman) reported that "many refined women are entering the profession."[41]

Throughout the first ten years the nurse's uniform underwent succes-sive modifications; the original was a blue and white striped floor-length gown with leg-of-mutton sleeves, stiff white collar and apron, and cap (first folded, then cup-cake).[42] The graduates of 1903 were the first to wear the cap with black band, and the folded cap that would be accepted as the permanent cap of St Michael's school of nursing was first worn by the 1913 graduates. Already by 1894 the graduation pin that would be worn by hundreds of St Michael's graduates had been adopted, a gold Maltese cross inscribed with the words *Quod Minimis Mihi Fecisti* (What you did unto the least of my brethren you did unto me).[43]

From the beginning, graduation exercises were festive occasions; for example, there were printed invitations, and the second class of graduates added to their uniforms "a pink sash from which depended [sic] bunches of sweet violets" – a touch that did not go unnoticed by the newspaper reporters of the day. Having no place large enough to hold a group, the emergency room was on occasion transformed into a reception hall for the early graduations, and red roses early became a graduation tradition. A typical sampling of the addresses to the graduates is that of 1900, with the archbishop exhorting the graduates to be compassionate, the medical superintendent emphasizing a sense of responsibility, and a senior sur-geon grasping the occasion of the assembled board to remark that, while the equipment in the Hugh Ryan wing was splendid, the surgeons had already outgrown their assigned space. One of the doctors usually enter-tained the graduates at his home; a yearly event was the annual sleigh-ride and oyster supper hosted for the whole school and for the house sur-geons by Dr Edmund King.

Ten years after the school's founding, the annals record that eight hun-dred applications had been received – "passing all expectations" – coming from Halifax in the east to Chicago in the west, and as far south as Texas. This may explain partially why there was not a predominance of graduates from Toronto proper in the early years; evidently the cream of the crop of applicants was skimmed, even from Chicago, Buffalo, New Haven, St Louis, and New York – all these appear as home addresses among those listed in the early graduating rosters. In 1904, the tenth anniversary of the first graduation, the Nurses' Alumnae Association was formed.

The sisters followed with interest and pride the careers of their graduates; in 1899 it was recorded that J. Keenan, an 1897 graduate, had received the gold medal for post-graduate work at the prestigious Polyclinic of New York City and in 1900 the annals note that five graduates had "obtained situations" as superintendents of hospitals in Canada and the United States. Meanwhile, right at home, Ellen O'Neill became the first St Michael's graduate (1898) to be placed in charge of the school.

Evidently the board also took a deep interest in the school of nursing; among the papers of the president of the board in 1903 (Archbishop O'Connor) is a list of the final marks obtained by the graduates of that year, ranging from a high of 91 1/2 to a low of 80 1/2, and with such fine distinctions as 90 4/5 and 86 1/10 in between. (The board was, ultimately, the body that vouched for the competence of those nurses the school graduated, there being as yet no external regulatory body.[44])

The Financial Picture

The ledger entry for the "Half-Year Ending June 30, 1894"[45] provides a context for examining financing in the early years:

Bal. on hand Dec. 31/93	65.41	
Payment by patients	1,890.39	
Payment by City	2,339.60	
Government Grant	3,104.58	
Out-door Nursing	164.00	
Donations	254.32	
Profit on Habits for Dead[46]	39.00	
Trust & Loan Co.	200.00	
Borrowed money	150.00	8,207.30

The following discussion offers a detailed look at these various sources of revenue.

Payments by Patients

In the first month of operation, July 1892, revenue from paying patients amounted to $108.50, increasing to $202 in August. While no details are available as to how these charges were levied, five years later the records show private patients paying $8 to $20 per week, depending upon the room, semi-private patients $6 per week, and ward patients $2.80. By 1906 the rates were revised to $15 to $17.50 per week for private patients, according to location, $7 to $8 for semi-private patients, and $10 for maternity patients.

Payment by the City and by the Provincial Government

As noted earlier, the city paid a per diem rate of forty cents to hospitals receiving indigent patients admitted by order of the medical officer of health. In October 1892 St Michael's received its first such payment, which included retroactive payments for July and August. (City council minutes of 13 July 1892 record that a communication was read "from the Lady Managers of St Michael's Hospital, asking to be paid the usual rate for the City patients cared for in that institution.") After the twelve-month suspension of this grant – August 1894 to August 1895 – payments resumed.

The provincial-government grant amounted to thirty cents per patient per day (Appendix B). City and provincial grants, therefore, constituted a significant part of the operating revenue, exclusive of loans.

In 1897 the four public hospitals (St Michael's, Toronto General, Grace Hospital, and the Hospital for Sick Children) made a joint appeal to the city to increase the grant to seventy cents a day. H.T. Kelly, secretary to St Michael's advisory board, testified to the effect that St Michael's would not be able to handle its expenses except for the fact that "its management is entrusted to people who do not cost one cent for salary" – a reference to the sisters' services. He continued, "All the salaries we pay are for minor services and nurses." Cost per patient per day at St Michael's was 80.9 cents.[47]

Ten years later, a large deputation from the same four hospitals was still asking for the increase to seventy cents; meanwhile, the average daily cost per patient had risen to eighty-eight cents at St Michael's, compared to an average of $1.13 at the other hospitals, H.T. Kelly explaining the difference in the same way as he had previously. In the absence of a response from the city to their appeal for an increase, the hospitals appear to have taken joint action in January 1908, notifying the city that "on and after that date the City will be charged seventy cents a day" for city-order patients.[48]

The question of provincial-government appropriations to hospitals was the subject of intense debate from 1904 to 1906. The catalyst for the debate was the government's award of $250,000 to the Toronto General Hospital to assist in its redevelopment; further, the government had suggested that the city match the grant. Not everyone at city hall supported the idea; interviewed on the subject, Dr Charles Sheard, medical officer of health, questioned the fairness of singling out the General for special funding. He pointed out that, of the seven hospitals receiving city-order patients, St Michael's stood second only to the General, having received in the past year $11,723.40. "St Michael's," he said, "as a public servant is but little behind the oldest and best-endowed hospital in the city."

The city finally voted $200,000 towards the General's redevelopment project, whereupon St Michael's, the Western, and the Grace made a joint approach to the city for a like grant, to be divided equally among them. In March 1909 St Michael's was awarded $50,000, an amount estimated to be the cost of the new wing about to be constructed. Arguing the case for St Michael's, H.T. Kelly drew attention to St Michael's excellent facilities for surgery and its intensive involvement in medical education.[49]

"Outdoor" Nursing

Ledger entries of "wages for outdoor nursing" (called special nursing after 1895) appear regularly from July 1893 until 30 June 1905; in 1905 the total of such receipts for the twelve months previous was $2,295.85.[50] While such entries do not appear after 1905, there is a possibility that they were included in the category "Other sources of Revenue." Apparently the school of nursing subscribed to the prevailing practice of assigning senior students to "special" very ill patients in their homes, a practice that was justified on the basis that this would be experience for the future private-duty role many nurses would assume.[51] From the ledger entries it is clear that the fee – if not all, at least in part – became revenue for the hospital. The wide fluctuations in the amounts recorded annually –$210.25 (1893), $189.75 (1895), $360.28 (1896), $186.65 (1897), and $967.00 (1898) – and the fact that some months yielded no revenue from this source, leads to the conclusion that the students were dispatched only when a bona fide need existed and were not routinely exploited as a source of income.[52]

Although we are dealing with revenue at the moment, there is another side of the ledger. An allowance for the "pupil nurses" was initiated in 1895, beginning with $3 per month per student, irrespective of seniority. This was increased to $4 in 1895. In 1897 the allowance was refined: $4 for first-year students, $5 for second-year, and $6 for third-year. These rates continued until 1919-20, the last year in which they appear on the financial statement. Historians of Toronto General, Kingston General, and St Joseph's Hospital (London) report a similar practice and similar amounts.

Private Donations

The first year's financial statement shows donations of $3,040.70, some of which were probably intended as one-time start-up gifts. While the next year's donations dropped to $254.32, there continued a steady trickle of small and medium-sized donations, amounting to about $6,000 annually by 1907. News of such were carried in the daily papers, for example, $1,000 in the will of Frank Smith, and "everything," which amounted to $2,525.17, in the will of one Ann Reynolds, who stipulated that $300 of this was to go towards erecting a chapel at the hospital.

Thus concludes our overview of the sources and levels of revenue in the early years, admittedly small but not so small as to hamper growth and obscure a vision of the future.

Land Acquisitions and Building Projects

A newspaper reporter described St Michael's in December 1896 as "the most homelike hospital ever built," with accommodation for 154 patients. The need for more housing was being felt, however, and was coming from two sources – an increasing volume of patients and a growing school of nursing.

In 1896-97 three small houses on Victoria Street, immediately to the rear of the hospital, were purchased for $5,824, of which Hugh Ryan contributed $3,000.[53] These were made into "one commodious structure" to serve as a nurses' residence, called the Margaret Ryan Home. A newspaper account predicted that the former backyards of the three houses would be transformed in the spring into a "magnificent lawn" for the patients. The same newspaper described the new nurses' home: two upper flats with ten bedrooms of various sizes, all handsomely papered and decorated; a large reception room and parlour on the first floor; nicely fitted lavatories and baths in the basement – the whole heated by hot water radiators. The ledger for February 1898 records an expenditure of $1,050 for "Nurses' Home Furnishings, Painting, Telephone, etc.," and one of $156 for bedsteads. A good beginning, yet as early as 1905, and repeatedly until 1921, provincial inspectors would call for a proper home for the nurses. (Over and over again, in the early records, one is struck by the brevity of the period of usefulness of those old buildings which were refurbished to satisfy an immediate pressing need.)

Reporting on a tour of the hospital in September 1899, a journalist noted "a beautiful figure of St Michael, set there in loving memory of a sister who had died." This sister may have been Sister Juliana Morrow, one of the pioneers, who died of cancer two years after the hospital's founding. One hundred years later the statue stands in the main entrance of the hospital at 30 Bond Street. It has a mysterious history. The sisters found it, dirty and blackened, in the back of a second-hand store on Queen Street and sometime between 1895 and 1899 they purchased it for $49 – a sum accumulated over the years from the sale of old newspapers. The statue had been sculptured in Carrara, Italy, out of that city's beautiful marble – the stone obtained from Pietra Sancta, the same quarry from which Michelangelo procured the marble for his famous Pieta. The date and the sculptor are unknown, but "Pietra Sancta" is clearly chiselled on the back of the statue.[54]

The reporter of 1899 also described a splint room, manned by a carpenter; a laundry equipped with a mangle, where semi-weekly washings were done, all in charge of a sister; a chapel capable of seating 100 and decorated with stained-glass windows; and a dispensary, where two sisters were working. Sister Columba Hayes (not to be confused with a later Sister Columba, also a pharmacist), a pioneer at the Isolation Hospital and one of St Michael's first graduating class of nurses, was in charge of the pharmacy for twenty-five years. To qualify for this position, it appears that she trained under the supervision of a physician, a practice both common and accepted at the time.[55] When Sister Columba was posted to Comox, British Columbia, in 1917, St Michael's sent two sisters, St Maurus Barry and Genevieve Farrell, to the Ontario College of Pharmacy to become "state-qualified." These two had served four years' apprenticeship, and after their year at the College of Pharmacy became the first of the sisters to receive their PhmB from the University of Toronto[56] and also the first of the sisters in health care to have a university degree.

Further property was acquired in 1902 – two houses on Bond Street north of the hospital, for $4,940 in January, and three more houses south of the Hugh Ryan wing for $11,250 that summer. In July of that year the unnamed hospital annalist wryly summed up the situation at the end of the first decade:

> Property has been added regularly to supply the demand for room, and although eighteen lots have been added at an expense of $37,000 many serious attempts to build have proved futile, always meeting with some serious obstruction before the plans pass through the hands of the Sisters, Superior, Mother Superior, her Council, the Archbishop, and the Advisory Board.
>
> Room appears more inadequate than ever, all branches demanding space – Outdoor Patients, Pharmacy, Office, Laundry, Wards, Sisters, Mortuary. We cannot keep up with its [the hospital's] rapid growth in a satisfactory manner.

It is interesting to note in the above the ascending order of authority and decision-making spelled out with some frustration by the writer, and the descending order of priority for space allocation – perhaps all unconsciously.

Plans for a new wing were evidently being pursued seriously, as referred to in the colourful report of a province-wide inspection of prisons and hospitals published in the summer of 1902. While the inspector declared one of the police stations with cells to be "an old rookery," and urged the removal of "lunatics" from the county jail, he had only praise for the city's hospitals. Of St Michael's he wrote: "St Michael's was found to be an excellent institution in all respects. The addition of a new wing will increase the accommodation available, and make it one of the best-equipped hospitals in the City."[57]

The following spring, on a fourth parcel of property on Victoria Street, houses were designated for the sisters' accommodation. It appears that this purchase included two houses on the front of the lot, and three in the rear, paid for – either in whole or in part – by $2,500 plus a mortgage for the same amount.

The following year (1904) a new $10,000 laundry was opened on a portion of the land mentioned just above, boasting machinery and apparatus of the latest and best, staffed by six to eight women, two men, and a skilled mechanic overseeing the new equipment. In future very little laundry would be done by hand, ironing would be by machinery and drying by large presses, with electric fans to carry off the steam. Those sisters still living who had carried water from King Street to do the laundry at the House of Providence would have marvelled at the progress.

A more ambitious building project was decided upon at the annual meeting of the board in July 1906 – a new three-storey wing, to be erected across Victoria Lane from the existing building, at a cost of $50,000. The starting date depended upon successful negotiations with the city for that part of the lane adjoining the hospital on the north.

In the meantime, the new maternity wing was opened, the need for which had become increasingly apparent over a space of ten years. The number of births recorded for the first decade was as follows:[58]

1892...0	1895...9	1898...43	1901...91
1893...1	1896...19	1899...65	1902...80
1894...3	1897...51	1900...78	

A notation, dated December 1902, records the sum of $5,000 for house and lot number 38 on Bond Street "to be used for the present as a maternity hospital." Prior to that, the top floor of the Hugh Ryan wing had been used for maternity patients.

It appears that the 1902 reference may have represented an interim step on the way to a maternity wing. At any rate, provisions were made for a dramatic increase in accommodation (from twelve to eighty beds) for maternity patients in 1907, when three large brick dwellings south of the hospital were converted into one building, connected by a covered laneway to the hospital proper.

Newly papered and painted from end to end, the wing had three large public wards of seven to ten beds each on the ground floor, with new bathrooms and medicine closets as well as kitchens at the rear of the building. On the second and third floors there were twelve private and eighteen semi-private rooms, the latter containing either two or three beds. A newspaper reporter remarked on "the wonderful taste in furnishing" and the "homelike atmosphere" which had also won congratulations from several American physicians. M.M. Crawford, "already one of Toronto's most skilled obstetricians," assumed charge of the new facility.[59] The provincial inspector of 1907 commended the hospital for the new facility, yet the inspector of just six years later (Dr Helen MacMurchy) would declare it "inadequate and unsuitable." Parenthetically, one might be inclined to fault the sisters for not having made this assessment themselves. However, there existed at the time no medium for the exchange of information and for making comparisons. The journal *Canadian Hospital* began publication only in 1924; prior to its advent there were no hospital journals in Canada and few in the United States.[60]

Dr Malcolm Crawford, an 1898 graduate of the University of Toronto, remained head of obstetrics until 1916, when he went overseas with the Canadian Army Medical Corps. In the university reorganization of 1909-10, Dr Frederick Fenton became chief of the combined obstetrics and gynaecology department, with Crawford his assistant in obstetrics. In 1926 Crawford became lecturer in medical jurisprudence at the university and chief coroner for the city of Toronto; at the time of his death in 1937 he was supervising coroner for the province of Ontario. Said to be full of energy and good cheer, Crawford worked tirelessly for extension of the city's playgrounds to reduce children's injuries as a result of playing in the streets.

This completes the account of plant development over the first few years – development consisting mainly of modest, make-do improvisations as the demands grew and all connected with St Michael's learned day by day the details that go into the making of a hospital.

Medical Staff and Medical Education

When St Michael's opened in 1892 there were schools of medicine for men students at the University of Toronto and at Trinity College, and for women students at the Ontario Medical College for Women. The faculties of Toronto and Trinity became one in 1903 under the University of Toronto, and the women's medical college closed in 1906 when women were admitted to the faculty of medicine at the university.

We have no record of St Michael's physicians, other than Dr Dwyer, until the letter to city council in June 1893 protesting Alderman Orr's charges.[61] How these men were recruited and appointed is not clear, but, as noted earlier, "a list of doctors" for the new hospital was tabled at the sisters' council before the hospital's formal opening. The earliest complete roster is that published when the Hugh Ryan wing was opened in 1895; it includes thirteen of the fourteen who signed the letter to the city council in 1893 (Appendix D).

The hospital advisory board under Archbishop Walsh's presidency, which would assume responsibility for medical appointments, was not constituted until 1895. However, some notes are found on Walsh's stationery, dated 1894, which may be considered rudimentary medical staff by-laws:[62]

> Dr. Ross* had an interview with me to-day on hospital matters. [Then follow some jottings]: How many are necessary? entitlement for promotion: service; consultation with staff to see if more physicians necessary; have a definite number, and then applicants can be told if number is filled; need a code of rules drawn up by a committee of the surgeons and doctors; possibility of re-election, and only by advisory board; appointments should be made irrespective of the medical schools and entirely on the merits of the men.

Further handwritten notes in the archbishop's file repeat the same principles, but add: "Resident doctor should not teach on any account at any institution or school; no preponderance of any school or institute should be allowed on staff; consulting staff – all who have served five years on active staff – the smaller the staff, as long as it is efficient, so much the better; staff too large, becomes unwieldy." The date of these latter notes appears to be around the time that the Toronto Western Hospital opened (under discussion from 1896, opened in 1898) for the notes say, of the person with whom the conversation was held, "Does not favour the Western Hospital – three is enough for this City." From the detail contained in these notes, evidently the archbishop, in his capacity as president of the board,

---

*Almost certainly Dr. J.F.W. Ross, who was president of the Toronto Medical Society from 25 May 1893 through May 1894. An 1879 graduate of the University of Toronto, Ross studied in London, Berlin, and Vienna after a year as house surgeon at the General. He later became professor of gynaecology and head of gynaecology service at the General Hospital. His name regularly appears in the admissions register of St Michael's over the first two decades. In 1895 he is listed as a specialist in gynaecology at St Michael's. (See Appendix D.) His son, Dr James Ross, was a prominent surgeon at St Michael's in the 1930s and 1940s.

was deeply involved in the first appointments to the medical staff.

From 1898 on, medical-staff appointments were regularly made at the meetings of the advisory board: on 3 October 1898, Drs J. Amyot and W. McKeown, surgeons (promoted from assistant surgeons); Dr A. Rose-burgh, ophthalmology; Dr J.G. Wishart, nose and throat; Dr G. Silverthorn, outdoor. Both Drs Roseburgh and Wishart held appointments at the General, the latter as chief and professor of otolaryngology at the university until 1922. Drs Amyot, McKeown, and Silverthorn would have long association with St Michael's.

A typical progression through the ranks is that of Dr F. Uren, who would spend many years at St Michael's. He was appointed as registrar in December 1899,[63] then to outdoor staff in June 1900, to assistant surgeon in July 1901, and to surgeon in June 1902 – to fill the vacancy left by Dr Leslie Sweetnam's death.[64]

Staff appointments at the annual meeting of the advisory board in 1902, the tenth anniversary of the hospital, were: visiting physicians (twelve) – Drs Alexander McPhedran, C. McKenna, M. Wallace, F. McMahon, A. Garrett, H.B. Anderson, G. Chambers, J. Guinane, R. Dwyer, A.J. Johnson, N. Allen, and J.H. McConnell; visiting surgeons (eleven) – Drs R.B. Nevitt, I.H. Cameron, W. Oldright, E. King, H.A. Bruce, G.A. Bingham, W. McKeown, A. Primrose, W.H.B. Aikens, and F. Uren; assistant surgeon – Dr G. Silverthorn. Several of these have been referred to earlier; new was Dr Alexander Primrose, professor of anatomy at University of Toronto at the time of his appointment, and later professor of clinical surgery from 1918 to 1931 and dean of the medical faculty from 1920 to 1932; Drs Bingham and Aikens were pathologists at the General Hospital in 1888 – Bingham operated regularly at St Michael's, and helped nurse Ellen O'Neill organize the necessary surgical instruments and equipment in the first operating theatre; Aikens was later active in treatment by radium therapy of a wide range of conditions.

In 1906 the newspapers prepared and published a comprehensive listing of the doctors of the city along with their clinical and teaching appointments. That listing shows St Michael's with eleven physicians, seven of whom held appointments at the university, and six of whom were also on the staff at the General; fifteen surgeons, twelve of whom held appointments at the university and ten of whom were also at the General; two specialists in eye, one in nose and throat, and one in obstetrics, all of whom had university appointments. The newspapers reported a proposed revision of Toronto General policies whereby no member of the visiting staff could hold a position on the visiting staff in any other hospital, except the Hospital for Sick Children which was considered a special, rather than a general, hospital – a proposal that, if doctors chose to remain with the General, would have halved the medical and surgical staffs at St Michael's.[65] However, the proposal appears not to have been implemented until 1913. In the meantime, St Michael's recruited new staff, as shown in the inspectors' reports of these years: in 1909 the number of doctors on staff at St Michael's was forty-seven, in 1913 there were fifty-four, and in 1918 there were seventy.

Some indication of the bond existing among medical staff at both St Michael's and the General, and with the university, is seen in the events surrounding the death of Dr Matthew Wallace in 1906. An honours graduate from the University of Toronto's faculty of medicine, Wallace went to New York for post-graduate work in obstetrics and in the treatment of cancer, following which he was among the most active of the medical staff at St Michael's until his death of cancer at age fifty-seven. Dr Wallace had had the first of his five children at age forty-four, and so left a very young family. His friends and colleagues, with Dr J.F.W. Ross, professor of gynaecology, acting as treasurer, immediately set themselves the goal of raising $10,000 for the education of the children. The subscriptions, ranging from $1 to $200, were regularly published in the newspapers and the target was soon reached.

The earliest reference to anaesthetists at St Michael's, and possibly illustrative of an expanding surgical service, appears in November 1901, when the advisory board appointed Drs M. Crawford, F.W. Marlow, R.N. Parent, and P.W. O'Brien to this service. Crawford had been housestaff in 1898, Marlow in 1900, and Parent and O'Brien from June 1901. The following newspaper notice of January 1906 provides evidence both of the efforts then being made to impose some order on the surgical service, and of the strains afflicting the emergency ward: "Patients suffering from minor surgical injuries will receive the first dressing at any time they present themselves at the Emergency Ward at St Michael's Hospital. All subsequent attendance to be at the Out-Patient Department at 9 a.m." A policy that would endure through the years was thus established, but the refinement of appointment times would not come until later.

Resident House Doctors

Dr Dwyer had one house doctor to assist him each year during the hospital's first six years. (Generally newly graduated doctors, these had living accommodations in the hospital and so were referred to as "housestaff.") When he moved out of the hospital after his marriage in 1898, two appointments to housestaff were made, Dr Malcolm Crawford and Dr W.P. McNulty, the latter an honours graduate of the University of Toronto who located in Peterborough following his two years at St Michael's. It appears that, beginning in 1899, three housestaff were appointed each year, some of whom stayed for a second year, at the end of which some were promoted to staff.

In June 1901, out of ten applications received, three housestaff – all male – were appointed, one from Trinity Medical School, the other two from the University of Toronto's medical school. Dr Helen MacMurchy, who had submitted applications to both St Michael's and the General, received an appointment at the latter.[66] The number of housestaff increased to four in 1904 (among whom was Dr Mary Callaghan, St Michael's second woman doctor) and to five in 1906.

St Michael's and Medical Education

The University of Toronto's faculty of medicine calendar for 1896-97 states with regard to St Michael's, "Clinical instruction is given in this Hospital by those members of the staff who are also on the teaching staff of the University." The calendar lists physicians J.E. Graham, A. McPhedran, and J. Caven, and surgeons I.H. Cameron, W. Oldright, and J. Amyot.

In May 1897 the university appointed Dwyer and Dr G. Boyd as lecturers in clinical medicine, subject to government approval; they appeared as such in the calendar of 1897-98.

As indicated, medical students came to St Michael's for clinical experience from the year the hospital was established. From October 1898 there appear regular ledger entries of student fees received ($275 in October, $282 in November), yet a year later a sceptical city council was questioning, through the medical officer of health, whether medical students really were using St Michael's.

Indicative of the interdependence of the hospital and the university, and foreshadowing the latter's future influence in hospital affairs, is an account of a meeting of the committee of the faculty on hospital facilities with St Michael's board of trustees in October 1903 for the purpose of "placing suggestions for the betterment of the work."[67] Having visited centres in New York, Boston, Philadelphia, Chicago, Montreal, and Baltimore, the committee tabled its views on a range of issues related to medical education in the clinical area, with particular emphasis on the importance of the public wards, out-patient departments, and pathology departments (including autopsies) in medical education (See Appendix E). These would become prominent issues in the hospital-university agreement to be negotiated in 1914.

A Few Summary Comments on the Early Years

The main players have been introduced, and the principal developments during the beginning years have been traced. In those early, heady times, a strong bond of respect and mutual support, and a depth of feeling and enthusiasm for the enterprise they were all engaged in, was evident among the sisters, board, medical staff, and nursing students. Board members and doctors, named and recorded, turned out *en masse* to graduations, receptions, and other occasions; sisters and nurses were there, too, but remained anonymous except for "Mother Superior," who was herself anonymous but for her role. Morale seems to have been high.

There were dark days as well; in 1899 a lawsuit followed after an eighteen-year-old girl died of poisoning, victim of the administration of carbolic acid from a poorly labelled magnesium sulphate bottle, filled by the sister in charge of the dispensary. From time to time the hospital was overcrowded, with sisters and nurses called upon to go the extra mile and relinquish their beds. We also catch the occasional glimpse of competition between hospitals, as when the Western Hospital opened in 1898 to serve the sick west of Spadina Avenue, and rumours were rife of others to be opened in the north end of the city. The medical officer of health, appearing before the city's board of control, recommended "reducing the number of institutions so that the general expenses of management, etc., would be proportionately lessened. [Where there are] various institutions, this leads to multiplication of officers interested in their respective work."

These words sound eerily familiar one hundred years later, as cash-strapped boards negotiate, amidst waves of nostalgia and protest, mergers of their once-proud institutions.

4
Growth and Growing Pains

The second and third decades of the new century, though deeply scarred by the First World War, were years of remarkable growth and development – in the city, in the Congregation of St Joseph, and in St Michael's Hospital.

Prominent among developments in the city were those in the transportation sector: these were the years that brought the automobile to Toronto, as well as the airplane, the motorcycle policeman, and even, in 1911, a proposal for a subway system to replace the inexpensive (eight tickets for twenty-five cents) but inefficient streetcar system. These years brought, also, the first skyscrapers to Toronto, and the first apartment houses. Population grew to near the half-million mark by 1918, and women won the right to vote.

Fiercely patriotic, Toronto proudly waved 70,000 of its young men off to war, then sickened with grief as every mail brought lists of those killed in action – 10,000 by war's end. Shipyards, munitions and aircraft factories, and ancillary services created unprecedented job opportunities. Many women went into the city's factories, a move that left the hospitals barely able to cope; but worse was to come, when an outbreak of deadly influenza accompanied the returning soldiers. At St Michael's, history was repeated as volunteers were called for and came – the sister-teachers from the motherhouse, supplemented this time by the alumnae of the academy (the sisters' high school) and the Sisters of Loretto.

Growth of the congregation continued, as did requests for extension of its hospital foundations – three requests in three years (Brampton, Ontario, as well as Manitoba and Alaska), all of which had to be refused; the congregation's emphasis was on the schools. Further, too few sisters were being prepared for hospital work to staff foundations beyond St Michael's. However, in 1913 the congregation founded St Joseph's Hospital at Comox, British Columbia, following this eight years later with St Joseph's Hospital at Sunnyside in west Toronto, and finally, St Joseph's Hospital, Winnipeg, in 1923. In each case some sisters were transferred from St Michael's to staff the new foundations. These were also years of intellectual vigour in the congregation; the teaching sisters took advantage of their proximity to the University of Toronto to pursue extra courses and degrees, and the hospital sisters began to travel to other centres (Detroit, Chicago, St Louis) and to conventions in order to keep abreast of developments. Formal post-basic preparation of the hospital sisters was, however, still in the future. Salaries for the teachers rose steadily, from $300 per annum in 1911, to $450 in 1917, and to $800 in 1920.

In 1918, in an attempt to estimate accurately the cost of its operations, the hospital devised its first complete salary scale (See Appendix F). For the sisters holding the various positions the scale merely represented the value assigned to their contributed services. The hospital moved from an annual cash-balance position in the years prior to 1916 to a deficit position for the next several years, with the "free" patients outnumbering the paying patients in 1917-18.

While the existing public wards and the outpatient departments were seen to be essential to the hospital's ministry to the poor (the archbishop having made his wishes known in no uncertain terms)[1] and to its involvement in medical education, these would soon be inadequate; as well, the university would demand more and better diagnostic services as a condition for including St Michael's among its clinical-teaching facilities. None of these three areas was revenue-producing to any significant degree; it was thought that a balance might be restored by providing more private and semi-private accommodation. All of this would mean new construction, more nurses, and more accommodation for nurses – major preoccupations for all concerned for a number of years.

The Machinery of Decision-Making

When Dr Dwyer left in 1902 for study in Europe, the decision was made by the General Council not to engage a medical superintendent to replace him. The superior became, in effect, the superintendent; the first official acknowledgement of this fact appears in the 1908 report of the inspector of prisons and public charities.[2] A markedly increased involvement of the General Council in setting policy and direction, making medical-staff appointments, and in addressing problems of all kinds – even in the details of day-to-day management – is evident for the next couple of decades.[3]

While momentous events were unfolding at the hospital, notable among which were an ambitious building plan and the negotiating of a formal agreement with the university with regard to medical education, the rotation of sisters from council to hospital and vice versa undoubtedly sparked council involvement in the hospital's affairs. In 1902 Mother Assumption Keenan, with nine years of hospital experience as superior behind her, was elected to council as assistant superior general. She was re-elected to council in 1905 and Sister Demetria MacGregor, with three years' service as superior at the hospital, joined her on the council. Sister Irene Conroy succeeded Sister Demetria as superior at the hospital, for a three-year term, and followed this with a six-year term as superior general, while Sister Demetria remained for a second term on council. Throughout all these years there were, therefore, sisters with considerable background in hospital work involved at the highest level of decision-making in the congregation. Archbishop Fergus McEvay in 1908 specifically directed that one councillor should have hospital matters as her major sphere of responsibility; the same arrangement had probably been in place less formally in earlier years.

One of the negative side-effects of the council's heavy involvement in hospital affairs was that the hospital board appears to have been bypassed, or at least under-utilized, for several years; too, the declining health of the board chairman, Archbishop O'Connor, and the short three-year term of his successor, Archbishop McEvay, probably led to council's directly assuming control. At any rate, when Archbishop Neil McNeil arrived on the scene, he urged the council in 1913 to consider setting up a hospital board of governors which would exercise delegated authority in certain areas and act in an advisory capacity in others. This would be an executive board, the powers of which would be more extensive than the current advisory board. Further, he suggested the composition of the board. Less autocratic than his predecessors, McNeil suggested that the council take a week to consider his proposal; promptly at the end of the week council made its decision – the board and the terms of reference were agreed to. But council by no means passed the reins over completely, either to the board or to the archbishop; several months later, the councillors informed McNeil that they would like to do the business of the hospital through their own solicitors (rather than the archbishop's) and that they wished to be informed of the conditions (payments, interest, and so on) of a recent property transaction he had made on behalf of the hospital. One can imagine the emotions that must have surrounded these two communications to the archbishop.

On another front, the landmark 1909 survey of medical schools in Canada and the United States (the Flexner report) had come out strongly in favour of the arrangements in place for medical education at the University of Toronto, and had placed Toronto on a par with Harvard and Johns Hopkins.[4] The report argued for control of the administration and financing of the university hospital by the university trustees, with medical conduct of the hospital and teaching in its wards to be left to the medical faculty of the university. These recommendations, if adopted, would have constituted a radical redistribution of powers between the participating institutions.

Earlier the Province of Ontario had passed the Hospital Act (1906), legislation that the university interpreted as giving it exclusive control over the clinical teaching at the Toronto General; the $300,000 that it had contributed to the General's building program was to secure for the university, for all time, exclusive rights and privilege of access to the hospital wards, and adequate provision – at the hospital's initiative – for clinical chemistry and such other subjects as would advance scientific medicine. Additionally, all public-ward patients must agree to be subjects for clinical teaching. Frequent references are contained in university-hospital correspondence attesting to the hospital board's difficulty in reconciling its responsibility for the care of patients with the university's aspirations for its teaching staff and its responsibility for medical education.[5]

In a draft agreement (1909) between the governors of the university and the trustees of the Toronto General Hospital, acknowledgment was made of the university twice giving $300,000 to the latter. The draft agreement stipulated that all appointments to the hospital staff would be made by the trustees only, on the nomination of the Joint Hospital Relations Committee, with the exception of heads of such departments as medicine, surgery, and obstetrics at the university, who would be *ex-officio* members of the hospital staff.[6]

It was against this background of the university's established relationship with the Toronto General that negotiations for a formal arrangement between the university and St Michael's were begun in June 1909. That same year a reorganization of St Michael's Hospital staff was announced in the university's faculty of medicine calendar. (There had been some movement earlier; Sister Irene Conroy, before finishing her term at the hospital in 1908, had had one or more interviews with President Robert Falconer on the subject, but no record remains of their talks.[7]) Dr Malcolm Cameron records that he and Dr Harris McPhedran, both of whom had been demonstrators of clinical-laboratory methods in the university's department of pathology, were transferred in 1908 to clinical medicine and clinical surgery respectively, and assigned to St Michael's.

The university took the initial step, indicating a wish to have the medical faculty make suggestions about the laboratory in the hospital's proposed new wing, and to discuss "what the University Medical Department will be prepared to do towards equipment of the laboratory, provided some definite relationship is established between the Hospital and the University Medical Faculty."[8]

Mother Victoria Devine, superior at the hospital, responded in January 1910 in a letter to Dean C.K. Clarke; she said that professors and students would be given as much room as possible in the new wing to be built, and she reminded the dean that 40 percent of the clinical experience for students was already being offered at St Michael's Hospital. Further, she proposed that the hospital purchase the lot at the southeast corner of Shuter and Victoria streets and erect thereon a special building for outpatients, as well as a pathological laboratory, on a plan to be approved by the professors of clinical medicine and surgery. The projected cost of lot and building was $80,000; she invited the university to pay the interest on the capital invested at 5 percent per annum, that is, $4,000 a year for twenty years, and further, to staff, equip, and maintain the laboratories.[9]

President Falconer replied on 18 February 1910 suggesting that a special committee of the Joint Hospital Relations Committee meet with representatives of St Michael's to consider the matter. But a week later hospital solicitor H.T. Kelly informed the archbishop and the superior general that the proposal for additional clinical facilities at the hospital (which had originated with Professor I.H. Cameron[10] of the hospital staff and Dean Clarke, and which President Falconer and Mother Victoria had begun to act upon) had never gone through the appropriate channels, namely the university board of governors. That body now directed that a communication be directed to its chairman, stating what had been proposed, and the board would appoint a committee to consider it. Kelly advised that "the proposal is likely to meet with some opposition, and any negotiations upon it will most probably involve a suggestion that the Hospital bind itself to appoint to its visiting staff those doctors who are Professors or Lecturers on the Medical Staff of the University."

The university's medical faculty, meanwhile, began its work, and in a letter of 5 April 1910 from Dean Clarke to the university's lawyer, the dean reported:

The heads of the departments (Medical Faculty) think that an arrangement similar to that existing with the General Hospital should be made with St. Michael's Hospital. There has been a change of opinion regarding the amount of room requested for the pathological work, and a building much less extensive than that first proposed will answer the purpose. This will materially reduce the cost of the outdoor department building .... If any sum of money is paid for privileges to be granted to us, we should clearly understand our rights and have them defined in such a way that there can be no misunderstanding.

As at Toronto General Hospital, the head of each department shall be ex officio head of each department at St. Michael's Hospital. We should have the right to nominate the staff in the same manner as at the General, and it should be clearly specified that our men shall have charge of all public patients .... We should have full charge of the outdoor department ... full clinical advantages for our students ....

In connection with the main wards, there should be a small room for our service devoted to clinical laboratory purposes. Our pathologist should be head of the pathology department, and have placed at his disposal all the pathological material available. These are the chief requirements, and the whole thing is much simplified by the fact that no elaborate or costly building is asked for; all we require will be a few rooms for laboratory purposes.

No reason was given for the considerable shrinkage in the amount of room required for a clinical program – one may speculate that, if the hospital had been going to provide it *gratis*, the medical faculty would have been inclined to dream a little; if the university were to be required to pay, needs then became more realistic.

Suddenly, on 1 September 1910, the university asked that arrangements between the two parties be delayed until the end of the year.[11] However, it appears that the property for a new wing which would accommodate the university's requirements had already been bought, whereupon the General Council took the position that, since the building was intended for university work, the university should pay the interest on the capital borrowed and invested for that purpose. On 26 September 1910 H.T. Kelly informed President Falconer that, although a committee was actively examining the proposal[12] with Mr Z. Lash (the university's lawyer), "the attendance of medical student classes at St. Michael's pending the University's decision ... is not to be considered as binding on the hospital to continue this accommodation." In December 1910 the General Council decided to call a meeting of the hospital board and lay before it the transactions in connection with the university; it appears that the council had been dealing directly with the university.[13]

Then followed a spirited one-on-one exchange between President Falconer and Mother Victoria which resembled nothing quite so much as a fencing match. In a letter to Archbishop McEvay, Mother Victoria said that President Falconer had called on her on 3 March 1911 and had asked that "a letter be sent him, stating what we want in the line of students' fees, and upon what basis we ask for such."[14] Each medical student paid the university a fee of $150 to cover one session's clinical facilities at Toronto General, St Michael's, and Sick Childrens' hospitals. Mother Victoria countered by asking Falconer to state in writing what the university proposed doing, and "to send it to Reverend Mother."[15] She said that the president "assured me that at no time did he think the University could afford to do without St. Michael's."

It appears that the archbishop then attempted to respond regarding the issue of student fees, for within a week Mother Victoria received a copy of his letter to the president, but it did not contain the information the latter had requested. Mother Victoria immediately wrote the archbishop that what the hospital wanted in student fees was "not anything extraordinary – but only our just proportion." Probably frustrated, she then wrote directly to President Falconer a not entirely gracious letter in which she attempted to answer his query as to the basis on which the hospital felt student fees should be based, lecturing him that it was the university's duty to provide for doctors-in-training and the hospital's duty to care for the sick, and that the hospital's revenue from students' fees was hardly worth mentioning.

The usually courteous Falconer replied by return mail, saluting her simply, and rather coolly, as "Madam." He admitted the university's duty as Mother Victoria had stated it, but also expressed his belief that it was "not asking too much to expect from hospitals which receive grants from the Government that they should be willing to do something to make this education possible and efficient." The president then specified the minimum requirements of the university, such as those related to staff appointments and privileges as well as a second operating-room theatre, a large demonstration room, and two units for pathology in addition to the two used for hospital purposes. He concluded with the assurance that "the Board of Governors of the University of Toronto desire to approach this matter in a fair and reasonable spirit, with a view to the making of a permanent

73

arrangement with St. Michael's Hospital which would prove to the advantage of both."[16]

While softening the tone of her response a week later, Mother Victoria continued to instruct the president: "The hospital simply receives grants in the same proportion as hospitals all over the Province where students do not attend, and therefore the grant should be left out of the discussion." She told him further that, as a result of the university's delay in answering the letter of January 1910, construction of the new wing on Bond Street (the D-wing) had advanced too far to include the requirements the president had stipulated. Then she extended the olive branch: "It will be absolutely necessary, in the new building on Shuter St., to arrange the plans so that professors and students may have a reasonable opportunity to do their important work." She concluded by naming Dr R. Dwyer and H.T. Kelly as St Michael's representatives to meet with a committee from the university.

Meanwhile, at its meeting of 31 March 1911 the General Council decided that the university should erect a building for its own use, at its own expense, on ground given for the purpose by the congregation, if necessary – terms similar to those arranged with the Toronto General.[17]

Finally, on 4 April 1911 a meeting of the special committee of the University of Toronto and St Michael's Hospital was held, attended by President Falconer, Dr I.H. Cameron, Dean Clarke, and Z.A. Lash for the university, and Dr Dwyer and Kelly for the hospital. It was agreed that a new building was necessary,[18] and Kelly suggested that the university contribute an annual sum based upon a rate of interest on the capital borrowed to erect such a building – a return to the proposal of January 1910. In exchange, the agreement would provide for "certain control by the University over the appointment of the teaching staff ... on somewhat the same lines as the agreement between the University and the Toronto General Hospital." The upshot of this meeting was that draft plans would be submitted to the university board of governors, which would set up yet another special committee to fashion a basis for the intended agreement.

Throughout the negotiations thus far, the hospital appeared distinctly wary about entering into a binding agreement with the university whereby it would surrender some of its autonomy. At the same time, it acknowledged the enhanced status that would accompany its formal affiliation with the university. While St Michael's was desperately in need of new facilities to replace ones condemned by the provincial inspector, it must have felt out-manoeuvred by the General, which had received from the university a total of $600,000 toward its splendid new facilities to be opened in 1913 in return for privileges similar to those being sought at St Michael's with no guaranteed money on the table. Further, the passage by the Province of the Toronto General Hospital Act in 1911 had established a special relationship between the government, the university, and the Toronto General – with twelve government and university representatives on the hospital's twenty-four-member board of trustees.[19]

The gloves came off, and the issues of money and institutional autonomy were addressed directly at a meeting on 30 January 1914 of the two parties.[20] The representatives from St Michael's quoted figures: the university's outlay for the acquisition of clinical material at the General, and the fact that 40 percent of the clinical material available to students (in the previous year) had been at St Michael's and had been given to the university free of charge. Furthermore, the university was assuming the right to appoint whomsoever it wished for the purpose of utilizing the clinical material available.

Returning to the issue of money, at a meeting of 14 May 1914 the university pointed out that, in view of the many obligations incurred by the university towards the General Hospital, the sum for St Michael's must be moderate, far below that suggested by representatives from St Michael's. President Falconer said that he regarded "an annual rental of $3,000 a not unfair remuneration for university use of St Michael's pathological building." St Michael's representatives then proposed some principles which would preserve the autonomy of each institution, and suggested that, for the university to fulfil its responsibility to its students at the hospital, the laboratories and such other facilities necessary for medical training should be established and staffed at the expense of the university – specifically, a hospital museum, a resident pathologist, a properly fitted post-mortem room, clinical laboratories readily accessible from the wards, and one or more rooms for clinics (Appendix E).

The memorandum drafted at the January 1914 meeting represents, for all intents and purposes, the first agreement with the university.[21] It appears that both parties perceived it as such, judging from the correspondence of 1914 and 1916 surrounding the appointment of Dr D'Arcy Frawley as chief of obstetrics at the hospital, with a university appointment as demonstrator in gynaecology.[22] Refinements in the parties' understanding of their relationship continued to be worked out over a period of years: in 1920 the university provided the hospital with a comprehensive document dealing with the development of young staff clinicians and teachers, and with staff appointments and organization, patient records, and staff regulations – the last items based upon "The Minimum Standard for Approval under the Hospital Standardization Program of the American College of Surgeons."[23] Finally, in a draft letter from St Michael's board to Sir Robert Falconer in March 1921, the hospital endeavoured to clarify further the "relations and scope of authority of the two organizations ... in order to avoid all sources of friction – our constant desire."

The outbreak of the war further complicated relations between St Michael's and the University of Toronto. In March 1915 Drs W. McKeown, G. Silverthorn, G. Wilson, J. Amyot, J.B. Elliott, and H. McPhedran volunteered for active military service through the university, which had offered to equip a base hospital.[24] A problem arose, however, concerning nurses who wished to volunteer for this Canadian army hospital: in a letter of 16 March 1915 to President Falconer, the secretary of St Michael's board charged that the board had been informed that "a certain party in close touch with the General Hospital had represented to the Minister of Militia that only graduate nurses from the General Hospital are qualified to do duty abroad," and that, as a consequence, only three graduates from St Michael's, out of twenty-six who had volunteered, were to be accepted.[25] The secretary wrote a second time, this time naming "the certain party." By return mail, President Falconer, though acknowledging that "someone was up to some mischief," assured St Michael's that the person mentioned had in no way used her influence to prejudice St Michael's, and that Dr Clarke, superintendent of Toronto General Hospital, had made the selection from names submitted. St Michael's board then assured Falconer that "[we are] fully conscious of the honesty of your motives, but we are equally aware that certain influences are at work to make an understanding between us difficult."[26]

In reviewing the negotiations with the university and the subsequent struggles over appointments, one is at first inclined to conclude that the hospital and its officials were being excessively leery and suspicious – disposed to see themselves in danger of being taken advantage of at every turn. Yet the quote from the last letter mentioned above, along with Falconer's earlier reference to "some mischief," suggests that their concerns may not have been groundless.

How the question of the nurses' applications was settled is not documented; however, the first contingent of St Michael's nurses, eight in all, went overseas in 1915. Before war's end, twenty-six nurses from this young hospital would serve with the armed forces overseas, and a further six at home.[27]

The Building of the North "D" Wing

The negotiation of an agreement with the university, while dominating the middle years of the period between the First World War and the Great Depression, was not the only project underway. From early 1906 the General Council was discussing plans for a new wing at St Michael's. These deliberations were complicated by Archbishop McEvay's proposal in late 1908 that another site be chosen for the building of a new hospital, with the present one retained as an emergency hospital. Council stood firm, maintaining that the present site had the advantage for professors and students of proximity to the university,[28] and of easy access for ward and outdoor patients living in the downtown core; later, another site might be chosen to erect a building for private patients and convalescents.

The starting date for construction of the new wing depended upon successful negotiations with the city for that part of the lane adjoining the hospital on the west. A direct communication from the old building to the new was desired, on each floor, and so the hospital wanted to acquire either the lane or the right to erect bridges over it from one part of the building to another. This would make possible the removal of the medical patients from the old north wing to the new one, which would have accommodation for 150 patients. The attendants would be moved from the houses on Victoria Street into the north wing, which would get a new slate roof. Mindful of the events of a few years previous, two new fire escapes would be added to the present building, which already had two.[29]

The building plans, including negotiations for the lane, were no doubt accelerated by recommendations from the provincial inspector, Department of Hospitals and Charities (replacing the inspector of prisons and public charities) who, with sharper criticism each year from 1906 onward, drew attention to the inadequate accommodation for public-ward patients.[30] Although acknowledging that the situation at St Michael's was no different from that of all the other Toronto hospitals, also overcrowded (the immigration of the early 1900s was being felt), the inspector declared it to be "quite intolerable in a public hospital receiving Government and Municipal Aid." Here one is struck again, when reading reports of inspections, of how quickly facilities deteriorated and had to be condemned. The situation would, nevertheless, continue until 1911-12 when the new wing was built; it appears that the hospital took some beds out of service, however, since the numbers shown in the inspector's report decreased from 250 in 1908 to 180 in 1911.

In November 1909 final plans were submitted for proposal of a new wing north of the original building. The presbytery part of the old Baptist church was pulled down, and the north (later called the "D") wing was built – an imposing three-storey structure that doubled the bed complement to 350. The architect was Albert Post of Whitby, who had earlier designed the Hugh Ryan wing. Each of the three floors was divided into large wards containing twelve to sixteen beds each. These provided minimum privacy for the patient but maximum opportunity for supervision by the nurse. Balcony rooms offered isolation areas for tuberculous patients. These floors would remain with little change until the 1950s. An x-ray machine was installed in the basement, and a technician was employed; later, two sisters learned to operate the machine and took the night and weekend calls.[31] The building was topped by a pleasant roof garden, overlooking the Metropolitan Church grounds. This became a favourite setting for patient outings and nurses' graduations, as well as for entertaining guests. A fourth storey, consisting of five operating rooms – two for major surgery, and one each for eye, ear, nose and throat; urology; and septic cases – would be added in 1921, displacing the roof garden.[32] On 19 March 1912 the formal opening of the addition took place, Sir John Gibson, lieutenant-governor of Ontario, officiating.

But there was still work to be done, and immediately. While the provincial inspector commended St Michael's for "the splendid new addition ... which greatly improves accommodation for public ward patients," he condemned the facilities provided for maternity patients. In 1913 the inspector suspended the provincial grant, pending provision of proper accommodation for these patients. To correct the situation, the hospital sisters proposed returning maternity patients to the top floor of the surgical wing as in previous years, and council, which had wanted to use the new wing for the maternity patients, acceded to their proposal, with an interesting proviso – the maternity patients were not to be allowed to work throughout the hospital, and their meals were to be served them in their own quarters.

The War Years, 1914-1918

Following the outbreak of the First World War, the hospital's advisory board moved quickly to clear with the university a plan to choose competent fifth-year medical students to act as residents. Outstanding among these was Dr Esther Harrison, who would later become the first woman to hold a staff appointment at St Michael's.[33]

In 1916-17 the university sent 170 of its medical students off to war, forty-two of whom were ordered home by the Imperial War Office to complete their course.[34] The aftermath of these interrupted years was felt later at St Michael's when, in 1923, the hospital had thirty-seven applicants for its nine intern positions.

The times called for flexibility and ingenuity, and in 1917 Dr E. King used his influence as president of the College of Physicians and Surgeons to have house doctors provisionally qualified to administer anaesthetics. But flexibility had its limits: after the advisory board had approved a plan to have fifth-year medical students attend obstetric cases in the homes of needy patients "provided one of the Hospital's *accoucheurs* remained available if required," Dr M. Crawford (head of obstetrics, but not a member of the advisory board) appeared before the latter body and held firm that this responsibility be reserved to the house doctor.

As mentioned earlier, in 1915 the university sent a 1040-bed hospital to the front, its forty-three officers drawn from the faculty of medicine. From St Michael's, Drs J. Amyot, I.H. Cameron, M. Crawford, W. McKeown, H. McPhedran, A. Primrose, W. Scott, and G. Wilson became part of the university's field hospital. Dr McKeown became president of the Standing Medical Board of England; Amyot was mentioned in dispatches and was decorated for distinguished service, as was Dr W.A. Scott.

The home front, too, had its heroes, for the departure of the senior men left large holes in the ranks. For several months in 1917 Dr F. Uren attended single-handed to the surgical, gynaecological, and emergency departments in this 350-bed hospital, an effort that led to his collapse when his colleagues returned.[35]

It was not only personnel who were in short supply: during the war years board members had to be pressed into service to use their influence to meet the hospital's urgent need for coal and for money, repeatedly approaching city and provincial authorities during 1917 and 1918 in efforts to have the per diem rates increased.[36] Apparently aware of the need to contain costs, the advisory board reviewed the doctors' use of expensive anaesthetics and expensive drugs, coming down on the side of respecting their colleagues' professional judgment and what was best for the patient.[37]

79

Finally, A Real Nurses' Residence

In February 1912, as finishing touches were being put on the new north wing, estimates were already being calculated for a new building on the corner of Victoria and Shuter streets, to include, among other facilities, a new pathology laboratory. (Earlier a pathology laboratory had been set up in the basement of the old church building, equipped mainly through the generosity of Eugene O'Keefe; Dr Robert Mann was appointed pathologist in 1908.)

However, a new nurses' residence would come first. In March 1914 General Council informed the archbishop that it had decided to purchase the Pellatt lot on Victoria Street for $80,000 on condition that it have the privilege of selling 60 x 70 ft. of the lot at Victoria and Shuter, reserving for the convenience of the hospital 60 x 46 ft. at the corner of Victoria Lane and Shuter.[38] (Victoria Lane ran north/south from Queen to Shuter.) Mother Victoria calculated the required capacity of a residence, based upon the number of nurses needed to staff the present various services, and successfully argued against carving up the property as suggested, which could result only in a residence too small to allow for future growth, as well as an unused piece of property also too small for any meaningful use.

Construction did not begin for six years;[39] the first steps were the razing of several one-storey cottages that had stood for almost a hundred years near the southeast corner of Shuter and Victoria streets, and the excavation of the land beneath and around them. Earlier, at a meeting of the hospital board on 12 October 1919, architect P.J. Hynes had reviewed the plans, and the tender of Russell Navin for $248,660 – exclusive of heating, plumbing, and elevators – had been tentatively accepted. Afterwards, however, Archibald and Holmes submitted a tender for the whole of the nurses' home, along with the new surgical theatres. Their offer of $292,277 were accepted, provided their firm's credentials and financial status were satisfactory. The city, acknowledging that "the Hospital's demands upon the City Treasury had hitherto been modest," awarded a grant of $100,000 towards the cost of the nurses' home.[40]

The residence – as well as the new operating rooms above the north "D" wing, planned by Sister St Philip Wanner, a member of the second graduating class – were blessed at formal opening ceremonies on 6 July 1921. The new nurses' residence was now the tallest building in the hospital complex – seven storeys, of which the six upper floors were bedrooms, capable of accommodating 150 nurses. While the bedrooms were spartan, the ground floor boasted a spacious reception room decorated with soft grey walls, dull blue curtains, and velvet-covered chesterfields. Exquisite Oriental rugs, the gifts of friends of the hospital, covered the floors of the reception room. Emphasizing its purpose as a school, not merely a residence, the new facility had a lecture hall capable of seating 300, and a library.

Close beside the new residence there remained, until its demolition a year later, a structure on that southeast corner of Shuter and Victoria streets that was then spoken of as one of Toronto's oldest landmarks. A church building over seventy years old and still well preserved, it was originally known as the James Beatty Church, after its founder, who was editor of the *Daily Leader*, and who preached there on Sundays. The church was taken over by the St Vincent de Paul Society, and was used successively by Italian, Syrian, and Maronite Catholics. The sisters bought the church from the St Vincent de Paul Society in 1910 for $30,000.[41] It was to be torn down the year after the new residence was built, and ten years later a ten-storey extension to the residence was erected on that spot.

Mother Victoria Devine and Mr Hugh Kelly

Two names are prominent in the records of these years of the hospital's development: Mother Victoria, superior of the hospital, and Hugh Kelly, solicitor.

Sister Victoria Devine, born in Renfrew, Ontario, was forty-two years of age and a teacher with several years' experience when she was appointed superior of St Michael's Hospital. She held the position through seven eventful years, 1908 to 1915, the superior's usual maximum term of six years having been extended for one year, at the request of the archbishop, because of the projects underway. The office of superintendent, vacant since Dr Dwyer's departure for Europe in 1902 but probably unofficially assumed by the superior, became merged with that of the superior during Sister Victoria's tenure.[42] Thus was initiated an administrative structure (the two offices of religious superior and hospital superintendent held by the one person) which would endure, with two exceptions, until 1968.

While Sister Victoria's correspondence with the university seems at times lacking in diplomacy, and even somewhat abrasive, it may reflect the inferior bargaining position she was in rather than the woman herself. New to the position, she was dealing with an archbishop/board chairman who was also new, and who would die within three years, but whose sometimes testy letters via his secretary would, in the meantime, add little to her good cheer.

As has been seen, Sister Victoria was heavily involved in building up the hospital's physical plant and in revising its administrative structure. In each of the three important positions she held – superintendent of the hospital, principal of the St Joseph's College School, and then superior general – Sister Victoria's leadership style was strongly collegial. She consulted widely with the hospital sisters, the teachers, and her council, and adjusted her plans accordingly.

Nothing daunted by her long struggle to conclude an agreement between the hospital and the university, Mother Victoria as superior general took on a similar challenge, this time with the Holy See, from which she sought papal approval of the Institute of Sisters of St Joseph. She had the happiness of seeing her prayers and her efforts rewarded when papal approval of the congregation was bestowed in perpetuity in 1925, together with interim approval of the constitutions; final approval would come shortly after she left office.[43]

Working tirelessly as legal adviser to Mother Victoria and the board throughout these years was Hugh T. Kelly. Born at Adjala, Ontario, grandson of immigrants from County Kildare, Ireland, Hugh Kelly was the first St Michael's College student to be awarded a BA degree from the University of Toronto. Active in church and city volunteer organizations, Kelly was also for thirty-nine years a member of the board of governors of the University of Toronto, in recognition of which the university awarded him the LLD. Appointed to the Supreme Court of Ontario in 1911, Mr Justice Kelly continued to serve for many years as the hospital's legal counsel; he died at his home in 1945, at age eighty-seven.[44]

The First Executive Board[45]

As mentioned, the advisory board was replaced in 1913 by an executive board, with power over all appointments to medical and surgical staffs, relations with the university, expenditures of bequests and donations, annual appointment of an auditor, and examination of plans and proposed contracts for new hospital construction.[46]

Archbishop McNeil assumed the chairmanship.[47] As called for by the terms of reference he had proposed, membership of the board consisted of the superintendent of Catholic charities, at that time the Reverend Michael Cline, and later the Reverend P.J. Bench; three sisters appointed by the General Council (but not to be members of the council) – in 1913, these were Sister Victoria Devine, Sister de Sales

Ryan, and Sister Mechtilde Lecour; A.W. Anglin, M.J. Haney, F.B. Hayes, and J.J. Seitz; and finally, a member to be appointed by city council. The four laymen were prominent business and professional men: Anglin was widely known as an expert on banking law; Haney had been involved with Hugh Ryan in railway construction and in the building of the Sault Ste Marie Canal; Hayes was president of the Toronto Carpet Manufacturing Company; and Seitz was president of the typewriter company Underwood Elliott Fisher, Limited.

The reconstituted board was intended to represent a significant change in the governance of the hospital, transferring the locus of much of the decision-making from the General Council to the board, and offering the opportunity for a voice to those sisters with experience and responsibility for the conduct of the day-to-day operations, as well as tapping into the broader experience and expertise in business and political affairs that interested laymen could bring. It is questionable what influence the sisters had, however, since for several years their names were not listed in the board minutes, which stated simply "three Sisters present."

The new board appears to have taken up its duties energetically, especially with respect to university relations and staff appointments. A board member signed the diplomas of the house doctors, and explained hospital rules and regulations to the housestaff.[48] Though there were occasional misunderstandings with regard to the university's and the hospital's respective rights, these appear to have been resolved amicably; a very cordial relationship between Archbishop McNeil and President Falconer is evident in their letters. Illustrative of McNeil's initiatives in his capacity as board chairman was his proposal to the council in 1914 that the sisters purchase the Wellesley Hospital as an annex to St Michael's. No specifics are contained in council minutes as to why the idea was not pursued, merely that "the purchase was not favoured."[49] The suggestion of linking Wellesley's destiny with St Michael's would resurface more than fifty years later in a major study of Toronto's four teaching hospitals commissioned by the Province of Ontario.[50]

The Board and the Hospital-University Agreement

The uneasy truce that followed the 1914 memorandum (Appendix E) did not last for long: in October 1916 the university made, without consultation, an appointment to the teaching staff at St Michael's, whereupon the board reminded President Falconer that *it* was the only authorized body to speak for the hospital, and requested that the appointee discontinue teaching at once.[51] While the university sent a letter of apology, a similar appointment was made two years later, the appointee having neither applied to the board nor been nominated by it.[52] This prompted the university to suggest that St Michael's board and its medical advisory board hold a joint meeting to clear the air.

To its embarrassment, a committee appointed by the board to review the matter reported that "correspondence (with the university) did not reveal any definite agreement between the Hospital and the University that would substantiate the Hospital's desire not only to nominate but, in the event of a deadlock, to appoint the teaching staff."[53] In the midst of subsequent meetings designed "to establish more friendly and mutually agreeable relations," the university – without so much as a by-your-leave – plucked out Dr Jabez Elliott, head of St Michael's tuberculosis clinic, placing him in the General's clinic, an action that prompted St Michael's board to dispatch two of its members to the university to demand Dr Elliott's immediate return.[54] Throughout all these misadventures one gets the impression that heads of departments within the medical faculty, and possibly heads of services at the hospital, were acting without reference to the upper echelons in their respective institutions.

Obviously weary of the recurring problems, Robert Falconer asked for a joint meeting to discuss closer relationships between the institutions and also the matter of appointments. The board appointed three of its members, headed by Sir Bertram Windle, to serve on a permanent university relations committee.[55] (The first task given the three was to ascertain what portion of Dr Magner's salary would be borne by the university, a task hardly guaranteed to start things off amicably.) To this new joint committee the university submitted a draft document containing its requirements for its teaching staff; the hospital amended the document to protect the rights of its patients and of its non-university attending staff.[56] A further breach of the collaborative approach – this time by the hospital, in appointing Dr Julian Loudon as chief of staff without reference to the university – resulted in the production by Sir Bertram Windle of a comprehensive memorandum that delineated the scope of authority of both the hospital and the university in the matter of appointments. President Falconer's reply to this latest effort is alluded to, but with no details, in the board minutes. It appears that the 1914 and 1920 memoranda contained the necessary elements of a satisfactory working relationship that lasted for many years.

It is of interest that the board, in the midst of manoeuvring *vis-à-vis* the university, did not neglect its responsibility to the patients, suggesting that a committee of three of its members make semi-annual visits to the wards, that a receiving nurse (preferably a sister) accompany incoming patients to their rooms, and that an expert be engaged to oversee dusting, window-cleaning, and such so as to ensure "scrupulous cleanliness in the Hospital, and everything pertaining to it."[57]

Clarification of the Nature of the Board

Sir Bertram Windle, a member of the faculty of St Michael's College, was prominent in the work of the hospital board throughout the 1920s. Physician, former president of the University of Cork, and world-famous anthropologist, Windle appears to have had easy access to President (by now Sir Robert) Falconer, and he used this friendship to advance the interests of the hospital, especially in the building up of the medical staff.[58] He was an enthusiastic admirer of Sister Juliana Mitchell, hospital superintendent from 1926 to 1928, repeatedly expressing his esteem for her in his letters to the archbishop.[59]

A weakness in the board's terms of reference, – as established at Archbishop McNeil's recommendation in 1913 – or at any rate in their interpretation, was highlighted in April 1928 when Windle suddenly resigned after eight years of able, energetic service. He alleged that, while outside funding agencies held the view that the board was responsible for the financial business of the hospital, the congregation sometimes entered directly into contracts that involved large expenditures, bypassing the board completely.[60] (The congregation had just borrowed $800,000 to finance the hospital building project then underway.) Among the options for resolving the conflict, Windle recommended that the congregation should obtain a charter incorporating the hospital as a legal entity. The same recommendation was made to the congregation from the board at its next meeting – specifically, that "a corporation within themselves and distinct from themselves," to be known as the St Michael's Hospital Corporation, be organized.[61]

The council sought advice from canon lawyers and civil lawyers. Archbishop McNeil attended the next council meeting, and appears to have concurred with the conclusions reached: the board's powers must be advisory, not executive; and the interests of St Michael's would be best served by the hospital operating within the present Act of Incorporation, backed, as provided therein, by all the resources of the Sisters of St Joseph.[62] The issues of ownership, and the rights and obligations accompanying ownership, were paramount in the discussion. Less apparent, but no doubt powerfully influencing events, was the frame of reference out of which these sisters operated: a perspective of faith that considered the work of St Michael's Hospital to be God's work – if He was calling them to launch out into the deep, they could trust Him not to withdraw His sustaining hand. The approach must have seemed risky to those who composed the board, businessmen all, who had the sisters' interests sincerely at heart; the archbishop undertook to carry an answer back to them. The proposal for separate incorporation was subsequently dropped.

The Evolving Administrative Framework

Following the restructuring of 1913, a growing sense of partnership in the management of the hospital was evident among the three chief players – the sisters' administration, the hospital board, and the advisory board.[63] This spirit of cooperation became especially clear as the board and administration, guided by the Reverend C.B. Moulinier, founder of the Catholic Hospital Association of the United States (and later, Canada), initiated a process of self-examination aimed at ensuring that the hospital meet "minimum standards."

Beginning in 1918 the hospital worked energetically to implement Father Moulinier's recommendations in areas of weakness: restructuring the medical staff to define and limit the range and sequence of authority; establishing ten committees of two or three doctors each "to work in conjunction with the Sisters connected with the various departments"; developing an improved system of record keeping; and drafting the medical staff's constitutions, by-laws, and rules "on instructions from Sister Superior."[64] In the March 1923 issue of the *St. Michael's Hospital Medical Bulletin* the editor expressed the view that "incorporation in the Catholic Hospital Association ... in 1918 ... more than any other single factor has stimulated progress."

The hospital received favourable reports on the site surveys carried out by the Committee on Hospital Standardization of the American College of Surgeons in 1924 and 1925, and in 1926 proudly hung a framed certificate from that body as testament that the principal standards had been met. To complete the requirements, the medical staff began twice monthly meetings in 1927; interestingly, the second of these meetings was devoted to management of drug addicts, with a decision to poll the other hospitals to see how they dealt with these patients.

Aside from collaborative projects, board, administration, and medical advisory board each had its own primary focus: the board heavily involved with the university, the superior and her council responsible for internal management of non-medical matters, and the medical advisory board serving as an effective forum for policy-making and for new initiatives in patient care.

Faculty and Staff Appointments

During the early years it was not unusual for a doctor to hold staff appointments at both the Toronto General and St Michael's, in addition to a teaching appointment at the university; some held, as well, a staff appointment at the Victoria Hospital for Sick Children (later called the Hospital for Sick Children). This pattern was particularly true of those in the emerging areas of specialization: pathology, gynaecology, ophthalmology, and otolaryngology.[65] Dr Dwyer held an appointment as registrar at the General in 1899-1900 and was on its outdoor staff in 1904-05. One gets the impression that Toronto was oversupplied with doctors at this time, making it necessary for clinicians to move beyond their base hospital (in order to make a living), serving in the prisons, refuges, and such, as well as in the small hospitals not connected with the university.

Besides the five university faculty members who accepted appointments at St Michael's from the outset (Drs J. Amyot, I.H. Cameron, J. Caven, Alexander McPhedran, and W. Oldright), Dr Dwyer was the first St Michael's man to receive a faculty appointment (lecturer, 1897-98), followed by Drs W. McKeown and G. Silverthorn in 1901-02, the former as demonstrator in clinical surgery, the latter as assistant demonstrator in pathology. By 1915-16 Dwyer was one of only seven with the rank of associate professor of clinical medicine on the faculty, and Dr McKeown one of only five with the rank of associate professor of clinical surgery. A marked increase in the presence of St Michael's on the faculty is noted in 1923, with the addition of Drs J. Loudon, Harris McPhedran, E.A. Broughton, Malcolm Cameron, and T.A. Robinson, followed by a further increase in 1929 with Drs W. Magner, F. O'Leary, W. Noonan, J.W. Ross, and G. Foulds – reflecting the recently improved facilities at the hospital for pathology, obstetrics, and urology.

The Medical Advisory Board[66]

The first six-member medical advisory board (not to be confused with the hospital's board of governors/directors) established in October

1914, was composed of two surgeons (Drs E. King and W. McKeown), three physicians (Drs R. Dwyer, J. Guinane, and J. Loudon), and Dr J.A. Amyot. Dr Amyot was assistant surgeon at St Michael's and demonstrator in pathology at the university at the time, and later became associate professor of pathology and bacteriology. In 1913 he and Dr John Fitzgerald were the first in Canada to prepare an anti-rabies vaccine. He went on to become provincial bacteriologist in Ontario, and later deputy minister of health in the federal government.[67] The board met faithfully once or twice a month, Dr King chairing the meetings over a period of seventeen years, and Dr Loudon recording the minutes in his neat handwriting. Of this group, Dr Joachim Guinane is new to the reader. A member of St Michael's staff from early days, and a holder of the degree MRCS (England), Guinane became chairman of the board after King's death in 1930; he died in 1936 after eight days' illness with pneumonia.

Membership remained unchanged until Dr D'Arcy Frawley joined the board in 1917; later Dr Magner joined in 1921 and Dr G. Wilson in 1927 – changes that followed upon Dr McKeown's death and Dr Amyot's move to Ottawa. Dr Frawley recommended in 1929 the inclusion of the chiefs of the eye and the ear, nose, and throat departments, but the motion was not immediately acted upon.

In the early years, applicants for internship appeared before the medical advisory board before being recommended to the board of governors. Much attention was given to defining the scope of practice of the house doctors, and also to developing policy around the administration of anaesthetics, with precise records kept of same.

Evidence of the developments within the clinical fields is contained in the clinics developed during the medical advisory board's early years: a dental clinic in 1915, a psychiatry clinic in 1917, a well-baby clinic in 1919, and a venereal disease clinic in 1922; a clinic for diseases of the lungs, staffed by a nurse from the city's health department, had been in operation since 1907. The medical advisory board made recommendations to the superior on a range of issues: that a sister be assigned to assist with sections (the specimens of tissue obtained for examination), cultures, and so on in the bacteriology laboratory after a course in some well-equipped laboratory;[68] and, as early as February 1918, that a convalescent home be secured, where chronic cases could be housed and attended by hospital staff, to relieve congestion at the hospital. And there were the less serious recommendations, as that of June 1923 referring to house doctors' uniforms: the duck should be shrunken before the uniforms are made!

The Sisters' Local Council

Those areas of management handled by the board of governors and the medical advisory board during these years have been discussed. There remains the work of the sisters' council, a three member-team appointed by the General Council, made up of the superintendent and two sisters, one of whom was usually the financial officer. Minutes of their meetings are available from 1924.

Precursor to the hospital's administrative teams of the 1960s and thereafter, the sisters' council initially handled personnel matters (including non-medical staff appointments and salary administration), renovations and space allocations, room rates and service rates, and even ambulance services.[69] An important part of its portfolio was the work assignments of the sisters, of whom there were thirty-three in 1924. At that time there was a sister in charge of every floor in the hospital, as well as in the various departments – laundry, purchasing, pharmacy, x-ray, admitting, business office, dietary, and school of nursing.[70]

There is a gap in the minutes of the board of governors from mid-1928 to early 1936. The sisters' council carried on during this time, years that were basically a period of growing to maturity in the expanded facilities and services of the new A-B-C wings.

The *Hospital Medical Bulletin*[71]

In 1922 the medical staff launched a periodical, the *St. Michael's Hospital Medical Bulletin*, with Dr Magner as editor and Drs Loudon and Malcolm Cameron as associate editors. Something of the energy and enthusiasm within the staff at the time can be caught from the introductory paragraph of the first issue. The *Bulletin* was to be

> a clinical journal devoted to the work carried on in our wards and laboratories. We realize that such a project is ambitious, but in view of the abundance of exceptionally interesting cases passing through our wards, the great advances which are being made in our organization, the development of our special laboratories, and the splendid spirit of cooperation among all connected with the hospital ... [a decision has been made to publish a journal].

The St Michael's Hospital Clinical Society, organized that same year under the chairmanship of Dr Loudon, provided articles for the *Bulletin*. Published twice a year, by 1931 the *Bulletin* was being distributed free to 4000 doctors in Ontario, as well as to 1000 hospitals, sanatoria, and institutions across Canada. It appears that the cost of publication was met, in large part, by advertising, which amounted to fifteen pages in the December 1931 issue.

Frequently the articles took the form of a review of the entire year's experience with certain disease categories: for example, appendicitis (Dr T.A. Robinson) in 1922, and again in 1929 (500 cases in eighteen months); pneumonia (Dr E.A. Broughton) in 1923 – 248 cases in twenty months, of whom eighty-nine died, a mortality rate of 35.8 percent. Some *Bulletin* issues were devoted to a single disease entity, for example the treatment of gonorrhoea by Drs W.T. Noonan and G. Foulds in 1927; disease of the brain, meninges, and spinal cord by Dr D. Pratt in 1928; the staff's early beginning experience with the use of radium for treating carcinoma of the cervix in 1928 and follow-up in 1931. (At its 23 August 1926 meeting the advisory board had recommended the purchase of 50 mgms. of radium, at an approximate cost of $3,500.) The clinical society continued Dr Dwyer's earlier emphasis on the autopsy and the pathology laboratory as indispensable to the growth in understanding of disease processes, supplementing these methods in 1930 by some modest beginnings in animal research.[72]

Scanning the *Bulletin* during its thirteen-year lifespan, one can assume what a boon it must have been to doctors practising in rural Ontario and in the small towns, isolated from peer contact and from the three university medical centres of the day. It appears that it was with the further needs of these doctors in mind that St Michael's medical staff offered between 1929 and 1939 its Annual Clinical Week, billed as "postgraduate instruction designed to give practitioners an opportunity to keep pace with modern research work."[73] Some indication of the need that was filled by these annual five-and-a-half-day clinics can be deduced from the attendance. With registrants coming from Kingston, Port Hope, Guelph, and even the border cities of the United States, attendance had to be eventually limited to 250. The Clinical Week was free of charge in the early years; a $5 registration fee was charged in 1938 and 1939.[74]

Developments in the Practice of Medicine

The first St Michael's man to use an x-ray machine was, according to Dr Malcolm Cameron,* Dr Edmund King, in 1898, a year after its discovery.

---

*Dr Malcolm Cameron, who was on the staff of St Michael's from 1908 to 1955, rising from clinical assistant through the ranks to consulting surgeon, has left an account of developments at the hospital between 1908 and 1922. His paper, ending mid-paragraph, is preserved in the hospital's archives; excerpts from his paper are here shown in quotation marks. Dr Cameron did extensive research into the history of medical practice in the seventeenth and eighteenth centuries and lectured on the subject. Four years before his death he wrote his own obituary, to save trouble for his good friend, Dr Harris McPhedran.

(An 1898 newspaper account of a brawl records that Dr King located the bullet "by means of the Roentgen process.") Dr Cameron describes Dr King as a man who "almost attained greatness." More than once elected to office in the various medical organizations, including presidency of the College of Physicians and Surgeons of Ontario, Dr King was also a busy surgeon and "a pioneer in operating on the prostate gland." He had his office at 61 Queen Street East – on the modern-day site of the St Michael's Hospital Health Centre, opened in 1989. Dr King was chairman of the medical advisory board from its formation in 1914 until his death in 1930, and in that capacity did valuable liaison work with the university. At the time of his death, Dr King was still physician to the Royal Grenadiers, with which regiment he had served, and he was buried with full military honours – gun carriage, riderless horse, reversed boots, and all.

Dr Frederick Fenton, a well-trained surgeon and an expert obstetrician, was, according to Cameron, "the first man in Toronto to combine the specialties of obstetrics and gynaecology. He performed a Cesarean section, a rare operation at the time, before a crowded amphitheatre at the hospital during the annual meeting of the Ontario Medical Association in 1906." Dr Fenton became St Michael's first chief of obstetrics and gynaecology in 1909. Four years later he died, at only forty-two years of age, following surgery for appendicitis at the Wellesley Hospital. Ironically, his fellow gynaecologist, Dr J.F.W. Ross, had been "one of the first to insist that a diagnosis of appendicitis demanded immediate operation, an idea which required a champion of Dr Ross's stature to overcome the conservatism of senior surgeons."

Quoting Dr M. Cameron again, "The man who brought science into the surgical practice at St Michael's as Dr Dwyer brought it into medical practice was Dr Gideon Silverthorn." A surgeon who had studied pathology at Strassbourg and Heidelberg, two years under the famous von Recklinghausen, Silverthorn read avidly and (being a bachelor until his fifty-ninth year) travelled extensively to other centres to learn and to assess new developments. He was assistant professor of surgery from 1901, and professor of medical jurisprudence from 1922, and became chief of surgery and professor of surgery upon Dr McKeown's death in 1925.

Dr Cameron records that "Dr Silverthorn expected his juniors to work and study on their own. When one of his young men displayed skill in anastomosis, for example, in gastroenterectomy, Dr Silverthorn might find that the preliminary practice had been done on socks for stomachs, tubular neckties for intestines, and chamoisette gloves to separate the layers for when peritoneum was to be sutured." A specialist in appendicitis, Silverthorn was himself to die a victim of that disease in 1926, having served as chief of surgery for just one year.[75] He left $5,000 in his will for the maintenance of equipment in the operating room.

Equipment for the surgeons was far from sophisticated during these years. Rubber gloves were private property. They were prepared by boiling and were applied wet after the surgeon had scrubbed his hands and rinsed with carbolic acid or bichloride of mercury. Blood transfusion was considered a formidable procedure before the First World War and for some time after. The treatment of fractures was improved with the introduction of overhead extension and the Balkan Frame, the latter constructed from odd ends of piping left by the plumbers as they built the north wing.

Not everything, however, lacked sophistication; on Sunday mornings the doctors arrived in formal attire – Prince Albert coat, striped trousers, and silk hat. Dr Clayton Bryan records that he bought the complete outfit at Tip Top Tailors for $25. On weekdays there was less decorum, as some of the doctors travelled by streetcar or bicycle.

The years 1910-20 marked the introduction of three new diagnostic tools –[76] the metabolometer for estimating basal metabolism, the electrocardiograph, and the cystoscope. The last was introduced by Dr Malcolm Cameron, who had gone to the Mayo Clinic in Rochester, Minnesota, to observe its use.

Anaesthesiology emerged as a specialty during these years. Dr Leo Killoran was appointed chief of anaesthesia about 1915. He used a McKesson gas machine, first with ethylene, then with cyclopropane. Dr Clayton Bryan, who had spent time in Chicago learning the technique of administering various gas mixtures, became chief following Killoran's death. He was joined by Dr Kenneth Heard, who soon gained an international reputation for his contributions to the study of anaesthesia and became chairman of the board of governors of the International Anaesthetic Research Society. A gifted scientist, Heard worked to correlate the art of anaesthesia with the basic sciences of physiology and pharmacology. According to Dr Cameron, Heard was the first to introduce pentothal anaesthesia to Canada and was considered an authority on spinal anaesthesia. Heard also pioneered the development of much of the instrumentation required for the intratracheal delivery of gases and the continuous intravenous delivery of barbiturates.

Doctors from the smaller hospitals came as post-graduate students to learn his method.[77]

Throughout these years, Dr Walter McKeown was chief of one of the two surgical services, then chief of surgery at the hospital and professor of surgery at the university from 1909 until his death in 1925. Already on staff in 1894, and a signatory of the letter protesting the cancellation of the city grant, McKeown later went to London where he obtained his MRCS. Those who knew him admired his cheery, jaunty presence, his liberality of mind, excellence of professional judgment, and his courageous, independent spirit.[78] A veteran of the Riel Rebellion and of the First World War, in which he distinguished himself as head of the Imperial Hospital at Brighton, England, and was granted the Order of Commander of the British Empire, McKeown did not hesitate to engage in local skirmishes if the future of his department was at stake – he is said to have shocked the General Council, at one point, by proposing that the congregation abandon its property on Wellesley Street, adjacent as it was to Queen's Park, and relocate the hospital to that site in order to facilitate its transactions with the university.

The Nursing Department

Enrolment increased and the number of nurse graduates tripled within a space of twelve years – from ten graduates in 1903 to twenty-nine in 1915 – in spite of cramped living quarters. After the new residence opened in 1921 the annual numbers of graduates increased further, reaching fifty-three by 1929.

The school continued to be in the charge of laywomen, several of whom served for one year only, until finally the six-year-term of Helena Graves, followed by the six-year-term of Julia O'Connor – both women of outstanding character and competence – gave continuity and stability to the teaching program.[79] Illustrative of the character and philosophy of these women is the section on the school for nurses in the hospital's *Rules and Regulations 1914*, where the necessary qualities of a nurse are spelled out, obedience being one of the pre-eminent qualities. As well, this material describes without apology the hierarchical order within the hospital community, noting, for example, that "senior nurses, junior nurses, and probationers are to bear in mind their relative position towards one another." O'Connor was receiving a salary of $50 a month in 1910, increased to $75 in late 1912. The nurse in charge of the school was in charge of the operating room as well, a pattern that probably developed out of Archbishop O'Connor's directives, referred to earlier.

By 1910 lectures and classes had become well organized, although material appears to have been covered more in breadth than in depth. Every student had class from 8:00-9:00 in the evening twice a week, one with her own class, the other with the full school. Only doctors are listed as lecturers, thirty-three in all entered on the 1910-11 timetable.

Note that some of the classes were held in the evening after what must have been difficult days on the wards, judging from a provincial inspector's report in 1911 – "public wards are greatly overcrowded, and the ventilation is wretched." Seeing the conditions under which the nurses worked, the inspectors wanted better for them when they were off duty, making strong recommendations in 1913 and again in 1918 for a new nurses' home, which finally came to be in 1921.

While sisters had been in charge of the wards from the first, it was not until 1915 that a sister took charge of the school, initiating a pattern that would continue uninterrupted until 1974. Sisters Mercedes, St Philip, Edana, and Hieronyme each directed the school for short periods until 1926, when Sister Amata Charlesbois assumed the position. Among these, one of the best-known figures was Sister Hieronyme Kennedy, an 1895 graduate of the old Toronto East General School of Nursing. Sister Hieronyme served mainly as night supervisor, for periods as long as nine years at a time. Friend of waifs and strays, to whom she regularly provided sandwiches when they straggled in to her ward from the street, and of policemen, firemen, ambulance men, and newspaper reporters – as night supervisors often are – she appears, also, to have been the friend of nurses, for at their own request uniformed nurses formed a guard of honour at her funeral.

Beginning in September 1918 and continuing apparently for at least seven years, the nursing students received the greater part of their class instruction at the university, a centralized lecture course having been established there "owing to the shortage of nursing instructors and for the sake of greater uniformity in training methods."[80] The plan was vigorously opposed by the medical advisory board on the grounds that it would be wasteful of nurses' time, and nurses would cease to be identified with their own hospital, an objection that would be raised again – some would say, accurately – in 1974 when the school was moved into a community college.

Sister Edana Ryan, superintendent of nurses in 1924, arranged that year for a formal inspection of the school by the New York State Board of Nurse Examiners. Chief among the inspector's recommendations were two: that the school's one nurse instructor (Sister St Philip) receive some special preparation for teaching, and that the students obtain three months' affiliation in paediatrics.[81] Sister Edana acted immediately upon the recommendations; arrangements for affiliation were made with the Hospital for Sick Children beginning in September 1925, and she began exploring opportunities at McGill University and at Marquette University (Milwaukee, Wisconsin) for a sister to be prepared for teaching. In October 1924 Sisters Amata Charlesbois and Stanislaus O'Connor enrolled at Marquette University, for that purpose.[82] Sister Amata returned home to become superintendent of the school, and Sister Stanislaus as instructor.

Energetic in her efforts to keep pace with an enlarged and improved hospital, Sister Amata invited a second inspection in 1928. Among other recommendations,[83] the inspector stated that more supervisors should be appointed to supplement the seven sister-supervisors who were trying to handle a 300-bed hospital, soon to double in size. The council approached the Sisters of St Joseph of London for the loan of two sister-nurses for one year to take charge of floors; their answer was sympathetic, but negative.[84] This marked the advent of lay nurses as floor supervisors, beginning with Augustine Bourdon, a graduate of 1926, who became supervisor of the 4th floor, D-unit.[85] While Bourdon's salary is not easily determined from the records, some idea of her expenses can be estimated: Corbett-Cowley, which became the principal supplier of nurses' uniforms, was in 1927 advertising "three quality uniforms for $10.00."

Other Professional and Support Groups

The first paid staff had appeared on the ledgers in 1893 (laundry helpers, housemaids, pantry maids, and charwomen); next a "scientific cook" in 1899 (Mrs Joy, at an annual salary of $25 – part-time, one would hope). A chaplain was receiving a salary in 1899; he was one of the priests from St Michael's Cathedral staff who served as chaplains for the first three decades. St Michael's was assigned its first resident chaplain in 1929, the Reverend Wilfred Smith, who served until assigned to a parish in 1938. Father Smith returned several years later to live in semi-retirement at the hospital.

The operating-room nurse's salary of $300 annually in 1901 had tripled by 1912 through several increases which may reflect the advances being made in surgery and the consequent responsibility of the operating-room nurse. The first anaesthetist appeared on the ledgers in 1904, with a salary of $200 annually. The first paid pharmacist appears in 1916, at a salary of $1,144; this was probably in anticipation of the transfer of Sister Columba in 1917, and the enrolment in the College of Pharmacy of the two sisters who had been serving their apprenticeship in the pharmacy. A *Pharmacopoeia of St. Michael's Hospital*, dated 1916, compiled by a committee chaired by Dr Loudon, is preserved at the Academy of Medicine, Toronto. It lists 282 compounds and their ingredients, all in Latin.

Finally, the Social Service Association was begun in 1918, in charge of Irene Foy, a St Michael's graduate nurse who had attended a one-year course at the University of Toronto on a scholarship awarded by the hospital to prepare herself for the position.[86] Foy took a position with the Provincial Board of Health in 1920 and her good work in the outpatients department was continued by Sister M. Eusebia, who had passed examinations to qualify for the work.

It is unclear what the early function of this association was; however, in 1928 it was asked to take over the task of admitting new patients to the outpatients department.[87] The confusion arises from the fact that public-health nurses from the city were already present in the outpatients department, beginning in 1907. It is possible that these formed the nucleus, if not the whole, of the Social Service Association.

To explain: in 1905 a tuberculosis clinic was opened at Toronto General, and in 1907 a nurse from the city health department was asked to take charge of it, along with the newly opened tuberculosis clinic at St Michael's.[88] Later, in 1910, one public-health nurse from the city became responsible for service at St Michael's clinic, along with the whole eastern portion of the city, while another nurse took charge of the Toronto General's clinic, plus the western part of the city. Neilson records that "compulsory reporting of diagnosed cases became law in the Province in 1911, but at first only Toronto's two chest clinics observed the ruling." St Michael's chest clinic was, then, a valued partner with Toronto's health department in disease control.

In 1912 the public-health nurses began to coordinate the city's well-baby clinics, including St Michael's; this included the "milk stations" where pasteurized milk could be procured. These efforts were undoubtedly an important factor in the dramatic fall in the infant death rate in Toronto, from 148.9 per 1,000 in 1910 to 37.3 in 1943. Following the passing in 1919 of the Act for Control of Venereal Diseases, venereal disease clinics were opened in six large public hospitals, including St Michael's, and public-health nurses were assigned to each.

Thus it was that the city's nurses became valued colleagues in St Michael's outpatients department. By 1945 these "Hospital Health

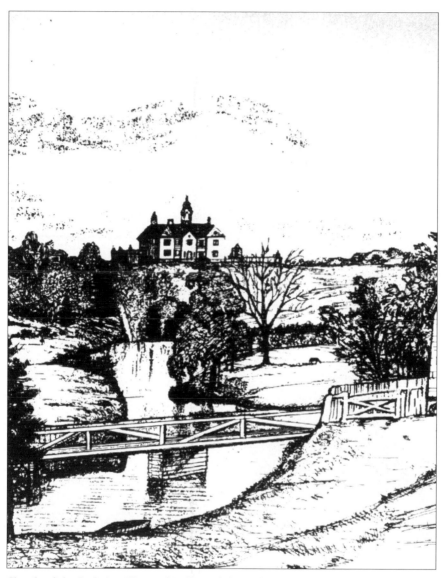

Sketch of the Isolation Hospital in Riverdale Park where the sisters went as volunteers in 1891 to take charge of the care of diphtheria victims. (Courtesy of the Baldwin Room, Metropolitan Toronto Reference Library.)

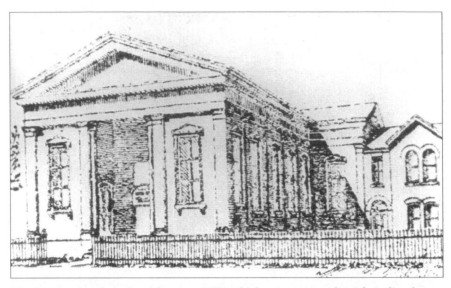

The Baptist church on Bond Street, *c.* 1897, which was converted to a boarding-house for girls called Notre Dame des Anges. The roof was subsequently raised and a storey was added.

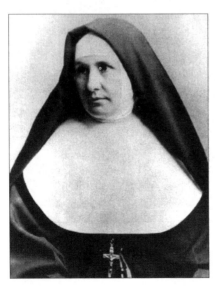

Mother de Chantal McKay, who directed the conversion of Notre Dame des Anges to St Michael's Hospital in 1892, and remained as its first superior/superintendent for one further year.

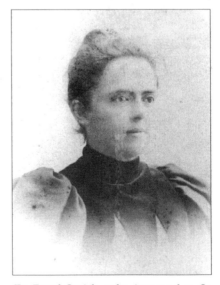

Dr Pearl Smith, who interned at St Michael's in 1895, is believed to be the first woman to do a medical internship in a Canadian hospital.

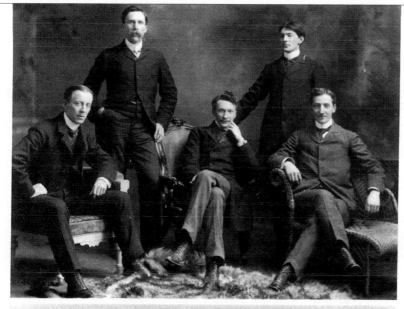

St. Michael's Hospital Medical Staff.

Dr Robert Dwyer (centre), medical superintendent from 1892 to 1920, with 1898 interns F.P. McNulty and Malcolm Crawford (who became St Michael's first head of obstetrics), on Dr Dwyer's left and right and 1899 interns H.C. Wrench and C.H. McKenna.

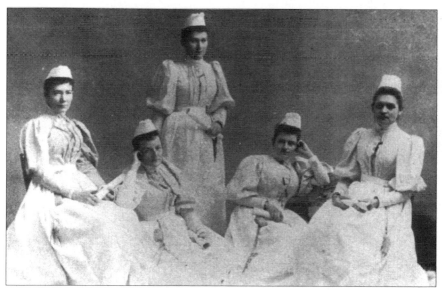

The first graduating class from the school of nursing (1894): Mary Murphy, Kate Madden, Annie Crysler, Lizzie O'Leary, and Mary Skinner. Not included in the photograph are Sisters Columba and Attracta, who also graduated in the first class.

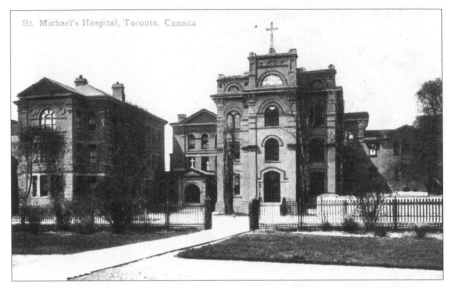

St Michael's Hospital *c.* 1895. The original hospital is on the right, the Hugh Ryan wing on the left.

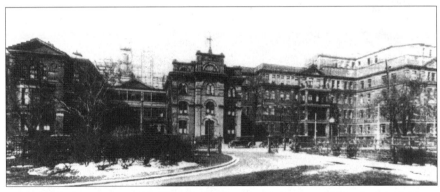

St Michael's Hospital *c.* 1912. The original hospital is in the middle, the Hugh Ryan wing on the left, and the 1912 addition (the D-wing) on the right. The original exterior walls of the 1912 addition are still doing their work in 1992, housing – among other services – the CV-ICU.

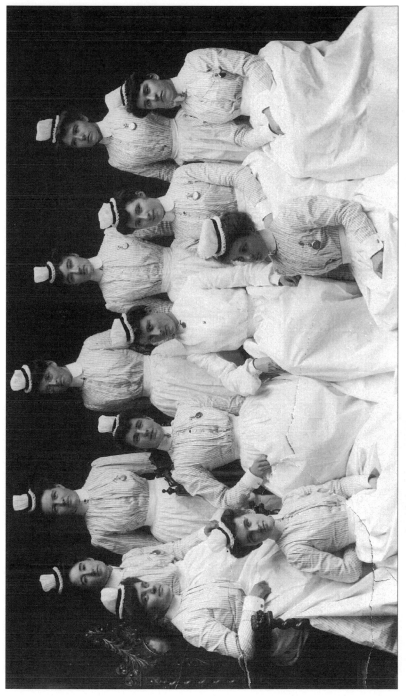

Graduating class of nurses in 1902 with head nurse Helena Graves who subsequently married Dr P W O'Brien, St Michael's first paediatrician. Their granddaughter, Joan Dewan, graduated with the 1960 class of nurses.

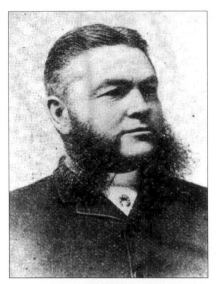

Hugh Ryan, who, with his wife, Margaret, donated in 1895 the money required to build and furnish an entire surgical wing. The Hugh Ryan wing was replaced in the 1926-28 building program (A, B, C wings) to comply with new fire-proofing standards that had been established.

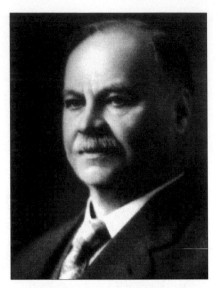

Dr Edmund E. King, surgeon and pioneer urologist at St Michael's, and first chairman of the medical advisory board, an appointment he held from 1914 to 1930.

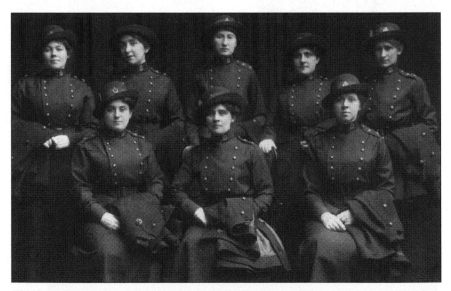

The first contingent of the twenty-six St Michael's graduate nurses to go overseas between 1915 and 1918 to serve in the First World War.

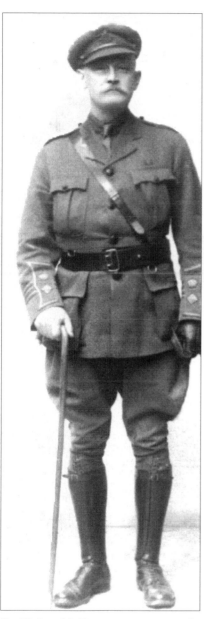

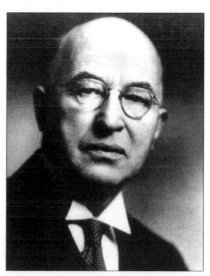

Dr Julian Derwent Loudon, St Michael's second physician-in-chief (1921-45) and a pioneer in the use of the electrocardiogram in Canada.

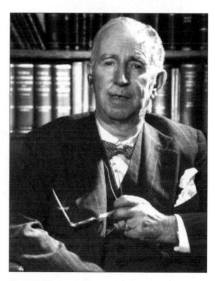

Dr Walter McKeown, surgeon at St Michael's from 1894 to 1925, veteran of the Riel Rebellion and of the First World War (president of the Standing Medical Board of England during the latter), and St Michael's first chief of surgery.

Dr William Magner, recruited from Cork, Ireland, in 1921 to assume the post of head of the laboratories, became one of the major pathologists in Canada and a powerful influence in moving St Michael's to full accreditation as a teaching hospital.

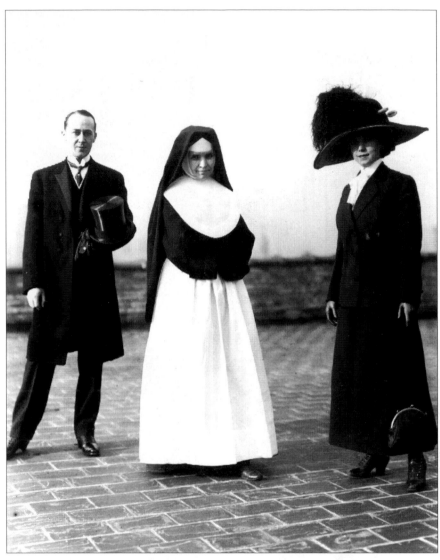

Sister de Sales Ryan, an 1895 graduate of St Michael's School of Nursing, with Dr Harris McPhedran, who became the hospital's third physician-in-chief, and Mrs McPhedran, on the roof garden of the hospital, *c.* 1912. (Courtesy of the City of Toronto Archives, James 1224)

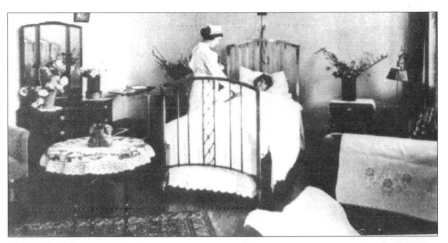

A private room, *c.* 1930.

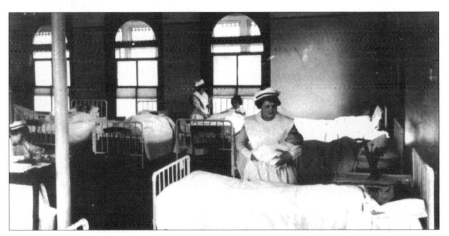

A public ward on the 7-C obstetrical unit, *c.* 1939. The ward was little changed until it was replaced by the new F-wing in 1964. The second and third-year student nurses are recognized by the absence or presence of the black band on the cap.

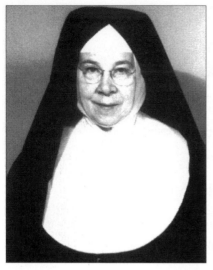

Sister Vincentia Mullen, the highly respected nursing supervisor of obstetrics from 1928 to 1956, was among the best known of the nursing sisters during those years.

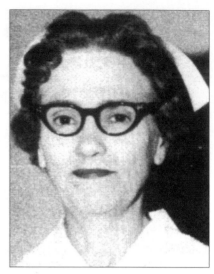

Marcella Berger, instructor and head nurse in the delivery room from 1930 to 1960. There she taught and supervised more than 3,000 undergraduates and assisted at 35,000 births.

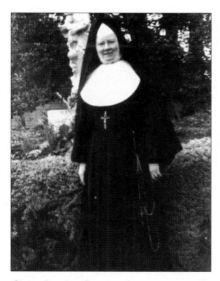

Sister Louise Carey, whose career at St Michael's moved from business-office manager, to secretary-treasurer, to superintendent, in a period that extended from 1922 to 1948.

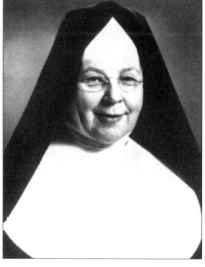

Sister Margaret Phelan, who emigrated as a teenager from Ireland, was twice superior/administrator of St Michael's (1930-32 and 1944-50). She initiated the post-Second World War building boom at the hospital.

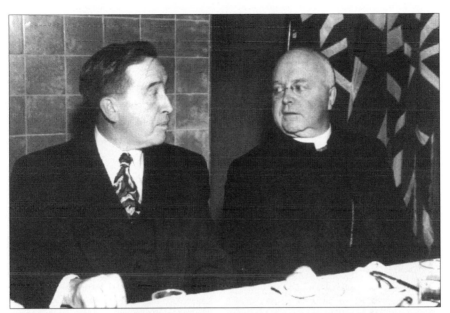

John J. Fitzgibbons, first layman elected to chair St Michael's board of directors, an office he held from 1940 to 1963, pictured here with James Cardinal McGuigan, honorary chairman.

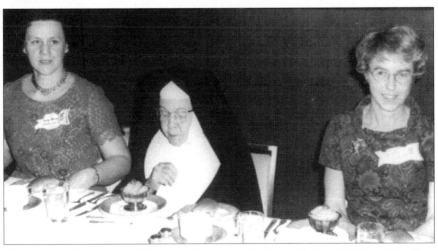

Sister Jeanne Barry, superintendent of the school of nursing from 1928 to 1940, then medical supervisor of a large public ward, and finally St Michael's first director of nursing service. Pictured with Sister Jeanne are nurses Mary Shaver and Jacqueline Mulcahy.

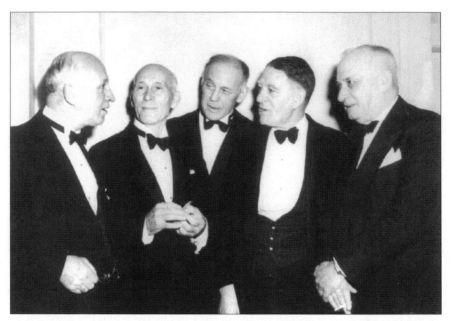

At the close of the Second World War four chiefs retired. Shown here, left to right, are Dr T.A. Robinson, senior surgeon, with chiefs George Wilson (surgery), Harris McPhedran (medicine), J.X. Robert (otolaryngology), and D'Arcy Frawley (obstetrics and gynaecology).

The new chiefs (1947) are pictured on the opposite page.

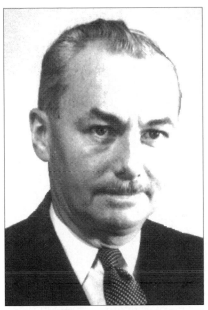

Dr J. Edward Brooks (medicine)

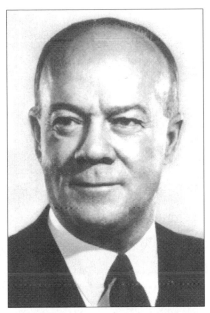

Dr Joseph Sullivan (otolaryngology)

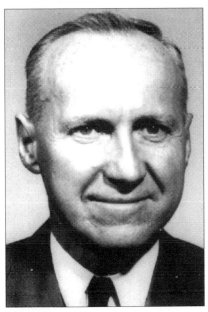

Dr W. Keith Welsh (surgery)

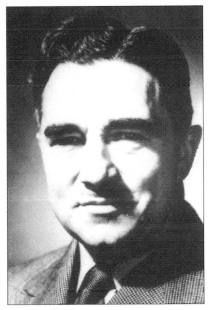

Dr Frank O'Leary (obstetrics and gynaecology)

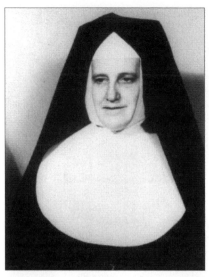

Sister Mary Kathleen Moore, superintendent of nurses from 1940 to 1958, was a leader in basic and post-basic nursing education – locally, provincially, and nationally.

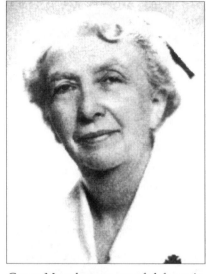

Grace Murphy, a powerful force in nursing and nursing education at St Michael's from 1928 to 1958, and a role model for students and graduates alike.

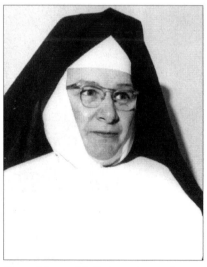

Sister Maura McGuire, who, as hospital superintendent from 1950 to 1956 and superior general of the congregation from 1956 to 1968, played a pivotal role in the changes in the hospital and the congregation during those years.

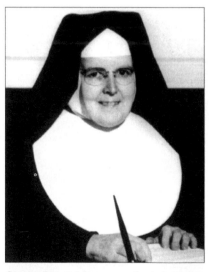

Sister Janet Murray, administrator from 1956 to 1963, who then chaired throughout a period of fifteen years the umbrella committee charged with coordinating more closely the efforts of all of the health-care institutions owned and operated by the sisters.

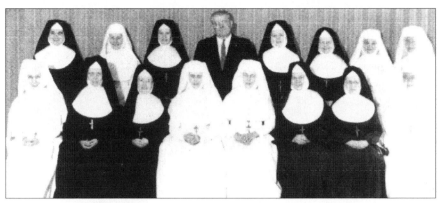

Hospital department heads in 1959. Front row: Sisters Georgina Stern, laundry and linen services; Mary Anthony VanBergen, general purchasing; Alice Marie McFarlane, laboratory office; Mary Avila Mulvihill, pharmacy; Mary Enda O'Connor, food purchasing; Mary Paul Biss, medical records school; Eugenie Skelton, secretary-treasurer; Mary Frederick Sheehan, dietary. Back row: Sisters Mary Zimmerman, admitting; Eucheria Smith, radiology; and Patricia Roddy, accounts receivable; Frank Benvenete, chief engineer; Sisters St Nilus Barnett, medical records; Angeline Coyne, surgical purchasing; Mary Regis Nelson, physiotherapy; and St Jude Doherty, laboratory supervisor.

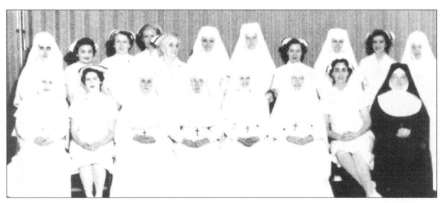

Nursing supervisors in 1959. Front row: Sister Marie Stella Emery; Shirley Young, Sister Eileen Bradley; Sister Albertine O'Connor; Sister St Matthew Reich; Sister Colette Delanty; Adele Johnston; Sister St Edward Rush. Back row: Sister Margaret Ann Hazelton; Sue Nagamatsu; Margaret Simpson-Ray; Kathleen Whalen; Augustine Bourdon; Sister Brigid Ann Payne; Sister St Hugh O'Leary; Mollie Trimnell; Sister Mary Brigid Vezina; Dorothy Shamess; Sister Florian Tattersall.

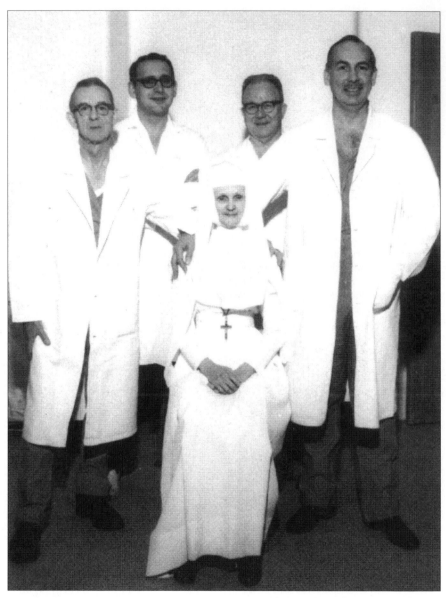

Staff of the division of urology, *c.* 1960: Sister St Matthew Reich, nursing supervisor, with Drs Stanley Lowrey, Vincent Colapinto, Dyce Duckworth, and J.L. Thomas Russell, chief.

Service" nurses had extended their range to include the chest, obstetrics, venereal disease, diabetic, and cardiac clinics, and provided a valuable link between clinic, ward, and district nurse. The hospital, for its part, became an early and active ally of the city's health department in its disease-prevention and health-promotion efforts, especially among the city's poor.

The Fund-raising Campaign, 1924

In 1924, with a view to entering upon another ambitious building project, the hospital made its first public appeal for funds. Frank Hughes (lawyer and crown attorney) served as chairman, Rabbi B.R. Brickner as one of three vice-chairmen, and Lady Edith Windle as head of the women's section, all headquartered in the King Edward Hotel which offered its premises without charge. Although highly organized and well publicized, the drive netted subscriptions amounting to just less than half of its $500,000 objective. The time-span and the timing may have contributed to the disappointing yield: the campaign was conducted over a single five-day period, and had the misfortune of coming immediately after a similar drive by the Western Hospital.

The campaign was followed up in 1925 by an effort to persuade individuals and groups to endow rooms or floors, as memorials to their loved ones, in the new wings about to be built. To endow a room would cost the subscriber from $1,000 to $4,000, depending upon size and location of room, and a whole floor would cost from $34,000 to $500,000.[89]

Poor as it was, the Nurses' Alumnae Association responded by furnishing Room 501A, a large private corner room. The overall success of the 1925 efforts is not clear, but there can be no doubt about the urgency of needs. Outpatient and laboratory facilities were required for the sake of patient care, medical education, and the advancement of medical knowledge. Since these facilities would generate little revenue, it was judged necessary to provide extra accommodation for private and semi-private patients, not only to increase revenue, but also to lower the maintenance rate to patients.

The Addition of the A, B, and C Wings[90]

The hospital now plunged into a vast expansion program that extended over a three-year period, adding a laundry and power plant (1926), 250 new adult beds and thirty-one infant beds (1926-28), and an outpatient department as well as emergency, laboratory, and x-ray facilities (1928). The resulting seven-storey structure was roughly L-shaped with one arm of the new construction extending along Victoria Street on five lots purchased by the congregation for $121,400,[91] and the other stretching across the property to Bond Street running just south of the original building. To finance the project, the congregation borrowed $750,000 and used the campaign subscriptions described above.[92] The city awarded a grant of $150,000, while the university granted $2,500 for furnishing the laboratories and provided, in addition, all material equipment;[93] what the latter consisted of is not specified.

The project necessitated disturbance of two landmarks, the one of emotional significance, the other of political. The Hugh Ryan wing had to go since it was judged impossible to renovate it to meet new standards for fireproofing. And a portion of Victoria Lane, the purchase of which St Michael's had pursued with the city for years, always opposed by the merchants on Queen Street, was finally sold to the hospital for $12,857.[94] The lane was diverted south of the hospital buildings to give access now to Victoria Street rather than to Shuter Street as formerly.

Prized, perhaps most of all, among the new facilities were those allocated to the laboratories and to x-ray. For more than fifteen years concern had been expressed over the difficulties under which the laboratory staff worked. Their statistics, however, were impressive – during one month in 1921 the laboratory handled a total of 275 Wassermann tests, 109 bacteriological and 75 pathological tests, and five autopsies. (Microscopy and the young science of biochemistry had been first brought into practice in the hospital in 1903 by Dr Fred Colling, who subsequently joined the staff in 1921 as biochemist under Dr Magner. Dr Colling was later recipient of the Order of the British Empire for his service in France and Siberia during the Second World War.)

It was to the existing laboratory quarters, housed as they were in two small rooms in the basement of the original building, that Dr William Magner came from Cork, Ireland, in 1921 to assume control. The speed with which this appointment was concluded is worth noting: on 21 September 1920 Drs McKeown and Amyot called upon the council and urged that a competent pathologist be engaged. Council immediately empowered a board member, who was about to visit Ireland, to negotiate with Dr Magner there, and before month's end Magner's appointment had been decided upon. By May 1921 Magner had arrived and, in company with the archbishop, Sir Bertram Windle, and Dr McKeown was discussing with the council plans for improvements at St Michael's Hospital.[95]

Dr Magner was given immediately a university appointment as lecturer in pathology; further, the university immediately contributed $1,800 annually towards his salary.[96] In 1929 he refused an offer of deanship of the medical faculty of Marquette University, preferring to remain in Canada. Considered one of the major pathologists in Canada of his time, Magner authored several books, including a 395-page *Textbook of Hematology* (1938), and more than forty published articles between 1916 and 1950.

One of his medical colleagues offers this assessment of Dr Magner, the man:

> He was outspoken, sometimes impatient, but with never any hint of meanness; a witty speaker and a superlative raconteur; he was "the medieval man" – in the breadth of his life, his profession, and his interests; a superb teacher – his lectures to the medical students were probably the best didactic lectures I ever listened to; he had an interest in medical politics, and was elected to presidency of both the Toronto Academy of Medicine and the Canadian Medical Association, bringing to both offices a degree of eclat.

Of particular significance to the historian is this speaker's summary comments: "Dr. Magner was a powerhouse in the evolution of his department and of this hospital. Along with Dr. George Wilson, Dr. Magner engineered our transition to a fully-accredited teaching hospital."[97]

So the laboratories were happily launched. The x-ray facilities, too, gained a welcome promotion from the basement to the fifth floor. Although diagnostic x-ray had been used at the hospital since 1901,[98] the first paid x-ray technician arrived only in 1911: he was B.J. Fenner, who had previously operated a portable x-ray unit out of the Toronto General Hospital.[99] Early in the 1920s the university organized a post-graduate course for doctors, leading to a diploma in radiology. Fresh from this course, Dr E.H. Shannon, one of the first two doctors to receive the diploma,[100] came in 1925 to take charge of the new radiology department and the adjacent physiotherapy department. The x-ray department was equipped with the most modern apparatus, including two of the latest Wappler machines, a portable x-ray outfit, and a fluoroscope.

Working with Dr Shannon was Sister Carmella Fischer, who had learned earlier to operate the first x-ray equipment installed in the basement. Handsome, intelligent, and largely self-educated, Sister Carmella spent forty-one years at St Michael's, most of it in x-ray, and contributed in no small measure to the hospital's growth and development.

The emergency department, too, moved out of its cramped quarters – two small rooms and two hallways – where more than twenty-five patients a day had been regularly received.[101] In 1926 a resident casualty officer was added to staff, Dr J.W. McConville, who came from Glasgow with impressive credentials in clinical surgery. The next year Dr J.A. Dietrich was appointed part-time to take charge of the dental clinic.[102]

The geography of the in-patient areas assumed a shape that would endure for several decades: urology on the second floor, workers' compensation cases on the third, and maternity on the entire seventh floor. In December 1929 – a year after completion of the new maternity facility – rates were published for its semi-public wards: a flat rate of $3 per day "in a 4-bed, bright, attractive, quiet room," with operating room, anaesthetic fees, all baby and nursery charges, and laboratory fees included in the one flat rate. The family doctor was allowed to attend in this ward, but the meals served were as for public-ward patients. Medical and surgical patients in the new building were charged $2.50 a day in the semi-public wards, but radiology and operating-room charges were extra.[103]

The completion in 1928 of these three additional wings, A, B, C, along with the still-new north wing, brought the bed complement to 600. It was the end of a long struggle and the beginning of a completely new era. Woven within the fabric of the improved and expanded hospital, however, there were threads of continuity: Sister de Sales, who had been with the hospital from the beginning, was still in charge of an entire floor, and Dr Edmund King, one of the original surgeons, was still sending his patients to her floor. The old Baptist church stood firm amidst the new growth but it would, itself, fall victim to the new needs of the coming decade.

5

The Emergence of Giants

Hardly had the ribbons been cut for the opening of the last of the new wings (which were to have been revenue-producing) when the stock market crash of 1929 plunged the world and St Michael's into the Great Depression with its tragic sequelae of unemployment, labour unrest, hunger and homelessness, crime, and despair.[1] The Depression spawned or furthered a number of major movements, all of which had their adherents in Toronto: the Communist Party, the fascist cells, the organized labour unions, and the birth-control movement.

The Catholic Church in Toronto responded to these developments by recalling and reviewing the landmark encyclical of Pope Leo XIII, *Rerum Novarum*, issued forty years earlier, the theme of which was the condition of labour – hours of work, wages, workers' associations, and the rights and duties of employer and employees.[2] The national Catholic newspaper, *The Catholic Register*, discussed the encyclical in a series of articles and inveighed against the growing advocacy of birth control as a partial solution to the country's economic woes.[3]

But the church in Toronto went far beyond theory and exhortation; Archbishop McNeil earned a hearty vote of thanks from the city council for his work in providing hostels during the winter of 1930-31, and in September 1931 he launched a drive for $200,000 to help Toronto's 30,000 registered unemployed through the winter they would soon face.[4]

Documentation is sparse regarding the effects of the Depression on hospital personnel and hospital activities. There are references to the difficulty in borrowing money to finance building projects; to cost-cutting measures; and to reduction of room rates, possibly to attract those patients who could still pay. Revenue from paying patients fell by more than 50 percent from 1931 to 1933, and did not recover to its pre-Depression level until the mid-1940s.[5] It appears that entry-level salary for new staff was lowered: a teacher in the school of nursing was hired in August 1931 for $100 a month – twenty-five dollars less than a new assistant instructress had received in 1925. Graduate nurses on staff were supplied with room and board, as a supplement to their salaries; cleaners, maids, and orderlies were given three meals daily.[6] In 1931 the Nurses' Alumnae Association established a "loan fund" to assist its needy members, and a year later it arranged to pay from alumnae funds for two days' and two nights' private-duty nursing to unmarried sick nurses, while the hospital undertook to provide such private-duty nurses with board. Some unemployed – or unpaid – private-duty nurses had to resort to the Salvation Army for their daily bread; others were glad to accept the sandwich slipped to them when they dropped in at the hospital. Of less human toll, but nonetheless indicative of the times, were the instances where bulbs were missing from overbed lamps after the patients' visitors had departed. The medical advisory board reviewed "the excessive amount of drugs said to be used in the hospital and outpatient department, and recommended that heads should confer with Sister St Maurus" (pharmacist). They also agreed that the amount of x-ray material could be curtailed by "making a more thorough examination of patients before obtaining help in diagnosis from the X-ray department."[7]

The Labour Unions

The first record of labour-union activity at St Michael's dates to November 1935, when circulars were left about the hospital announcing a meeting to organize employees. The fliers spoke of the working conditions that needed to be changed in hospitals – the poor food, the ten- to twelve-hour shifts, and the caste system whereby "we are expected to stand at attention every time a doctor, a graduate nurse, or some other official passes."[8] Nothing came of this first overture to St Michael's employees, nor of another drive in 1940,[9] but when further invitations were extended by organized labour in 1945 Sister Louise Carey, superintendent, called a meeting of the service staff and, with them, organized an employees' association with elected officers, payroll deductions for a fund for expenses such as gifts and celebrations, and regular employee-management meetings.[10] This in-house association, after the pattern proposed in *Rerum Novarum*, exists to this day despite frequent drives by organized unions to replace it.

The Congregation

Requests continued to come from the archbishop of Toronto to undertake additional works: to take over the Welland General Hospital in 1930 and to buy the Wellesley Hospital in 1935 – both refused, as was a similar request from Port Alberni, British Columbia, because of existing financial obligations and too few sisters.[11] The rapid expansion of the past thirty years (eleven new foundations) was slowed, only two new foundations being made in the period from 1929 to 1945.[12] The 1929 flurry of appointments to university for summer school (two to a New York college for art, two to Columbia University for classics, two to Quebec for French) ceased abruptly and did not start again until 1939, when two sisters went to Harvard for English courses. The congregation did, however, contract for a $15,000 addition to its academy on Wellesley Street in 1934 (and at the same time lowered the rates for its resident pupils, as well as the tuition of its day students), and for a nurses' residence at St Joseph's Hospital.[13]

Governance of the Hospital

It appears that the board which was in place at the time of Sir Bertram Windle's resignation in 1928 disintegrated or was dissolved.[14] The council seems not to have acted on its own decision, made in 1931, "that St. Michael's Board be re-organized," continuing instead to deliberate on issues which ordinarily would have been board matters: installation of extra elevators at the hospital, insurance on the boilers, and plans for the new E-wing, including the choice of architect and contractor.[15]

Three major committees (building, cooperative purchasing, and hospital management), struck by the council in 1926, carried on. Sister Irene Conroy, formerly superior at St Michael's and now on the General Council, together with the superior and secretary-treasurer of each of the congregation's institutions as well as the superintendents of its member hospitals, constituted the membership of the committees. It cannot be denied that this superstructure accomplished much, guiding important developments at St Joseph's and Our Lady of Mercy hospitals and at St Joseph's College School. However, St Michael's had attained, by dint of hard struggle, a recognized place within the Toronto hospital community and the university, and required more than governance-by-committee.

From late February 1936 the board was again sitting on a regular basis. Several men who would give long and valued service were, or soon would be, among its members: J.J. Fitzgibbons, president of Famous Players Theatres, who became in 1940 the first lay chairman; Frank Hughes, justice of the Supreme Court of Canada; F.J. Crawford, president of the Toronto Stock Exchange; Charles Gillooly, active in charitable and welfare work; Duncan McDougald, head of his own investment company (his son "Bud" McDougald would in 1955 serve as chairman of the hospital's very successful fund-raising campaign); and Dr Peter Moloney, assistant director of Connaught Laboratories.[16] The board took up again its duties with regard to the university and with funding bodies, all of which will be commented on later, and handled some delicate negotiations concerning staff appointments. In 1939 new by-laws were drafted for presentation to the lieutenant-governor. Courtly and perhaps paternalistic, the board, in a policy illustrative of the times, was careful to assign its members to represent the sisters at evening meetings held outside the hospital.

Sister Louise Carey

Quietly prominent in the life and development of the hospital in this period was Sister Louise Carey, who, after four years in the main office, served as secretary-treasurer from 1926 to 1944 and as superintendent (with Sister Margaret Phelan as superior) from 1944 to 1948.

Sister Louise participated in 1923 in the introduction of a manual system of accounting acceptable to chartered accountants, a system that was replaced in 1931 by a bookkeeping machine costing $3,000 – "a marvellous thing, one of the first in the city."[17] When income tax was introduced ten years later, a second bookkeeping machine was installed to handle the payroll and accounts receivable – a mammoth instrument that years later could be relocated only by means of a crane inserted through a double window.

Ever alert to developments in the hospital field, and possibly moving out to the public arena more than did her contemporaries at St Michael's, Sister Louise established and maintained contacts with the management of other Toronto hospitals. She was active in the Ontario Hospital Association from its inaugural meeting in 1923, and was invited to stand for the presidency; because of the travel requirements of the position and the congregation's rule at that time which required that sisters be accompanied by another sister when travelling, she had to decline, but served several terms as vice-president.

Trained on the job as were so many hospital administrators of her day,[18] Sister Louise nevertheless qualified for fellowship in the American College of Hospital Administrators in 1954, the first of the congregation to do so. In 1948, with twenty-five years of hospital experience behind her, and with vital contacts at city hall and at Queen's Park in place, Sister Louise accepted an appointment to be administrator at St Joseph's Hospital, Sunnyside. There she successfully managed the reclassification of St Joseph's from a Group B to a Group A hospital (eligible for increased grants, but non-teaching).

Yet Sister Louise was not merely a capable and forward-looking administrator. When the author asked a contemporary of Sister Louise to name the people who were an inspiration to her during her years at the hospital, she answered without hesitation, "Sister Louise – in the way she dealt with people, especially the poor, the alcoholics, the down-and-out." Sister Louise's example in this regard influenced successive young sisters who came to the main office to be "trained" by her or to sort out their interest and suitability for the business field. Her niece, Sister Anne Marie Carey, became the first director of St Michael's detoxification unit.

The Changing Face of the Medical Advisory Board

During its first two decades this board remained small (three or four members). In 1933 the chief of otolaryngology (Dr F.X. Robert) was added; the chief of ophthalmology, Dr H.A. McCullough, had been recommended for appointment also, but apparently declined.

From 1930 to 1936 the board, now under Dr Guinane's chairmanship, dealt mainly with appointments, as distinct from the situation in Dr King's time (1914-30) when it had been more widely involved. In 1937 a standing committee on interns was struck to review intern applications and to report to the medical advisory board on their suitability. The Clinical Society remained active; the proceedings of its weekly meetings were printed and distributed for a $2 fee. The annual post-graduate week continued.[19]

Following Dr Guinane's death in 1936, Dr D'Arcy Frawley was elected chairman. It had been on his motion that the chiefs of the eye, and ear, nose, and throat departments had earlier been nominated to the medical advisory board; now it was during his tenure as chairman that Dr L. Sebert, the new chief of ophthalmology, and Dr L. Killoran, chief of anaesthesia, were added to the board in January 1938; Dr Eugene Shannon, chief of radiology, in May 1938; and Dr A.J. McDonagh (dentistry) in October 1938. Beginning in March 1939 Sister Zephyrinus Lyons, superintendent, is shown in attendance *ex officio* for just two meetings – after which the medical advisory board appears to have adjourned sittings during the whole of the Second

World War.[20] When the meetings resumed in 1945 both Sister Margaret Phelan, superior, and Sister Louise, superintendent, attended, but the membership included only the chiefs of medicine, surgery, obstetrics and gynaecology, and pathology.

Women As Medical Interns

In December 1931, out of fifty-three applicants for internship, twenty-one applicants (all male) were recommended for internship. However, from 1933 there were generally one or two women accepted each year, and even three in 1936 – out of what was for several years an intern roster of twenty-one. It is possible that the minutes are a reflection of the secretary's personal style, but it is also possible that they may reflect some discomfort and less-than-hearty support of the idea of women doctors; in any case, the women applicants are listed in the minutes as Miss So-and-So, without an initial or first name, although frequently three initials are given for the male applicants.

Earlier, in 1930, Miss (not Dr) Evelyn Breslin had been recommended as an extern in the outpatients department, her duties restricted to that department only, and with no responsibility for inpatients. In 1938 Dr Geraldine Moloney, complete with name and qualifying title, became the first woman to be advanced to senior internship at St Michael's.[21]

Surgery, Medicine, Biochemistry

Growth and reorganization of the medical services, together with a more disciplined approach to patient care, teaching, and the development of the young medical staff followed upon the provision of the improved physical facilities described in Chapter 4.

In 1927 Dr George Ewart Wilson became chief of surgery, in full charge of all surgical activities including the various special departments which had no university heads. Wilson resolutely took command, appointing four well-qualified men (Drs Wallace Scott, M. Cameron, T.A. Robinson, and James Ross) as senior surgeons, while a number of junior surgeons, each associated with a senior, were given charge of the outpatient department. New to the reader are Dr James Ross and Dr Wallace Scott. Ross was the son of Dr J.F.W. Ross and holder of the fellowship in surgery from the Mayo Foundation in 1922; he would serve for more than twenty-five years in the department of surgery. Wallace Scott was a silver medallist upon graduation in medicine from the University of Toronto, and fellow of the

Royal College of Surgeons in 1904. For several years Scott held faculty appointments in surgery and in obstetrics and gynaecology, and from 1909 he served on Dr W. McKeown's surgical service at St Michael's. Scott was acting head of surgery between the time of Dr McKeown's death and Dr Wilson's appointment, the latter's superior administrative skills having been recognized when it came down to the point of choosing a chief.[22]

In 1931 the department of medicine announced its reorganization, dividing its staff into three units under its chief, Dr Julian Loudon. The beginnings of some major medical specialties are evident: Unit I was in charge of Dr Jabez Elliott (whose clinical interest was in pulmonary disease), with five assistants, including Drs E.A. Broughton, Roderick Smylie, and H.A. Snetsinger; Unit II was headed by Dr A.J. Mackenzie (whose area of concentration was internal medicine), with five assistants, including Drs G. Glionna, W.B. Edmonds, and G. Chambers. Unit III was under Dr Harris McPhedran (whose clinical interest was heart disease), with five assistants, including Drs A.R. Hagerman, D'Arcy Prendergast, and E.C. Tate. Consultation, supervision, and teaching were built into the new structure, as evidenced by the rounds held once a week in each unit, "at which the chief physician and all those concerned with the work of the unit under review must necessarily be present."[23]

All of the doctors just mentioned had long years of association with St Michael's. Dr Alexander Mackenzie had degrees in arts and law, as well as medicine. Described by his contemporaries as scholarly and forward-looking, Mackenzie was president of the Ontario Medical Association at the time of his death in 1939. Dr Jabez Elliott made significant contributions to St Michael's, and far beyond it. Gold medallist in his graduating class of 1897, Elliott was, within the year, physician-in-charge of the Muskoka Cottage Sanatorium for patients with tuberculosis; he went on to become prominent in the tuberculosis field in both Canada and the United states. In 1931 Elliott was appointed the first professor of the history of medicine at the University of Toronto, in addition to his clinical work as chief of the tuberculosis services at St Michael's and at the Hospital for Sick Children.[24]

It was during these years that the first mechanical respirator appeared at St Michael's – the "iron lung" donated by Lord Nuffield, the immensely wealthy owner of an automobile-manufacturing industry in England.[25] Occupying the greater part of a room in the 3-D medical ward, and infrequently used, it defied the efforts of many a night supervisor to set it in motion; the one sure person to whom it would respond was Kathleen (Kay) Whelan, supervisor of that floor. The second piece of new technology in those years was the fever machine, a favourite for ten to fifteen years in the treatment of syphilitic patients; it was installed on 2 D-E, at the request of Dr E.F. Brooks who advised the board to accept it lest the special clinic be relocated out of St Michael's.[26] Primitive and cumbersome by today's standards, these inventions were nevertheless representative of a stage of the growth in medical knowledge and medical appliances.

Meanwhile, the new laboratories were beginning to make their presence felt and appreciated. Michael O'Sullivan, MA, came in February 1941 at a salary of $175 a month to set up a separate department of biochemistry – a branch of the laboratories formerly supervised by Dr Colling, under Dr Magner, but without a qualified biochemist since Dr Colling's death in 1939. O'Sullivan credits Sisters Zephyrinus and Emerentia O'Brien, together with Dr Peter Moloney of Connaught Laboratories, with arranging for him to study for a time under Dr E.P. Joslin, the world-famous diabetic clinician in Boston.

As director of the department of biochemistry for thirty-two years, O'Sullivan would guide it through a time of spectacular growth – in methodology, in volume of work, in physical facilities, and in numbers and qualifications of staff. His arrival was significant in that a non-medically qualified scientist was now a recognized member of the medical team, and his technicians could take over blood-collecting and analysis – duties previously the prerogative of the doctors and interns. The motto adopted by his department, "Laborandum est; non progredi est revehi" (We must work; not to go ahead is to go back), tells much about this man and explains in no small part the respect in which he and his department were held.[27]

The Obstetrics Department

Though not as fully documented in the hospital records, these years saw steady, rapid growth in the obstetrics department. This was the first department to have a senior intern (Dr H.J. Shoniker, 1924);[28] staff paediatricians were first appointed in 1925 (Drs P.W. O'Brien and F.F. Tisdall); and by 1928 the department had grown to such a size as to require three interns. In 1934 it recorded 1,324 births, double the total of 1928 and, among the hospitals in Toronto, second only to the combined Toronto Western-Grace hospitals which had reached a total of 1,458 births that year.[29]

Dr Frank O'Leary

Among the staff at St Michael's during many of these years none was better known than the team of Dr Frank O'Leary and Sister Vincentia (Mullen), chief and nursing supervisor respectively of the obstetrics department. The confidence these two enjoyed as specialists in maternal and infant health, as well as the sheer force and richness of their personalities, extended far beyond "their" 7th floor.

When he had just finished his first year in the school of medicine at the University of Toronto, by which time he was already a qualified pharmacist, Frank O'Leary went overseas in 1915 with the Canadian Army Medical Corps. He served in the field-ambulance unit in the bloodiest of battles – Flanders, Somme, Vimy, Passchendaele – losing a leg at the last-mentioned and winning the Military Medal. After obtaining his medical degree in 1922, O'Leary did post-graduate work at New York Women's Hospital and returned to the obstetrical staff at St Michael's, becoming chief in 1945. In 1951 he resigned his position as chief and devoted himself entirely to his private practice, one of the largest in the city. He attended his last delivery just two hours before his death of a heart attack on 3 February 1952, in his sixty-second year.

The outpourings of respect, gratitude, and love contained in the countless tributes to Dr O'Leary are convincing testament as to how one life, lived with vigour, generosity, and joy, can influence for good the lives of other human beings met along the way. Medical colleagues and students spoke of his fine mind and the quality of his lectures as associate professor at the university. All, from medical man to layman, rejoiced to recall his moments of high drama as when, for example, he removed a mother from an iron lung at Riverdale Hospital for thirty seconds, just long enough to deliver a six-pound baby girl. Struggling young couples told of their hospital bills mysteriously paid, and the doctor bills never even received. The Newman Club at the university spoke of O'Leary as the tireless worker on its executive and the life of every party, his artificial leg not only no impediment but even an occasion for merriment. In addition to all this, O'Leary was a patron of writers and the theatre, each year buying blocks of season's tickets at the "Royal Alec," dispensing them liberally among interns and nurses. A bachelor until his fifty-fifth year, O'Leary – always youthful – in 1945 married a nurse many years his junior but lived to share with her only seven years of married life.[30]

Sister Vincentia Mullen

Hardly less prominent than Dr O'Leary was Sister Vincentia, who for almost thirty years was nursing supervisor of the obstetrics department. After graduation from St Michael's school of nursing in 1922, Mae Mullen earned a diploma in public-health nursing from the University of Toronto, nursed with the Victorian Order of Nurses and the provincial Department of Health in Cobalt, Ontario, and finally entered the Sisters of St Joseph, taking the name of Sister Vincentia.

Assigned to the obstetrics department in 1928 (sisters did not choose their area of practice, and were rarely asked their preference), Sister Vincentia was to care for approximately 60,000 mothers and babies during her career there. Although widely credited with being the one responsible for the department's reputation for excellence,[31] Sister Vincentia was always quick to dismiss it all as "just a matter of cleanliness, efficiency, and good technique." In pursuit of these qualities, she herself designed a stainless steel-and-glass-enclosed bassinet which was capable of being sterilized each day and which made each baby self-sufficient in terms of its bathing, clothing, and feeding supplies.

To Sister Vincentia every mother was precious, and in her presence parents were awakened to their dignity and responsibility as parents. In her, perfectionism and idealism lived side by side with an earthy realism, and she was equally at ease with prelate and senator, public-ward patient or prostitute. Most of all, Sister Vincentia believed in herself and in her mission, and in so doing inspired many to rise to their potential – sometimes, admittedly, through fear, for woebetide the doctor or nurse who dared to offer a shoddy performance in this very special department. Almost forty years after her death one of her former interns left a generous bequest to St Michael's to commemorate the life of Sister Vincentia, "from whom he had learned so much."[32]

Development of the Surgical Staff

The board of governors, "recognizing that every piece of machinery from time to time requires overhauling and tightening up," recalled Dr George Ewart Wilson in 1927 from his position as surgeon in charge of emergency and outpatients at the Toronto General to become surgeon-in-chief at St Michael's. Wilson had been on staff earlier, having been appointed in 1909 immediately after obtaining his FRCS in England. His return appointment followed "an exhaustive canvass of medical centres in Canada, part of the United States and all of Great Britain."[33]

Wilson moved quickly to carry out the board's mandate, including that of seeing that experienced surgeons groom the junior men for senior positions as these became available. Several among those who served on the surgical staff during Wilson's tenure had long, even illustrious, careers, pioneering in a number of surgical specialties. Among these was Dr Gordon Foulds, senior urologist from 1923 to 1943. A fellow in urology from the Mayo Foundation, Foulds published widely on this emerging specialty, producing seventeen articles in a four-year period. Dr Harold Armstrong, holder of fellowships in surgery from the Royal Colleges of England and of Edinburgh as well as the American College (1937), was a specialist in thyroid surgery. His career was cut short at fifty-six years of age, after only fourteen years of senior practice. Dr Laird Alexander, who had studied in Boston (Massachusetts Eye and Ear Infirmary and Peter Brent Brigham), was one of the first of St Michael's doctors to use the bronchoscope (1930), removing a tooth aspirated and embedded in the lung of a four-year old boy brought down from northern Ontario.

At least two among the surgical staff did pioneering work in their fields. One was Dr David Pratt, who graduated from the University of Toronto in 1926, recipient of the Ellen Mickle Scholarship[34] which enabled him to study in Freiburg, Germany, for one year. He was given an appointment on St Michael's surgical staff in 1927, and later qualified for fellowship in the Royal College and the American College of Surgeons. In 1934 Pratt, working with Dr Edward Brooks, made history: Brooks made the first-ever pre-operative diagnosis of cancer of the pineal gland, and Pratt devised an original successful approach to its removal. In order to satisfy themselves of the complete recovery of their patient (a twenty-five-year-old woman), Pratt and Brooks waited for three years before presenting their report at the 1938 convention of the American College of Surgeons.[35]

The second pioneer of this era was Dr Joseph Sullivan, a 1926 graduate of the University of Toronto and of subsequent study programs in New York and several European centres. Sullivan began practice in St Michael's department of otolaryngology in 1930, and quickly leaped into prominence: in 1936 he presented to an international convention a new technique for transplanting a thigh nerve into the face for the cure of facial paralysis; four years later he was awarded the international gold medal in ear surgery for his pioneering work in the treatment of deafness.

In the course of his post-graduate studies Sullivan had gone to Sweden to study the surgical technique known as the fenestration (the creation of a passage through a bone in the inner ear to allow the transmission of sound waves and thus relieve deafness), and became, it is believed, the first man in Canada to perform this delicate ear surgery. After that first nine-hour fenestration in 1938 – done under a microscope, with the aid of a high-speed drill – Sullivan would, over his long career, "open a window for sound" for more than 4000 patients from all over North America. During this time he trained two younger men, Dr K. McAskile and Dr Brydon Smith, to also perform this surgery.

Sullivan was chief of otolaryngology at St Michael's and associate professor on the university's faculty of medicine from 1946 to 1956. During this time he established the hard of hearing clinic, assisted by a grant from the Atkinson Foundation. In 1956 Canada's first vestibular clinic was established at St Michael's under his leadership, with Walter Johnson, BSc, PhD, in charge. (From his experience as consultant to the RCAF during the Second World War, Sullivan had developed a keen interest in two problems widely suffered by pilots – hearing loss and dizziness; the vestibular clinic would address the problem of dizziness.) Johnson became director of research for the department of otolaryngology, serving at the same time as consultant to the United States Space Agency, NASA. The eminent British otolaryngologist Sir Terrence Cawthorne described Johnson's vestibular clinic as the finest in the world.[36]

Sullivan was the recipient of a whole range of honours. He was named to Canada's Senate in 1957, received an honorary fellowship in the Royal Society of Medicine, London, and was made honorary surgeon to the Queen in 1964 (a distinction in which, it is said, he took a boyish pride). He also received the highest papal honours. A singularly gifted man, Sullivan gave back abundantly to charity; among his gifts to the hospital was the large crucifix that hung over the chapel's main altar from the time the E-wing was built until the changes of Vatican II required its relocation to the rear wall over the entrance.

These are a few of Dr Wilson's staff, but there were many others whose careers, because of limitations of space, can only be mentioned. Among them was Dr W.G. Carscadden, a chest surgeon, who developed the use of colour slides and photography in the operating room, and Dr Clifford Watson, who in 1938 introduced an ultraviolet lamp for killing microorganisms in the air and around the wound during surgery – an innovation that was a highlight of the convention of the American College of Surgeons that year. There was Dr

Hoyle Campbell, who pioneered in the treatment of burns and in plastic surgery at St Michael's, and Dr J.T. Danis, whose success rate with rectal surgery was widely recognized. Lastly there was Dr J. Brennan, a skillful general and orthopedic surgeon, and Dr W.D. Smith, whose unfailing kindness and patience with the nervous beginner made him every nursing student's favourite surgeon.

The records of these men, while attesting to each one's giftedness and to his commitment to his patients and students, are testament as well to the discipline and skill with which Dr Wilson fulfilled the board's mandate and his own vision for the department of surgery. Early in his term he published a 415-page textbook on fractures; towards the end, he negotiated St Michael's participation in the Gallie Course – a three-year program designed by Dean W.E. Gallie to prepare surgical residents to sit for the Royal College examinations, a training previously available only outside the country.[37] Between these two dates Wilson – professor and chief, skillful surgeon, and able administrator – was a familiar figure on the teaching wards where he would often startle the junior nurses with the abrupt question, "Do you know who I am?" and was never too busy to teach and question the senior nursing staff, nor to receive a carnation for his buttonhole.[38]

Funding

With the onset of the Depression in 1929 there were fewer private, paying patients, simply because few people could afford the cost of a hospital stay.[39] Fortunately, in 1928 the Hospitals and Charitable Institutions Act had been amended to increase government's contribution for indigent patients from 50 cents to 60 cents a day, and municipalities' contribution from $1.50 to $1.75 a day.[40] These rates were arrived at through consultation with the Ontario Hospital Association, founded five years earlier with the express purpose of pressuring government to provide more money for hospitals.[41] The city had already, in 1925, raised its contribution to $1.75 for city-order patients, after a joint appeal by the city's hospitals.[42]

In 1933 an amendment to the Hospitals' Act was introduced in the legislature, whereby grants would be cut by 10 to 15 percent and municipal liability for babies reduced from 90 cents a day to 60 cents. The newspapers carried the hospitals' anguished reaction: St Michael's spokesman said that the hospital already had many indigent patients for whom it received nothing; Sick Children's commented that most of the hospitals, including theirs, had cut salaries. At St

Michael's it was apparently the salaries of the hospital sisters, of whom there were fifty-one in 1935, which were counted on to help finance operations. In a 1939 letter to the bishop of Saskatoon, who had asked for assistance, the superior general wrote: "In order that St Michael's Hospital and St Joseph's Hospital might be able to meet their payments, the salaries of the Sisters engaged there have been wholly absorbed since 1930, and that will have to continue for some years."[43] Throughout these hard times the hospital, nevertheless, offered a special 50 percent discount to nursing alumnae who required hospitalization.

With the memory of these hard years still fresh, the Ontario Hospital Association in 1941 introduced Blue Cross – a prepaid insurance plan under the direction of the association – which covered up to twenty-one days of hospital room and board, general nursing, operating-room and anaesthetic charges, laboratory work, and ordinary drugs.[44] Although the plan was not without its opponents,[45] it provided welcome relief both to the hospitals and to the subscribers, for the relatively inexpensive premiums, often handled in the workplace, posed little financial burden in the improved wartime economy.

In August 1945 the Toronto Hospital Council (an association of all the hospitals of Toronto, formed for the purpose of exchange of information and of coordinated approach to hospital problems) recommended to all Toronto hospitals that they implement the same 7 percent to 10 percent salary increases as had been agreed upon among the Toronto General Hospital, the Ontario Department of Labour, and the Service Employees' International Union (which had been threatening a strike at the General). To meet the cost of such increases to their service staffs, all Toronto hospitals raised their room rates; at St Michael's the new rate was $3 for public ward, from $4 to $5 for semi-private, and from $6 to $9 a day for private accommodation. The professional staff, too, were given increases, "floor duty nurses to receive $125 a month, and teaching nurses $135 a month, less Income Tax."[46]

In the midst of all this, the congregation was considering acquiring the property south of the hospital, "lest some objectionable building go up there," but hesitated "to add to the already heavy burden of St Michael's."[47] However, not many years would elapse before this property would be acquired and the hospital's own building, the new A-South wing, would be erected there.

Nursing: The Move into Post-Basic Education

Mention was made earlier of two sisters going off to Milwaukee in 1924 for a post-basic course in nursing education. They were in the forefront of what was to become an almost standard career pattern for the sister nurses at St Michael's, as well as for many lay nurses. Indeed, those first two were even ahead of their time; preparatory to the launching at the University of Toronto in 1928 of an extension course to prepare graduate nurses for hospital administration and teaching, university officials conducted a poll to assess the need for such a course. This poll found that, of 512 graduate nurses engaged in teaching in the schools of nursing polled, only ten had special training in teaching.[48] With the opportunity for further preparation now brought almost within walking distance, the post-basic preparation of the sister nurses at the University of Toronto began in earnest, with Sisters Jeanne Barry and St Albert Mattimoe in 1929, and continuing thereafter with generally two sisters at a time for several years.

Until 1934 St Michael's had no nurses specifically trained in operating-room (O.R.) technique, although Sister Edana Ryan had had extensive experience in this area and had as early as 1926 undertaken an intensive study of operating rooms in several outstanding American hospitals. In 1934 Sister Amata Charlesbois (O.R. supervisor, 1931-41) went for a short time to the Mayo Clinic, Rochester, Minnesota, to study O.R. nursing, as did Marion Topham and Aileen Birns, who stayed for the full five month course – and returned wearing short-sleeved uniforms, an innovation.

With the leadership of Sister Amata and Marion Topham, St Michael's began in 1936 to offer a post-graduate course in O.R. nursing; in 1939 the nurse inspector from the provincial Department of Health wrote, "In the three years since its inception there has been no dearth of applications. This appears to be a well-organized and valuable course."

In 1940 Sister Mary Kathleen arranged for Marion (Topham) Finegan's theatre instruction to be supplemented by formal classroom lectures. Sister Angeline Coyne (O.R. supervisor, 1941-48), Finegan, Jenny Jankowski, and other senior nurses continued to do extensive teaching in the theatres. The course was formalized still further in 1952 when Sister Eileen (Helen Bradley), O.R. supervisor from 1952 to 1962, appointed Jean Watson to assume responsibility for it. For the next twenty years Watson directed this highly successful and popular course, which twice a year attracted ten to fifteen registrants from all across Canada and from as far away as Palestine and Peru. The course was absorbed into George Brown College in 1974.[49]

A similar post-graduate course was offered in obstetrical nursing. The exact year of its beginning is uncertain, but it is known, from the nurse inspector's report, that there were four students in a four-month course in 1936. There were ten graduates a year in 1950, by which time the course had increased to six months, offered twice a year, with the sisters offering three scholarships each year to members of the graduating class, as they did also to students interested in operating-room nursing – a practice that continued well into the 1960s.

Nursing: The Guiding Philosophy

The prevailing philosophy of nursing during these years can be deduced from notes for a course on ethics given by Sister St Philip Wanner in 1925.[50] The notes reveal an understanding of psychology and of educational and organizational principles quite remarkable in a teacher who had little formal education in these areas: "The essence of nursing is personal service to the sick and helpless .... the nurse herself will have a large part in the training and developing of her own powers .... anything that helps her know herself better is of real importance."

The rationale for the rules of the school is given, and while there is a strong emphasis on obedience to authority, this is presented in such a way that obedience, far from being demeaning, emerges, rather, as ennobling – a vital link in the hierarchy of persons in the hospital community. All members of that community directed their efforts to the one goal: the patient whom they served; "the highest authority in the institution, the governing body, is itself bound by certain laws, and is accountable to the public and to those who contribute to the support of the institution."

In addition to the emphasis on obedience, there was strong emphasis on self-control, defined as "the full command of yourself ... a great conserver of self-respect." Nevertheless, "anger has its place. The man or woman who can't get angry when occasion arises, who can't feel deeply indignant, is made of poor material."

These were the principles offered to the nursing students by Sister St Philip, sixty-one years of age at the time. A tribute written after her death ten years later, signed simply "A Doctor," reads: "Gentle, tolerant, and wise, her person moved in an invisible aura of kindliness which enveloped all whom she met. She leaves behind in those who knew her a sense, not so much of loss or regret, as of warm and pleasant memory, a feeling of joy at having known at least one soul so truly great, and an abiding knowledge that with her all is well."[51]

Among the nurses who exemplified to a marked degree the professional qualities enjoined upon nurses of this era, few were as deeply involved in the hospital and school of nursing, and for so long, as was Grace Murphy. A graduate of the school in 1928, and of a post-basic course at the University of Toronto, Murphy was a medical supervisor for ten years and then the acknowledged "dean" of the nursing faculty for more than twenty years. It is almost impossible to portray in capsule form this sterling character. An expert practitioner and critic of nursing, with a warm, ever-youthful sense of humour, she was totally loyal and reliable. She was also possessed of high principles, mature judgment, and vision. None wore St Michael's cap and pin, uniform and cape with more pride and dignity than did Grace Murphy, who crossed Bond Street each morning for more than thirty years to attend an early Mass at St Michael's Cathedral.

Coming out of the same era in the school's history, and sharing with Grace Murphy the same three decades of development in nursing and nursing education, was Marcella Berger, head nurse and instructor in the labour and delivery rooms.

At the time Berger completed her training (1926) Ontario had the third highest rate of maternal deaths to total births in Canada – 7.2 per 1,000 live births.[52] The rate at St Michael's is not known, but the first thing Sister Vincentia did when Marcella Berger joined staff in obstetrics in 1928 was to pack her off – not without protest – to the Women's Hospital, New York, for a two-year post-graduate course in maternal-infant health.[53] Berger returned in 1931 and over the next thirty years taught, in the classroom and delivery room, a total of more than 3000 undergraduates and 104 post-graduate nursing students, and assisted at approximately 35,000 births. She kept herself always abreast of, often beyond, the current knowledge in the field, and in her later years maintained an open-mindedness to new concepts not always found in those possessed of tried-and-true methods.

Clear, direct, and authoritative in her guidance of nervous students and uncertain interns in the delivery room, Berger could be the tenderest of mothers to the woman who had come through a difficult delivery. Offering a rare glimpse into the most intimate depths of her own philosophy, Berger told the graduating class of 1971, "Tenderness towards the sick or weak strengthens the heart to life itself." She exemplified in her own conduct what she taught the nurses, namely that "every mother is a national asset, and entitled to the highest standards of care," and her high standards contributed much to the hospital's record of performance in obstetrics.

Nursing Developments

The first specific legislation for Ontario nurses had been passed in 1922 – the Nurses' Registration Act. Authority to administer the act was vested, not in the professional association (the Graduate Nurses' Association of Ontario, formed in 1904, which became the Registered Nurses' Association of Ontario in 1925), but in the office of the provincial secretary, representing the Ontario cabinet. In 1924 the authority was transferred to the Department of Health, and an inspector was appointed to assume responsibility for the nurses' registration division in that department.

The act regulated the specific requirements for conducting a training school (length of program, content, eligibility of applicants). Examinations based on the provincial minimum curriculum were held at designated centres once a year, leading to registration and the use of the title of registered nurse.

The content and the scope of practice of nurses during these years can be deduced from a review of the seven examinations they were required to pass before becoming eligible for registration.[54] The progression from simple to more complex instruction, and consequent growth in the nurse's responsibility, is evident in these examinations. So is the development of new medical-treatment modalities and of new disease patterns. For example, in 1926 the nurse was simply asked to locate a particular bone; in 1941 she was asked to describe the process by which a simple fracture heals. The advances being made in medical treatment are reflected in questions regarding administration of insulin (1928 examination), hypodermic injections (1929), blood transfusion (1930), intravenous infusion (1935), intramuscular injection (1936), and oxygen therapy (1941).

In children's nursing there was much emphasis on diet and a remarkable stress on the prevention and symptoms of rickets (contained in eight examinations between 1926 and 1941). As early as 1926 nurses were questioned on the care of a patient pre- and post-thyroidectomy or tracheotomy. In obstetrical nursing there was constant emphasis on the nurse's responsibility in the health teaching of expectant mothers. In preventive medicine the strongly recurring themes were the pasteurization of milk and ventilation of patients' rooms. An emerging insight in public health is evident in nurses being examined (1943) on the relation of fatigue to health and to the resistance to disease.

Other examinations highlight the impact of war. A 1941 examination questioned nurses on caring for air-raid victims, and in a 1945 examination a question begins with "venereal diseases are a serious health hazard at the present time ...."

Developments within nursing, medicine, and society as reflected above placed demands upon those hospitals that conducted schools of nursing. At St Michael's, the number of full-time instructors increased during the years under study, from the superintendent of nurses and two instructors in 1929[55] to five instructors in 1945. Yet the real, and necessary, increase was as yet in the future.

The nurse inspectors from the Department of Health observed and assessed not only the program of the school but also the quality of nursing care on the wards. For many years Ontario was fortunate in having experienced inspectors, blessed with wisdom and insight of the calibre, for example, of Edith Dick and Dorothy Riddell. These two were able to offer to the superintendent of nurses and the hospital supervisors the benefits of their observations on the field at large, and they became catalysts for improvement and change on a wide scale.

A continuing concern of the nurse inspectors was the heavy burden of the class and ward duty of the nursing students. Recommendations, which became almost warnings ("student hours far exceed provincial legislation," 1941), were made at every visit from 1936 through 1947.[56] Student hours could be reduced only by the introduction of general-duty nurses and auxiliary staff, a change that came slowly: in 1936 there were thirty-six general-duty nurses, most of whom lived in the hospital residences; by 1943 there were still only forty-nine, but by this time most had moved out.[57] These, along with the nursing students, staffed the 600-bed hospital of the time. No doubt recruitment to the armed forces (107 St Michael's nurses served in the Second World War)[58] decreased the pool of potential graduate nurse staff. In the 1945 review, the inspector noted that students did all the night duty, with the exception of a night supervisor and one graduate nurse in emergency and one in obstetrics.

Throughout all this, valiant efforts were made to offer sound basic and continuing education. As early as 1936 there was a monthly staff-education program underway, held in the evenings, with papers prepared and given by graduate-staff nurses. That same year students were doing case studies, and ward nursing clinics were just beginning, with doctor and dietitian contributing. By 1945, fifteen St Michael's nurses were in post-basic courses at the university, for which the federal government was offering $300 bursaries. All at St

Michael's must have felt rewarded and encouraged by the summary remarks of the senior nursing inspector in 1947: "This school has a valuable contribution to make in nursing education."

The superintendent of nurses through many of these years was Sister Jeanne Barry, assisted by Sister Colette Delanty as instructor in the fundamentals of nursing. Both were graduates of the University of Toronto's course in teaching and supervision. After some time in the school, Sister Colette supervised a private surgical floor for several years, and was highly respected for her knowledge and judgment and for her attention to patients' individual needs.

Attentive to current legislation and open to the recommendations of the nurse inspectors, Sister Jeanne pioneered what would be some enduring features of the school: among them, the establishment of the recommended committee on nursing (1932),[59] and the affiliation of nursing students at the Toronto Psychiatric Hospital and in Toronto's Public Health Department (1937). She earned commendation from the nurse inspectors for arranging for supervisors from the medical, surgical, and obstetrical wards to contribute to their respective clinical courses in the classrooms of the school.

Sister Jeanne made some progress in reducing student hours and extending their vacation (to eight weeks in three years). Equally important to the students, and despite her reputation for strictness, she successfully placed the case before the sisters' council in 1934 for the floor-duty nurses and the senior students to hold a dance in the residence from 9 p.m. to 12 midnight, and to invite the interns – a first!

After nine years in the school, Sister Jeanne assumed charge of 1-D, the large public medical ward where, again, an admiring senior nurse inspector noted that Sister Jeanne "sets an excellent example for students through her recognition of the social needs of the patient." In 1952 Sister Jeanne became, and remained for ten years, the first director of nursing service at St Michael's,[60] after which she spent her remaining years where her heart always was – visiting the public-ward-patients as a member of the pastoral-care team.

Sister Mary Kathleen Moore, fresh from St Louis University with her bachelor of science degree in nursing education – the first of the nursing sisters, and the first St Michael's graduate, to hold such a degree – came in 1940 to take charge of the school she had graduated from nine years earlier. She was to become the school's longest serving chief nurse, first in her capacity as superintendent of nurses from 1940 to 1952 and then as director of the school of nursing from 1952 to 1958.

Within five years of Sister Mary Kathleen's coming, nurse inspectors were commending the developments that had been effected: all students now had public-health experience; a well-qualified science instructor had been engaged; ward teaching and supervision had been improved; the numbers of general-duty nurses had been increased and their post-graduate study greatly encouraged, and finally, a form of student government had been established.[61]

But there was still work to be done; for example, the students' night term in the second and third years was nine weeks long, more than double the recommended standard. As a result, arrangements were subsequently made for students to have two hours off each night, and later they were given a night off weekly. We shall return to Sister Mary Kathleen's accomplishments in a later section.

The Dietetic Internship Program

St Michael's engaged its first qualified dietitian in 1924 and just four years later began a training program in dietetics. Graduates of any home-economics course were eligible for the program, which was three months long at first and increased to six months in 1930. The later program attracted graduates from colleges and universities all across Canada. Those enrolled in the program taught the nursing students at both St Michael's and St Joseph's hospitals, planned the therapeutic diets, and instructed both inpatients and outpatients, even going out to the homes.[62]

In 1935 Margaret McCarthy, the hospital's chief dietitian, began negotiations with the University of Toronto and the Canadian Dietetic Association to have the program formally approved for the training of dietitians. Under negotiations continued by Sister Mary Francis Peck (director of dietetics, 1936-50) and Sister Emerentia O'Brien (biochemistry department), St Michael's became in 1936 the first hospital approved by the Canadian Dietetic Association for the training of dietitians.[63]

At the time there were just three staff dietitians, together with the student dietitians, to supervise the now-centralized service for preparing the patients' trays in a 600-bed hospital, and also to handle the therapeutic diets and the teaching. For the student dietitians it was a demanding regimen: fifty-weeks of twelve-hour days, with only every third weekend off and no pay![64]

The doctors, followed by the nurses, had been the first of the health professions to standardize their teaching, certify their graduates, and form their own associations. Now the dietitians, followed by the medical-record librarians, were in the forefront of that wave of other professional and technical groups that followed the same route to recognition in the health field in the 1930s and 1940s.

Medical Records

The increasing volume and complexity of activities through the years to the 1940s is illustrated in the matter of patient records. Probably the most extensive records in the very early days were those kept in the operating room, where a loose-leaf binder held a record of all operations performed, with a space for pathological findings to be recorded.[65] By 1915 the medical advisory board ruled that the surgeon should dictate notes at the end of each operation, such notes to be recorded by the anaesthetists with the ward notes of the patient. That same year a special committee was elected at a meeting of the whole staff to "investigate and report on methods of recording and filing in-patient and out-patient records."[66]

In 1920 the record forms proposed by the committee on hospital standardization of the American College of Surgeons were adopted by the medical advisory board. A giant step forward towards complete and good records was made in 1926 when a recording stenographer was provided surgeons at the completion of their operations.[67] The perennial difficulty in getting charts completed was, nevertheless, evident in 1927 when registrars were instructed to endeavour to have incomplete charts for the month completed by the doctor in charge and, if unsuccessful, report him to the medical advisory board.

Throughout all this time there was no organized medical records department. Beginning in the early 1930s efforts were made to systematize the records; with the adoption in 1937 of the Standard Nomenclature of Diseases and Operations there evolved a method of securing, filing, and retrieving the medical records.

Coincident with this latter development was the establishment at St Michael's in 1936 of the first school in Canada for medical record librarians; its founder and director was Sister Mary Paul Biss.[68] The school flourished, expanding from a graduating class of one in its first year of operation to a class of twenty-three in 1965. More important, the school became fully approved by both the Canadian and American Associations of Medical Record Librarians.

Construction of the E-wing

As happens when one or more new wings are added to a hospital, former ones suddenly appear outdated and shabby. So it was with the original hospital, the old Baptist church, after the A-B-C-wings were built. In 1936, in preparation for building a new central wing, fronting on Bond Street to link the medical unit (D-wing) with the A-B-C-wings, the old church was demolished and its stained-glass window was donated to the Park Road Baptist Church "in keeping with the dignity of its history."[69]

Eight storeys high, the new E-wing provided administrative offices; doctors' staff room, assembly hall, and library; central sterilizing room; handsomely furnished private and semi-private rooms, which increased the bed capacity to 690; additional operating theatres;[70] and, finally, improved living accommodations for the staff of fifty-one sisters. (Previously their bedrooms had been scattered throughout the hospital, some even over the laundry.) The wing was officially opened on 8 September 1937 by Lieutenant-Governor Herbert Bruce, who had, as a young surgeon, held a staff appointment at St Michael's.

The important construction of the 1920s had been solid and utilitarian but was, with a few exceptions, unimaginative. By comparison, the E-wing was more grandly conceived, more tastefully decorated, more expressive of the status St Michael's was in the process of assuming among the teaching hospitals of Canada, and more evocative of pride and renewed commitment within the hospital community.[71]

The centrepiece of the new wing was the Gothic chapel, the fitting of which into the space available required all the ingenuity of the architect and contractors, W.L. Somerville and the Pigott Construction Company. Situated on the third floor, running two storeys high, it incorporated features of the Gothic design in the vaulted ceiling, the several arches with their overlapping leaf effects, and the tall perpendicular stained-glass windows. Steps of antique green marble led up to altars of creamy-yellow Sienna marble.[72]

Second only to the chapel as a source of pride was the new entrance. Flanked by lamps on either side, bronze double doors opening from Bond Street led to a wide rotunda decorated with black and gold marble base and dado, and pillasters of creamy marble – the whole considered "a splendid example of the Art Deco Style."[73] Mounted on the exterior wall, above the bronze doors, was an eight-and-one-half-foot figure of St Michael the Archangel, sculpted by Torontonian Frances Loring. This sculpture brought its own problems: the city's legal department warned the sisters that the Archangel's right toe and the tip of his nose encroached on city property! While the Civic Works Commission apparently approved the sisters' request to maintain the encroachments,[74] it appears that the decision was subsequently reversed for as late as July 1973 the hospital was paying the city $224.43 annually for "area rental" in connection with the statue.[75]

The superintendent of the hospital during these years was Sister Norine Pollard. An elementary-school teacher prior to this appointment, Sister Norine nevertheless soon became "a hospital person."[76] While the E-wing would be the crowning achievement of her tenure (1932-38), she established, as well, the first paediatric department (a three-room unit on 5-B) and the first medical library. A favourite with the Nurses' Alumnae Association, Sister Norine in 1935 initiated annual spiritual retreats for the graduate nurses.

A departure from the usual administrative structure occurred in 1938, when Sister Mary of the Nativity Sullivan was appointed superior, with Sister Zephyrinus Lyons assuming the post of superintendent "to relieve the Superior of much of the hospital administration, and to allow her to concentrate more on helping the Sisters."[77] It is difficult to assess how the duties were divided or how effective the arrangement was. Both sisters sat on the three-member sisters' council and both attended board of governors' meetings, but only Sister Zephyrinus attended, as an *ex officio* member, the two medical advisory board meetings in March 1939. No medical advisory board meetings were held between 1939 and 1945; consequently, little record remains of Sister Zephyrinus's involvement there before she went on to be elected assistant superior general of the congregation. Dr Arthur Hudson, who interned during those years, spoke of Sister Zephyrinus's "witty humanity." When medical advisory board meetings resumed in 1945 the new superior (Sister Margaret Phelan) and the new superintendent (Sister Louise Carey) both attended. Medical advisory committee meetings of these years document Sister Louise's direct involvement in intern affairs and in arrangements with the dean and the faculty of medicine at the university. Sister Louise spoke of Sister Zephyrinus's tenure as superintendent (1938-44) as an "experiment," and of her own time (1944-48) as "difficult"; she was not on the sisters' council but reported to it on financial matters. The single superior/superintendent role in the person of Sister Margaret Phelan resumed in 1948 when Sister Louise was transferred to St Joseph's Hospital.

A First-hand Account

The flavour of life in St Michael's just prior to, during, and following the Second World War can be caught from the edited reminiscences of one doctor whose association with St Michael's, beginning in 1937, spanned these years:

> The E-wing was the only really new section. As junior internes we knew the D-wing best; it had creaky floors and ancient fittings, but the feeling was homelike and the atmosphere generally comfortable. There were a couple of rooms in which disturbed patients, often with general paresis, would be secured. The windows of these rooms had bars, and the patient would sometimes open the inside window and call out to startled passersby that he was being incarcerated in St. Michael's Hospital.
>
> Dr. Bill Hall was the most compassionate of men when it came to dealing with internes. Also Dr. Harry Gibson Hall always had time to teach and to listen to you, in spite of running a very busy Medical Out-Patients. Dr. Eddie Brooks was a junior staffman, full of fun, and busier than a squirrel in autumn – a great favourite with the residents. Dr. Harris McPhedran (Haggis McBagpipes, we called him) ruled with a somewhat heavier hand. And who could forget Grace Murphy's maternalistic attitude toward the internes on 3-D. She used to test the morning diabetic urines herself, ostensibly to save the internes, but in reality to satisfy herself that they were done correctly. The emergency rotation was an extravagant learning process for juniors, presided over by Sister Florian, Marie Meehan, and Rita Moore. This experience gave us a greater appreciation of medicine as a whole than is now obtained.
>
> Dr. O'Leary, Sister Vincentia, Marcella Berger and Miss Gibbons ran a smooth Obstetrical Department and nursery. Sister Vincentia was the epitome of a giant cannon that fired marshmallows, not shells. There was not a mean bone in her body, but you always knew what was on her mind and where you stood. Dr. Stuart Mac-Donald and I were close friends, and internes together on Obstetrics. When I was called to the R.C.A.F. he kept my pet spaniel in his room on 2-A until he could find a home for it – the only time I know of that St. Michael's ever had a dog in residence. The lab. was Dr. William Magner, and his big booming voice pervaded the whole hospital. It was his communications satellite and he simply bellowed if he wanted you or any of his staff. One of these was Miss Janet Hutchison, a magnificent personality, who ruled bacteriology, serology, haematology and the animal laboratory on the roof. By far the most exciting laboratory work for me was assisting at the autopsies with Dr. Magner. I will never forget the exhilaration of having my findings accepted by this giant of a man of medicine .... There is nothing to compare with my early years at St. Michael's, not only medically, but in friendships made with so many of the Sisters and nurses.[78]

The Second World War

Apart from the human tragedy of injury, loss, death, and destruction that affected directly or indirectly everyone connected with St Michael's, the most immediate effects of the Second World War were the shortages – of personnel, of food, and of medical supplies and equipment. Detailed records of these years at St Michael's are few and scattered.[79] However, enough has been written about the war years in general for one to reconstruct partially the hospital scene.

First, there was the rationing, especially of food. Canada shipped to Britain vast quantities of wheat, flour, meat, eggs, cheese, and fish, leaving these and other foodstuffs (sugar, tea) in short supply at home.[80] In the hospital, problems connected with the shortage of food were compounded by the shortage of personnel; when the sister in charge of the kitchen was fortunate enough to get a truckload of fruit, the sisters from the offices (including the superintendent) were commandeered to sort and peel fruit for preserving, late into the night. As well, the sisters from the offices were drawn upon regularly to deliver patients' trays and to wash dishes, for auxiliary help was difficult to recruit as more and more women chose to serve in the better-paying war plants or in the armed forces.[81] Out of concern for the sisters' health because of these and other demands, the congregation purchased at this time a summer residence on Lake Simcoe, which remains today a favourite place for retreat, rest, and recreation.

In the midst of wartime hardships, the hospital took time in 1942 to hold modest celebrations to mark its fiftieth anniversary (its twenty-fifth had also fallen during war years). In 1944 the school of nursing celebrated the golden anniversary of its first graduating class, with two of the 1894 pioneer graduates in attendance. The number of staff doctors serving with the military climbed from sixteen in 1941 to twenty-seven by 1943, and although the government had its eye on Dr Magner for a military laboratory he was not called up.[82] Dr McPhedran, of St Michael's staff, chaired the Procurement and Assignment Board of Ontario, a body mandated to maintain a satisfactory balance between physicians in the armed forces and in civilian practice. Two St Michael's physicians, one of them Surgeon-Lieutenant William Lyon MacKenzie King, nephew of the prime minister, perished when their ships were torpedoed in the North Atlantic in 1943. Two St Michael's nurses were rescued after the 1944 torpedoing and bombing in the Mediterranean of the ship carrying them to that theatre of war.

The armed forces were to have 107 graduates of St Michael's school of nursing in its ranks by war's end. Most were attached to the 1200-bed Canadian General Hospital, recruited in Military District #2 (Toronto and Hamilton).[83] For the first two years this hospital was based in England, where the nurses were involved in routine care of sick or injured Canadian service personnel, while also receiving instruction in new methods of treatment of casualties from the air-raids. Their first actual contact with battle casualties came in August 1942, when they received 230 injured survivors of the Dieppe attack. Less than a year later #15 Hospital (the Canadian General Hospital) was ordered to the Mediterranean theatre, and was based first in North Africa and then relocated to Italy. The author of the official record states that there, although the hospital's capacity was increased to 1600 "through the procurement of additional tentage," its resources were from time to time "severely taxed."

At St Michael's the hardships of serving on the home front must have been made somewhat more bearable by the word pictures from the war zone published regularly in the *Alumnae News*.[84] Writing at Easter 1944 one nurse said: "15th Canadian General Hospital has quite a representative St Michael's group .... I am enjoying a leave at a Rest Home on the Adriatic, my first leave since leaving England last June." Another writes from Italy, acknowledging Easter greetings received: "We have had fresh eggs three times since Christmas. All I would like now is a quart of milk."A third nurse appears to take it all as a great adventure: "I was fortunate in being loaned out to Field Dressing Station, right up behind the lines ... a wonderful, but dreadful experience ... we get the direct battle casualties."

Paralleling these stories of youthful bravery and endurance overseas, there were the less colourful, but nonetheless heroic, examples of aging personnel making do with scant resources and with aging equipment at home. At war's end the four chiefs of surgery, medicine, obstetrics and gynaecology, and otolaryngology were all due to retire, and the sisters' council was considering the purchase of stretchers and wheelchairs which had been impossible to procure during the war years. A new chapter was about to begin.

6

Adult Stature, Adult Headaches

The exhaustion of the Second World War's closing months was quickly replaced by a surge of post-war energy and optimism as St Michael's, with the congregation and the city, plunged into a decade of unprecedented growth.

Following fast upon the return of the servicemen (and in many cases their brides) came an influx of immigrants from Britain and Europe, including the "displaced persons." By 1956 post-war immigrants to Ontario had reached almost the half-million mark,[1] a large proportion of whom settled in Toronto. Soon these would alter the composition of St Michael's staff, as well as its student and patient populations. More significantly, they would alter St Michael's way of viewing and responding to its world. Henceforth there would be a new respect – not just tolerance – for the scholarship, giftedness, and human qualities of newcomers from abroad; there would also be evident a greater self-confidence on the part of St Michael's people to move beyond any parochialism, and to risk taking their place as professionals within a wider circle, first in Toronto, in Ontario, and in Canada, and then, as will be seen, within the whole family of nations.

As in earlier times, with the influx of immigrants there came a shift of former residents to Toronto's rapidly growing suburbs. A more efficient transportation system became essential, and in 1954, after five years of construction, Toronto presented its citizens with their first subway – clean, fast, and a source of tremendous civic pride. In terms of social services, the growth in population generated a need for more hospitals and schools. No fewer than seven new hospitals opened in Toronto between 1950 and 1956.

Responding to the city's changing demography and its own flourishing novitiate, the congregation opened a new high school at Islington in 1949, a modern "village" for disturbed children at Scarborough in 1951, and a total of six other new foundations from Montreal to Vancouver within the space of twelve years (1944-56). Speaking at the opening of the high school, Toronto's Cardinal Archbishop James McGuigan spoke of "the burden the sisters shouldered." Prudent in its risk-taking, General Council enlisted the help of five prominent gentlemen to meet with it from time to time "for the purpose of discussing business problems and aiding us by their advice."[2]

Medical Staff: Change and Development

The major changes initiated at St Michael's in the post-war years included ones affecting the chiefs of staff. The resignation of the chief of medicine occurred in 1945, and was followed by that of his replacement and of the chiefs of three other services in 1947.

Dr Julian Derwent Loudon, St Michael's second physician-in-chief, had held that appointment through twenty-four eventful years (1921-45), years that raised scholarly enquiry, medical education, and practice at St Michael's to a new level. Loudon, with Dr Magner and others, was in the forefront of those developments, especially through the Clinical Society, the *Medical Bulletin*, and the annual Clinical Week. Son of Dr James Loudon – the first Canadian-born president of the University of Toronto and the first Canadian to occupy a professorial chair in Canada – Dr Julian Loudon received his medical degree at the University of Toronto in 1903. Following five years of post-graduate study in London, where he earned his MRCS and LRCP (Loudon was given a staff appointment at St Michael's in 1912. The next year he persuaded St Michael's board of governors to purchase an electrocardiography machine, an import from Cambridge, England. Believed to be the first electrocardiography machine to be bought by a Canadian hospital,[3] the acquisition was, according to Loudon, "a formidable-looking machine, filling almost the whole of a large room."

In 1914 Loudon became the first Canadian to publish an article on electrocardiography in a Canadian journal.[4] He authored, as well, one of the earliest systematic schemes for examination of the nervous system, a copy of which is preserved in the hospital's museum. The breadth of his interests, illustrative of the expanding medical knowledge of the times and his grasp of it (Dr Loudon earned fellowships* in both the Royal Canadian and the American Colleges of Physicians during his tenure at St Michael's), may be glimpsed in two 1938 articles for the *Clinical Society*, one on disseminated sclerosis and the

---

*Fellowships in the Royal College of Physicians or Surgeons, and in its American counterpart, is granted to those doctors who have undertaken preparation – usually of several years' duration beyond their basic medical degree, specializing in some branch of medicine or surgery – and have passed the required examinations.

other on recent advances in medical diagnosis and treatment, where he touches on the sulphanilamides, the new insulins (protamine zinc), the serum treatment of pneumonia, the bronchoscope, and other topics.

Described by his contemporaries as an excellent physician, thoughtful of others, soft-spoken and unassuming, Dr Loudon may have been by temperament less fitted for administration than for the life of the scholar and clinician. Faced with the university's call for reorganization of his department (he had several non-university men on his public-ward teams where the teaching was done), and with a heavy teaching load that could only become heavier in the booming post-war era, Loudon stepped down in 1945. Noted for his commitment to the poor, whose hard lives he had come to know first-hand in his duties as coroner – an appointment he held for several years – he continued to serve them after his resignation from St Michael's. Another group for whom he showed special concern was the nursing students, for whom he served as attending physician for more then two decades.

At the 10 September 1945 meeting of the hospital board, Dr J. Harris McPhedran accepted appointment as physician-in-chief, and at the October meeting the board and Dr McPhedran agreed on the written terms of his appointment. This marks the beginning of a new, more formal arrangement between the hospital and its medical staff. The university's policy regarding the retirement age of teaching staff (normally at sixty years of age) is mentioned for the first time, as is the provision of office space and secretarial assistance for the chief.

The new chief at St Michael's and assistant professor at the university had had a long association with both institutions, as staff physician at St Michael's since 1908 and senior demonstrator at the university since 1924. But Dr McPhedran's interests and activities extended well beyond the hospital and the university: he had been instrumental in persuading the Department of Health to give diphtheria toxoid to school-age and pre-school children; his wartime activities with the Procurement and Assignment Board have already been mentioned; and after the war he served on a national commission set up to prepare a bill for compulsory national-health insurance, in the course of which he made on-site studies of the operation of the state-financed health system in the United Kingdom.

Holder of an honorary FRCP as well as an honorary LLD from Dalhousie University, McPhedran occupied for a term the highest office in both the Ontario and Canadian Medical Associations, and was admitted to the latter's select company of senior members.

Described as a strict disciplinarian, McPhedran was, nevertheless, admired by many medical students as "the best teacher I ever had"; in his short two-year term as chief he apparently also demonstrated a gift for leadership, for, in the words of a contemporary, "the medical staff came alive [under him]."[5]

A Fresh Start: 1947

In 1947 Drs E.F. Brooks, W.K. Welsh, and Frank O'Leary became chiefs of the departments of medicine, surgery, and obstetrics and gynaecology; a year previous Dr R.G.C. Kelly and Dr J. Sullivan had been named chiefs of ophthalmology and otolaryngology. These five would provide St Michael's with vigorous, youthful leadership for the post-war boom.

With the appointments came hard-and-fast understandings about future staff appointments, promotions, and dismissals, and clarification of the duties and privileges of the incumbent chiefs. Particularly painful, in the wake of the new initiatives, must have been the resulting restrictions, or even dismissals, which followed for those staff members who held no teaching appointments. Obviously the university was prepared to demand that the hospital meet its standards for clinical teaching, and nothing in the records suggests that the hospital disagreed.[6]

In a broad review of teaching appointments presented to the board in April 1947, appointments to medicine included Drs Brooks, W.E. Hall, D. Moran, E. Broughton, A. Hagerman, A. Anglin, and A. Doyle; appointments to surgery included Drs Welsh, W.D. Smith, C. Day, and P. McGoey; to obstetrics and gynaecology, Drs O'Leary, W. Noonan, W. Murby, F. McInnis, S. MacDonald, and W. Apted; to otolaryngology, Drs Sullivan, A. Henry, and A.H. Veitch. Readers familiar with the subsequent twenty years will recognize how firmly the hospital's foundations were strengthened by those 1947 appointments – young men all, with the exception of Drs Broughton and Hagerman, most of them broadened, tested, and toughened by their experiences in the armed services.

The major architects over those twenty years, major from the sheer size and importance of their departments as well as from the significance of their personal accomplishments, were undoubtedly Dr Brooks and Dr Welsh. They first met in England in 1931; Welsh, an honours graduate (1926) from the University of Toronto, had just obtained his fellowship; Brooks, a silver medallist in his class at the University of Toronto (1928), had just obtained his MRCP (England).

Brooks returned to a staff appointment in medicine at St Michael's in 1932, and Welsh to a staff appointment at Toronto General in 1933, where he remained until his 1942 enlistment in the Royal Canadian Navy. During the war Welsh rose to the rank of Surgeon-Lt. Commander, and he was awarded the Order of the British Empire in 1945.

Dr Welsh was no stranger to St Michael's; as a medical student he had studied there under Drs Silverthorn and Wallace Scott, whom he described as "colourful clinicians and effective teachers." In his years at the Toronto General, he had studied under Dr Norman Shenstone, acquiring a basic and thorough knowledge of general surgery before specializing in head and neck surgery.[7] Interviewed after his retirement, Welsh spoke with special satisfaction of the development of the divisions of plastic, orthopedic, and neurosurgery during his tenure as chief.[8] The first of these to be developed was plastic, under Dr Hoyle Campbell (1948), followed by neurosurgery under Dr W.J. Horsey (1954), and finally orthopedics under Dr Paul McGoey (1957). Other important appointments made during Dr Welsh's tenure were those of Dr J.L.T. Russell as chief of urology (1950), Dr C.B. Baker (1953), Dr L.J. Mahoney (1954), and Dr D. Currie (1956). Drs Horsey, Mahoney, and Currie had all done their residencies under Dr Welsh. All of these appointees would have distinguished careers at St Michael's.

Reserved in manner, Welsh left no doubt, however, about his expectations of staff. He maintained withal a considerateness towards colleagues, appreciated especially by the operating-room nurses, who share with the surgeon the day-by-day tensions "under the lights."[9] Upon his retirement from the teaching staff, Welsh became in 1968 chief of surgery of the new North York General Hospital.

With an increase in the number of surgeons came a necessary expansion of the department of anaesthesia. Dr J. Vining was appointed chief in 1952, and within the next two years he secured the appointments of Drs S. Zeglan, A. Dunn, P. Bailey, and Margaret Dewan – the latter the first woman to hold an active* staff and faculty appointment (1954).

Paralleling Dr Welsh's building of the surgical staff was Dr Brooks's development of the department of medicine. In the seven years between 1949 and 1956, ten appointments were made and lines of specialization drawn:[10] Dr David MacKenzie (1949), internal medicine and

---

*An active staff appointment carried with it wider hospital privileges than did the outdoor attending staff appointment, the most significant of which was that of attending and treating patients on the standard wards of the hospital.

all venereal disease services; Dr Charles Bardawill (1950), whose special interest was haematology and cancer research; Drs Arthur Hudson, Paul O'Sullivan, J.K. Wilson, J. Alick Little, and Donald M. Finlayson, specializing in dermatology, gastroenterology, cardiology, endocrinology, and chest diseases, all appointed in 1954; and Drs J.A. Marotta, P. Higgins, and K. Butler, specializing in neurology, endocrinology, and haematology, all appointed in 1956. That same year, Dr Brooks obtained Dr David Lewis, who joined Dr A. Doyle as a second appointment to psychiatry. The department of medicine was, obviously, greatly strengthened and even transformed by Dr Brooks's recruitment of these highly qualified physicians.

A specialist in neurology, Brooks has been described as "a brilliant physician and brilliant teacher."[11] In addition to his heavy administrative duties, he was an examiner for the Royal College of Physicians and an acknowledged expert in the field of forensic medicine. An enduring testimony to the esteem and gratitude that he earned in the hospital community is the Edward F. Brooks annual memorial lectureship, established in 1977.

Following Dr Frank O'Leary's sudden death in 1952, Dr William T. Noonan, a graduate in medicine from the University of Toronto and Member of the Royal College of Physicians (Ireland), was appointed chief of obstetrics and gynaecology. A fine surgeon, Noonan was also the craftsman who designed the tables used for several decades in St Michael's delivery rooms. During his seven-year term several long-time appointments, all with fellowship standing, were made to his staff – among them, Dr John Harper, whose practice and teaching career at St Michael's extended from 1955 to 1991.

Medical Education: Undergraduates and Interns

From the first, Drs Brooks and Welsh established the principle that the public-ward patients would be solely in the care of the teaching staff and that the public wards themselves would be totally reserved for the teaching program.[12] Four years after he had taken over as chief, Brooks was able to report that final-year teaching in medicine would begin at St Michael's in September 1951. (Evidently students from the first three years only had been taught at St Michael's before this date.)

Through the late 1940s and early 1950s concern was expressed from time to time about providing appropriate guidance and discipline for the junior interns.[13] Earlier, during the terms of Sister Zephyrinus (1938-44) and Sister Louise (1944-48), the superintendent had been very involved and quite effective in these areas. After the war, however, the interns displayed a new assertiveness, and this development called for a different kind of supervision and dialogue.[14] In 1947 the intern committee, chaired by Dr Hagerman, was empowered to act as a disciplinary body, in cooperation with the superintendent.

Predictably, two issues causing restlessness in the intern ranks were those of time-off and of pay. In 1946 there was no regular remuneration for juniors or seniors at any of the three teaching hospitals, although the university paid the residents at the Toronto General.[15] By October 1947 St Michael's was paying its residents in medicine, surgery, and obstetrics $75 a month, soon to be increased to $100; an additional $1,000 annually was paid by the university as a fellowship to the resident in surgery. Keeping in step with the Toronto General and the Toronto Western, St Michael's began a salary of $100 annually for junior interns in 1948. At the same time, seniors in anaesthesia were given monthly salaries of $25, $50, and $75 in their first, second, and third years, and the resident received $100 – a scale somewhat "richer" than that of other seniors, but defended by the dean who said that anaesthetists were "fewer in number, harder to obtain, and up a good deal of the night."[16]

After repeated attempts, a policy covering time-off for interns was established in 1949: juniors and seniors would have two nights off a week and one weekend off every three weeks; time-off for residents in medicine and surgery would be flexible, with no definite rules.

Throughout all of these developments St Michael's maintained close collaboration with the Toronto Interne Board, created by the university in 1947. In 1951 Dr Welsh assumed chairmanship of the intern committee at St Michael's, an indication of the importance attached to this body and its mandate.

Medical Education: Post-Graduate

When the new chiefs took over in 1947 only the department of surgery was recognized for fellowship training. Before year's end they had applied to the Royal College for approval of post-graduate training in the departments of medicine, pathology, and obstetrics and gynaecology. The department of obstetrics and gynaecology was approved by the American College of Surgeons for post-graduate training in 1948.

Earlier, with Dr R.G.C. (Gordon) Kelly's appointment as chief of ophthalmology in 1946, the university had expressed its wish to develop graduate training at St Michael's in this service, leading to certification by the Royal College. Dr Kelly would begin by giving a course in clinical biomicroscopy at St Michael's to graduate students.[17]

In 1948 the university initiated a two-year post-graduate course for general practitioners; students from the course rotated through St Michael's departments of medicine and obstetrics. The hospital itself resumed the earlier three-day refresher courses for general practitioners,[18] and participated in the refresher course offered to eye surgeons.

By 1953 a resident was being proposed for anaesthesia for the first time at St Michael's, as also at Toronto General and Sick Childrens'. Two years later Dr Brooks reported that the dean would be recommending to the Royal College that St Michael's be approved for post-graduate training in neurosurgery, plastic surgery, radiology, and psychiatry. Truly the years 1947 to 1955 were years of spectacular growth in medical education at St Michael's.

Ongoing Relationships with the University

The agreement between the hospital and the university continued to claim much attention from St Michael's board, as well as from the university's president, Dr Sidney Smith, and Dean William Gallie (and later, Dean J. MacFarlane). Among the contentious issues was that of the rank of St Michael's department chiefs within the university faculty – the board proposing in 1946 a rank of associate professor, the university offering only assistant professor, but promising to reopen the discussion in two years' time. In 1948 the chiefs of medicine, surgery, and obstetrics were raised to the rank of associate professor.

The second issue concerned medical-student fees: each term, the Toronto General received from the university $25 per student, whereas St Michael's, Toronto Western, and the Hospital for Sick Children received only $5 per student each term. Further, the Toronto General was allocated $8 per student on the obstetrical service as living-in allowance, the other hospitals receiving nothing whatsoever. The president of the university conceded that St Michael's was justified in its request for equal treatment but "the arrangement had been of very long standing" and he was "having difficulty adjusting it," the chief obstacle being a powerful member of the General's board.[19]

Nursing

The quickened pace of the post-war years was reflected in the school of nursing in enrolment, student population, faculty growth, and curriculum change.

By 1951 enrolment in the undergraduate program numbered 332 students; the courses in post-graduate operating-room and obstetrical nursing graduated a total of forty-nine students in 1950. In addition, the University of Toronto regularly arranged field experience for its students in teaching and supervision at St Michael's, prompting the senior inspector from the Department of Health to urge that the school continue to improve its program "so that experience is readily sought in this Centre by other universities."[20] St Michael's own graduates were streaming to university (thirty-four enrolled in 1947), the Nurses' Alumnae Association awarding one scholarship annually to a graduating student and one to an experienced graduate. Several of these returned to teaching and supervisory positions, where they created an excellent climate for student experience, especially on the D-wards.

By 1950 the students were on an eight-hour day and on "block class assignments," without ward duty, repeated twice yearly.* While this was a significant step, the inspector estimated that students were still giving 50 percent of the nursing care. The number of nurse instructors had increased to ten, while priest-professors from St Michael's College taught (as they would for the school's remaining twenty-four years) the courses in religion, ethics, sociology, and psychology. The influx of post-war immigrants began to be reflected in the school (and eventually in the hospital staff). Among the places of birth listed in the 1955 student roster were Lithuania, Germany, Jamaica, Finland, Shanghai, British Guiana, and Ireland.

The change in the student program necessarily had ramifications for general-duty staffing, and yet the shock seems not to have been as great as one would expect: in 1941, out of a staff of seventy, all but two were St Michael's graduates. Fifteen years later, the senior inspector wrote in her report: "It is five years since our last visit .... here is practically a new hospital because of expansion and renovation. Here is a staff which give greater stability than is found in many institutions; 60 percent of the total hospital staff have been here more than ten years. Here many of the practices of the hospital have been long established. All these give a feeling of stability and general well-being."[21]

This efficiency and *esprit de corps* was very probably the result of the shared values and the strong bonds of trust and loyalty existing

---

*Previously students had spent a larger proportion of their day on the wards, and the remaining two or three hours in classroom lectures. In the block class assignments, groups of students were either in class *or* on the wards all day for a block of time – an arrangement which, it was judged, would eliminate the divided attention which they gave to the two facets of their training under the previous arrangements.

between the general-duty staff and the two persons – Sister Mary Kathleen Moore and Sister Jeanne Barry (by this time director of nursing service) – under whom most of them would have studied.

Sister Mary Kathleen was director both of the school and of the nursing service from 1940 to 1952, and served a further six years as director of the school alone. There can be little doubt that it was her own enthusiasm for learning, her astuteness in detecting and nurturing potential, together with her acknowledged position as a leader in nursing – locally, provincially, and nationally – that inspired so many of St Michael's students and graduates "to dream dreams."[22] Skilled, but always prudent, in public relations,[23] she made nursing and the possibilities it held for personal growth and public service an attractive option for the young.[24]

Valued by the University of Toronto as a strong supporter of its graduate programs (she was among the first to develop a planned field experience for its students), Sister Mary Kathleen was recognized, too, farther afield: repeated attempts were made to recruit her for schools and universities, not just in Toronto and Ottawa, but also in Brazil, Yugoslavia, Iceland, South Africa, and India.[25]

After guiding St Michael's school of nursing through eighteen years of dramatic change and growth, Sister Mary Kathleen returned to the hospitals, serving for five years as a nursing supervisor, followed by eleven years in senior hospital administration at Our Lady of Mercy Hospital, St Joseph's Hospital, and Providence Hospital and Villa – all of which are located in Toronto. Not surprisingly, Sister Mary Kathleen – teacher, mentor, and friend of countless nurses – is still, at the time of writing, the person most looked for at alumnae events.

New Drugs, New Treatments, New Departments

New Drugs

The impact of the cost of the newly developed drugs (penicillin, streptomycin, aureomycin, heparin, progesterone) on the hospital budget, and policies surrounding their use were recurring subjects of discussion at meetings of the medical advisory board during these years.

An interesting facet of a policy adopted in 1946 was the inclusion of the nursing staff in its development: in directives covering intramuscular injections, a line was drawn between those preparations that nurses were permitted to administer, and those that only the intern might give – including all doses exceeding 3 c.c. in volume. This marked the beginning of a greater tendency on the part of hospital administration and medical staff to involve nurses in the formulation of policies that affected their practice.

But the old deference to the physicians and the old pre-eminence still lingered: in 1948 the medical advisory board agreed that "the floor supervisor might suggest to the attending physician the discontinuing of an antibiotic, for his consideration and action." Six years later, Sister Maura McGuire, superintendent – concerned about the cost to the hospital of antibiotics, amounting to $4-5,000 a month for patients unable to pay – asked if it were "proper for the nurse in charge to bring to the attention of the internes" instances where patients had been on an antibiotic for several weeks. In reply, the pharmacy committee recommended an automatic stop order for antibiotics after five days, but the advisory board chose rather to have the nurse supervisor bring it to the attention of the doctor. (The automatic stop order was eventually adopted.[26])

New Departments and Services

Late in 1950 Dr J. Sullivan was awarded a grant from the Atkinson Foundation for the establishment of a hard-of-hearing clinic. Apart from the obvious significance of this clinic in terms of its contribution to assisting the hearing-impaired, it was important in that it underlined a new need and a new approach in patient care – the team concept – bringing together, as it did, the otolaryngologist, the speech therapist, the psychologist, and the electronics specialist. Diagnosis and treatment were, then, not only becoming more complex; there were also more resources at the physician's disposal.[27]

Among the requests made when he accepted his appointment as chief of surgery in 1947, Dr Welsh had asked for the aid of a photography service. In 1952 the hospital recruited Arthur Smialowski, who had immigrated to Canada from Poland after the Second World War and had worked in Ottawa under Yousuf Karsh. It was a most fortunate appointment: for the next twenty years Smialowski was a respected colleague of the doctors – and indeed of all the hospital services – especially in their teaching and research publications. He himself published from time to time, alone or with one or more doctors, most frequently Dr Donald Currie of the division of general surgery. In 1957 he joined with Dr Paul O'Sullivan and Hans Reinecke, the latter a microscope and camera technician, to develop a tiny camera to fit within the tip of a flexible gastroscope to assist in the diagnosis of stomach disorders.[28]

Prompted in part by the new legislation that required all nursing students to have three months' experience with psychiatric patients in a segregated unit,[29] the hospital opened in 1953 a thirty-bed psychiatric unit on two floors of the newly opened D-north wing. The division was headed by Dr Arthur M. Doyle, who had held an appointment on the indoor staff of the department of medicine since 1945, and Kathleen (Kay) Whalen, previously supervisor on a medical floor.

After obtaining his medical degree at the Universityof Toronto in 1931, Dr Doyle had done post-graduate study in Toronto and Boston. In 1946 he acquired a diplomate from the American board of Psychiatry, and certification as a specialist in psychiatry and neurology from the Royal College of Physicians (Canada). Between the American and Canadian awards, Dr Doyle practised in the Ontario Psychiatric Hospitals in Kingston, Hamilton, and Toronto, and saw five years of military service, most of it in the Mediterranean theatre where he attained the rank of lieutenant-colonel and was decorated for distinguished service. Although Doyle had patients referred to him from far and wide, he remained a humble man, always approachable and tolerant of those who still had little understanding of or appreciation for this emerging specialty. Kay Whalen supplemented her short period of post-graduate work by several years of close working relationship with Dr Doyle; nurses who worked with her commented on the remarkable effect her very presence had on calming many a disturbed patient.

The occupational therapy service, which would become a valuable adjunct in the treatment of psychiatric patients, was established in 1954 under the general aegis of the physiotherapy department. Although psychiatry's other important partners, psychology and social work, were still in the future, Dr Brooks was confident enough of the new psychiatric division to recommend it in 1955 as a site for post-graduate training.

Addressing Medical Problems, Old and New

While the emergency ward and the public wards were no stranger to the alcoholic patient, serious research into alcoholism and its treatment began at St Michael's only in 1950. Dr Brooks had expressed his disagreement with the idea of admitting patients for antabuse therapy, but in 1951, urged on by the university, whose cooperation the Province had solicited for the biomedical and medical investigation of alcoholic patients, the medical advisory board agreed that up to, but not more than, two patients at a time would be admitted to St

Michael's for medical investigation, then referred elsewhere for treatment. Brooks appointed Dr W.E. Hall to supervise the admission and treatment regimen for these patients.[30]

Policy decisions had to be made, as well, with regard to the victims of the poliomyelitis outbreaks in 1953 and 1954. (Salk Vaccine, a preventative to poliomyelitis, was not developed until 1955.) Although the Department of Health had included St Michael's on a selected list of general hospitals to which polio cases might be referred, and had assured the hospitals of funding to cover this treatment, questions were raised at the medical advisory board concerning the appropriateness of a general hospital with a school of nursing serving as a treatment centre during the acute phase of polio. It may be that the doctors felt that nursing students, who had limited experience with communicable diseases, might be at greater risk than other staff; an equally safe conjecture may be that this was just one more instance of the protective attitude senior doctors, in general, had towards the nursing students. It was decided, finally, to confine St Michael's participation to the treatment of chronic cases in the physiotherapy department.[31]

Among the newest of the questions to emerge in these years were ones concerning precautions to be taken where patients were being treated with radioactive isotopes, an issue resolved only with the help of the Banting Institute.[32]

The above developments, and the ones about to be described, highlight a period of rapid evolution when the large general hospitals ceased to be "all things to all people" and accepted a supporting network of outside agencies and services specializing in various activities – many of which the hospitals had previously begun and conducted on their own.

Influences from Without and Tensions Within

High on the agenda for the new chiefs at their marathon first meeting of the medical advisory board were decisions relating to blood transfusions – the how, who, when, and where of obtaining donors and of finally transfusing the patient. In 1948 Dr Magner began to train laboratory technicians to do blood typing and grouping; Sister St Jude Doherty, their supervisor, would take the night calls well into the 1950s, rising at 5:15 a.m. after an interrupted sleep for morning prayers in the hospital chapel – her Irish jauntiness only slightly lessened by her hours in the blood bank while others slept. That Dr Magner felt keenly his responsibility for patient safety comes through loud and clear in the records – in his selection and training of personnel, in his frequent exhortations to physicians to verify labels and other documentation, and in his instruction in the meticulous care necessary for the preparation of the rubber tubing used for the administration of blood. (A proposal to use plastic tubing was rejected in 1948 because of its expense.)

When the Red Cross Society invited St Michael's participation in its proposed blood transfusion service, Dr Magner was strongly opposed to "centralization and control of such an important service by a non-medical body."[33] Appearing before the hospital's board of governors in April 1949, Magner asked, "Why should we hand over to the Red Cross a well-managed service it has taken a number of years to bring to its present efficiency?" The board, hearing also Magner's doubts concerning the Red Cross's ability to maintain a supply of blood, and his projections of revenue lost to the hospital by contracting out this service, decided to carry on with the hospital's own blood bank. However, the discussion was continued by Dr Magner's successor and by Sister Maura's successor as superintendent, and finally in 1957 the board approved a contract with the Red Cross that had been eight years in the making.[34] This contract would relieve the hospital of the responsibility of procuring donors to supply its patients' needs.

While the laboratory was wrestling with the question of ceding a part of its territory to an outside agency, a similar situation was developing with regard to the scope and depth of its treatment of patients with cancer. In 1949, the establishment of a Radiotherapy Centre for Toronto (the future Princess Margaret Hospital), under the direction of the Ontario Cancer Research Foundation, was announced. Initial concerns about this development, among which was that of a possible loss of patients to the new facility, appear to have been eased by the appointment of one of the members of St Michael's board of governors to the board of the new agency and of Dr Welsh to its consultant staff. That the volume of patients being treated for cancer at St Michael's remained substantial is evidenced by the establishment of its tumour registry in 1955, assisted by a grant from the Cancer Foundation.[35]

Following fast upon its negotiation with the Red Cross of a contract for blood-bank services came the hospital's collaboration with the Canadian National Institute for the Blind in the 1956 development of an eye bank, with the CNIB providing the necessary equipment and the hospital collecting enucleated eyes for transplants.[36]

The Department of Health, meanwhile, was maintaining and extending its initiatives in direct patient care. In addition to its financial support since 1922 of a venereal disease clinic at St Michael's, it began in 1947 to provide for pre-natal examinations – free to the patient, but for which the hospital received $5 per examination. Standing firm on the principle that the intern years were a continuation of the educational program, the medical advisory board ruled that the money so collected would go, not to the examining intern, but into a fund to be administered by the hospital and the obstetrics department.[37] In 1948-49 the ministry introduced routine admission chest x-rays of all patients, installing free of charge to the hospital an x-ray machine for this purpose.[38]

Continuing an earlier pattern set when nurses' salaries were under discussion,[39] the teaching hospitals kept in close touch with one another and maintained what appears to have been a common front. Several issues confronted them in the post-war decade, one of the most contentious revolving around the increasingly popular pre-paid medical insurance carried by the public-ward patient. This issue appeared on the agenda of the medical advisory board no fewer than twenty times from 1947 on before finally being resolved in 1956. It was not unique to St Michael's; others among Toronto's teaching hospitals were grappling with the question of whether third-party payment should alter policies regarding the billing of public-ward patients.[40] (It had been a tradition that no medical fees were charged to the public-ward patient, who was expected to participate as subject in the clinical education and practice of medical students, and to accept one of the teaching physicians, rather than his/her own private physician, to supervise the medical care.)

Eventually, the medical advisory board proposed, and the board of governors approved, a plan whereby doctors' fees paid by insurance companies for the care of ward patients would be paid into a medical staff fund, to be used to assist doctors' special training and to defray convention expenses.[41] It was hoped this would settle the issue, but three years later Sister Maura, as superintendent, reported that several doctors were still putting to her their case that insurance companies' payments should go to them as individuals. The board of governors, acting on a formal recommendation from the medical advisory board, finally decreed that no member of the medical staff was to accept remuneration for services rendered to public-ward patients.[42]

Meanwhile problems had arisen concerning the formal establishment in January 1956 of a medical staff organization, the purpose of which was "to discuss problems and procedures relative to medical staff of the hospital."[43] Elected officers for the new body were Dr Hoyle Campbell, chairman; Dr W.E. Hall, vice-chairman; and M. O'Sullivan, secretary. The organization drafted its constitution, which was promptly rejected by the medical advisory board as not appropriate to a teaching hospital and in conflict with the board itself "which forms medical policy for this hospital," and with the by-laws of the hospital and of the university.[44]

The board of governors concurred with the medical advisory board. Not satisfied, the chairman of the medical staff organization asked for and was granted a hearing before the board, where he and his steering committee presented their case and the board confirmed its earlier ruling that the constitutions as drafted were unacceptable.[45]

Ironically, the hospital's success in having received full accreditation, and its efforts to comply promptly with accreditation survey recommendations,[46] may well have been a factor in fanning into flames the unrest that had long been smouldering around the issue of collecting from public-ward patients. The controversy makes clear that the medical advisory board played a central role in the analysis of issues and the establishment of policy throughout these years. The strong leadership given the board by Drs Brooks and Welsh is evident in the records. Dr R. Ross (pathology) and Dr J. Vining (anaesthesia) became members in 1953, and Dr E. Shannon (radiology) in 1955.

As the issues became more complex, especially around the new problem of a proliferation of expensive drugs and the old problem of incomplete and tardy medical charts, at Sister Maura's suggestion two standing committees were struck to study the problems and make recommendations to the medical advisory board. The resulting pharmacy committee (1952) and medical records committee and related tissue committee (1953) quickly became valuable supports – alleviating not all, but many, of the recurring irritants in this less-than-perfect working environment.[47]

From 1947 the chairman of the medical advisory board was an *ex-officio* member of the board of governors and provided the necessary medical perspective at the latter's deliberations. The board of governors' intense involvement in non-medical projects – especially in building projects and fund-raising during these years – will now be examined.

The Post-War Building Boom at St Michael's

Working with the board of governors as superior of the hospital from 1944 to 1950 was Sister Margaret Phelan. Sister Margaret had earlier

(1930-32) served in this capacity, left to serve a twelve-year term as the elected superior general of the congregation, and returned directly from the heavy responsibilities of that position to a hospital about to undergo a metamorphosis. True, the administrative responsibilities were shared for part of this second term with Sister Louise, but after Sister Louise's departure Sister Margaret planned and saw through to completion several important projects.

As a teenager, Sister Margaret had left her parents in Rathdowney, Ireland, to complete her education in Toronto, following in the footsteps of two aunts (one of them Sister Francis de Sales) and a Basilian priest-uncle. Prepared initially as a teacher, Sister Margaret now set herself to learn the ins and outs of hospital administration; in this she was acting upon the precept she had earlier, in her capacity as superior general, enjoined upon the congregation: "`Real fervour' implies putting our best into the task assigned, because we are doing it for God."[48]

Her deep Irish faith, together with her gifts of vision, judgment, and executive ability, enabled Sister Margaret to accomplish much for St Michael's and for Catholic hospitals in general. She was among the earliest to recognize the need for and the value of collaboration among the Catholic hospitals throughout Ontario, Canada, and the United States. She was a charter member and on the executive of the first Catholic hospital organizations in Canada, and was active as well in their American counterparts.[49] At St Michael's, she was in a position to influence strongly the hospital's development over a period of twenty-three years in all. Her successor (Sister Maura, who served as secretary-treasurer during Sister Margaret's second term) said of her, "She was determined to keep St Michael's on a par with any hospital in Toronto."[50] Sister Margaret spent her retirement years in pastoral visiting among the patients at her beloved St Michael's and died there on 21 January 1964.

Among the physical improvements effected during Sister Margaret's 1944-50 term at St Michael's were the new power-house, the first cafeteria, and the AS-wing stretching along Bond Street to Queen Street. Early in her term, Sister Margaret moved to secure property for the latter – foreseeing, correctly, that the end of the war would bring an influx of post-graduate medical students and a consequent need for housing.[51] In addition, Sister Margaret initiated the long-range plans for the new nurses' residence on the north side of Shuter Street and the north addition of the D-wing.[52]

Such is the large picture of the expansion program of these years; the details now follow. By war's end, St Michael's Hospital was beginning, in the words of Sister Maura, "to wear out"; it was also in debt (the net operating loss in 1948 was $136,436). Sister Margaret estimated that a considerable saving would result from replacing the five staff dining-rooms with one cafeteria. In 1948 she instructed Sister Maura (secretary-treasurer) to begin to work with W.L. Somerville, architect, and J. Pigott, contractor; these three came up with the plans for "not an elaborate cafeteria, but a functional one," at an estimated cost of $125,000.[53] The project was quickly approved and within a month the shovel was in the ground in an angle between the A and B wings. By the summer of 1949 the project was completed, coming in at $15,000 less than estimated; Sister Margaret was right – the operating costs for staff dining were reduced by $30,000 a year.

Having in mind the need for housing and other facilities for increased post-graduate training, Sister Margaret also recognized that the existing capacity for supplying power – twenty-five-year-old boilers in precarious condition – was totally inadequate. In 1950 a new power-house was completed, at a cost of $502,000. This in turn paved the way for the proposed new seven-storey wing which Sister Margaret "announced" to the board in early 1949.[54] The wing would run south along Bond Street to within thirty feet of Queen Street. It would provide two floors for interns and residents (the numbers had increased from twenty-one to sixty-eight), three floors for medical and surgical private and semi-private patients, one floor for post-partum patients, and a fifty-bassinette newborn nursery on the whole top floor. An up-to-date diet kitchen to serve the new patient rooms would occupy the basement level, and physiotherapy was to be relocated from 5-C, to become the department of physical medicine on the first floor.

The completed building, with its curved solarium windows on each floor, facing Bond and Queen streets, was a handsome addition at a cost of $1,020,000. It was formally opened by Premier Leslie Frost, and the admission of patients began on the Feast of St Joseph, 19 March 1951.

The allocation of a whole floor to the department of physical medicine was evidence of the growth that had taken place in this department, much of it under the direction of Dr J.R. McRae as physiatrist. As early as 1941-42 it had been separated out as a division in its own right and forming part of the training field for University of Toronto students.[55] A substantial contribution towards the cost of equipping the new facility was made by Famous Players Theatres and J. Fitzgibbons, the chairman of St Michael's board of governors.

With 139 new beds about to be put into operation, and new governmental regulations in effect relative to nurses' residences, property was purchased in 1949 at the northwest corner of Shuter and Bond streets, at a cost of $30,000, for a second nurses' residence. On this site a seven-storey building with 104 private rooms for senior students, classrooms, dietetic and chemistry laboratories, and demonstration rooms was erected – the cost was $830,000. A tunnel underneath Shuter Street connected the new building to the hospital. The residence was officially opened on 2 July 1952 – the Diamond Jubilee year of the hospital.

The ground floor of the new building was a welcome addition to residence living. It included a new 300-seat auditorium that was large enough to accommodate the student body and was easily convertible to a basketball court, where inter-nursing school tournaments would, in time, become a feature of the school year.

The second building completed and occupied during 1952 was the D-north wing, a seven-storey extension on Bond and Shuter streets diagonally across from St Michael's Cathedral. It provided sixty-one new patient beds (including the thirty-bed psychiatric department), as well as a research laboratory where Dr C.J. Bardawill would later do some significant early research in leukaemia,[56] and where the first radioactive studies at St Michael's would be carried out by Dr H.P. Higgins. To complete the picture, there were locker- and change-rooms in the basement and – adjacent to the existing fifth-floor operating rooms – six new operating theatres, which were probably a factor in pushing the cost of this wing up to $1,100,000. The top floor, used as a less-than-ideal large patient ward while the D-wing was being renovated, eventually became the occupational therapy centre for the psychiatric patients. For the first time two surgical subspecialties would now have a home of their own – neurosurgery and plastic surgery, the latter equipped with a large saline bath, at that time the treatment of choice for burns. These were housed on a mezzanine level between the psychiatric unit and the operating rooms.

Two further projects completed the 1952 expansion/renovation undertakings: new admitting offices with cubicles that provided a quasi-private space for gathering admission information, together with an ambulance entrance to accommodate four vehicles, entering from Victoria Street; and a major overhaul of the three floors of the outpatient department, which had had little attention since 1928. (However, an important appointment to that department had been made in 1946, with the designation of Dr Hagar Hethrington as its well-qualified medical director.) Here the patient volume had increased by one hundred patients per day in the past ten years, reaching 350 daily by 1956. The average cost of one patient visit in this area was $2.75; towards this, the hospital received seventy-five cents in grants. The sisters, as a result, were absorbing daily $700 of the cost of treating the city's poor – amounting to approximately $210,000 per year. There was, then, ample scope for living out the hospital's motto, *Quod Minimis Mihi Fecisti* (What you did unto the least of my brethren you did unto me), and evidently the sisters, as well as attending physicians (who gave their time without charge), generously grasped the opportunity.[57]

Accompanying the renovations of the outpatient department were those of its neighbour, the cystoscopic department, which acquired four air-conditioned operating rooms – the two projects costing, in all, $201,277.

Next to receive attention (1953) was the bustling emergency department. A comparison of the three adult teaching hospitals in the 1949-50 calendar of the university's faculty of medicine showed St Michael's heading the list for numbers of outpatients and emergency patients treated the previous year. In fact, the number of emergency patients at St Michael's doubled in a space of five years, increasing from 14,894 in 1945 to 30,192 in 1950. The capacity of St Michael's to respond quickly and competently to mass disaster had been tested in the early hours of 17 September 1949 when a call came alerting the hospital to prepare for victims from a fire on the *S.S. Noronic*, docked in the port of Toronto. The ship was totally destroyed; of the more than 600 passengers on board, 125 lost their lives. St Michael's and the Toronto General received most of the survivors who required emergency treatment. Seventy-seven patients came by ambulance or taxi to St Michael's, dripping wet, burned, bruised and lacerated, and in a state of shock; thirty-two of these arrived at 3 a.m., the remainder straggled in until noon on 18 September. One can imagine what such an influx must have meant to the still-cramped emergency quarters, staffed by the usually sparse night staff. (Betty Anne Phelan, an excellent emergency nurse, was the nurse on duty at the time.)

Dr Paul McGoey was then on his tour of duty in emergency; five years earlier he had been in attendance at the Coconut Grove fire in Boston which claimed more than 200 deaths. Dr McGoey, soon joined by Drs Welsh and Brooks, organized the emergency department into a casualty clearing station, and the victims were given first aid and passed on to minor and major operating rooms where doctors and nurses, who had been called in, were waiting. Teams of sisters contacted relatives of the victims, the vast majority of whom were Americans from as far away as Kentucky; other sisters hauled beds from the storerooms and set them up in the corridors to receive the twenty-five victims who had to be hospitalized, all of whom survived.[58]

So the emergency department, which had coped successfully with the *Noronic* and other lesser disasters, received a major expansion and update – private examining cubicles, an operating room, a room equipped to resuscitate patients, its own facilities for sterilizing supplies, a room for the on-call intern, and a recovery room for observation or for the inebriated patient. These facilities would serve the public well for thirty years, virtually unchanged during all that time.

Finally, to complete the revamping of existing facilities, work was begun on the D-wing. Although the wooden floors had been taken up in the large wards in 1946 (they remained in the smaller "hall rooms") and around-the-bed curtains had replaced some of the clumsy portable screens in 1947, little else had been done to update a structure that dated from 1912. A review by the inspector of hospitals and the Fire Department in 1953 condemned the building as not meeting current standards for sanitation and fire; among its shortcomings, this wing had too few washrooms and deteriorating balcony rooms for its tuberculosis patients, as well as fire hazards in the form of ample wooden trim and flooring and a broad open staircase climbing from the basement to the operating rooms.[59]

After complete gutting of the four-storey interior, this teaching wing was radically remodelled at a cost of $1,264,000. The twelve- to fifteen-bed wards disappeared, replaced by wards of no more than eight beds, as well as single and double-occupancy rooms. The deficiencies noted above were corrected, three-quarters of the equipment in use was replaced, and the decor was much improved by window drapes (a "first" on the D-wing), improved lighting, and new furnishings. An extension was built on the east side facing Bond Street which provided twelve new beds and a solarium at each of the four levels. The remodelling project was not without its difficulties or its drama. Patients continued to be admitted to the partially completed new facilities, as staff dodged ladders and tarpaulin. Outside, scaffolding ringed the building; the author (who was night supervisor at the time) recalls one summer night when a young male patient decided to escape to freedom via the open window and the scaffolding. An intrepid Irish nurse, fearing Sister Jeanne's wrath, scrambled down the scaffold in hot pursuit. A passing police cruiser scooped the two up and returned them to the ward, none the worse for their little escapade.

Paralleling the growth in patient beds were the increased demands on all the service departments, especially the laundry. In addition, the issue of parking space for the doctors was not going to go away, having recurred periodically on the medical advisory board's agendas since 1922. The logical site for new construction for parking was on the northeast corner of Victoria and Shuter streets, adjacent to the new nurses' residence. Wooed over a period of three years, Spee-D Auto Wash finally sold the lot to the hospital in 1955, and work began on a combined laundry/covered parking space, topped by one floor of residence for post-graduate nurses and dietetic interns. The building was opened in July 1956; its cost, including land, construction, and equipment, was $1,300,00. Obviously, this expansion program represented a tremendous financial outlay; how it was all paid for will now be outlined.

Funding for the Capital Expenditures, 1945-54

Speaking of the 1949 cafeteria construction – her first venture into financing hospital building projects – Sister Maura said, "The only way the Congregation had known was to borrow money ... but we were always careful not to take on a debt where we couldn't afford the interest."[60]

Faced with finding money for several mammoth projects, Sister Maura understood that something more than borrowing was required and so she placed the problem, in person and by letter, before the board, the city, and the provincial and federal governments. The response was heartening; a grant of $500,000 was awarded by the city; a commission on grants, composed of board members J. Fitzgibbons, Sir Charles Gillooly, and Harry Roesler, was successful in obtaining from the Province a grant of $800,000 and a promise of more between 1950 and 1954, more than one-quarter of this being towards the new psychiatric beds; and the federal government matched, fully or in part, some of the provincial grants, to the amount of $595,000.[61] In addition, the salaries of the sisters, of whom there were fifty-five on staff at the time, were totally designated for capital purposes.[62]

While substantial, these grants were clearly going to be inadequate to cover the more than seven million dollars' worth of projects completed or in progress. Consequently, the board decided in 1954 to go to the public, launching a fund-raising campaign with a target of $5,105,000.

The hospital was fortunate in recruiting as campaign chairman John A. ("Bud") McDougald, partner in the investment firm of Taylor, McDougald and chairman and/or director of many Canadian companies. His father, Duncan J. McDougald, had earlier served as member and one of the rotating chairmen of St Michael's board.[63]

McDougald himself recruited his co-chairmen, including M. Wallace McCutcheon, vice-president and managing director of Argus Corporation; Charles McTague, QC; John J. Fitzgibbons, president and managing director of Famous Players Theatres; Major-General A. Bruce Matthews, president of Canada Permanent Trust; W. Preston Gilbride, of Great West Life Assurance Company; J. William Horsey, president of Dominion Stores; John S. Proctor, vice-president and general manager of the Imperial Bank of Canada; James Stewart, president of Canadian Bank of Commerce; and G. Peter Campbell and C.E. Jolly. These, along with Sister Maura and hospital board members Frank Hughes, F.J. Crawford, and Frank Shannon, made up the campaign management committee; the services of the John Price Jones company were retained to assist in the conduct of the campaign.

The gala-opening of the campaign took place on 31 January 1955 with a concert in Shea's Theatre, where prominent artists (Lois Marshall, the Leslie Bell Singers, and others) contributed their talents free of charge and the minister from Yorkminster Baptist Church was the keynote speaker. Throughout the campaign that followed, statistics were employed convincingly to prove that St Michael's was for people of all denominations – including the hospital's own doctors, of whom 65 percent were non-Catholic.

In the month of February, readers of the Toronto newspapers were reminded almost daily of St Michael's campaign and the hospital's urgent needs. The public was told all – what had been done, what was yet to be done and at what cost, and how they could "Buy Shares in Humanity."[64] McDougald compiled and had published figures to show the impact on the city's population and its health-care needs if St Michael's did not exist. Pictures of cuddly newborns and fresh-faced nursing students, accounts of some recent breakthroughs by St Michael's doctors,[65] stories of grateful emergency patients (for example, one "knight of the road" who insisted on leaving twenty-five cents towards the campaign) – all were grist for the mill of the campaign committee. Some of the coverage was unabashedly affectionate, such as the *Toronto Star's* declaration on 31 January 1955 that "few people in Toronto have not been touched and blessed by St Michael's Hospital."

Within three and one-half months of the opening events, a jubilant board was able to pronounce the campaign a resounding success;[66] in fact, it was over-subscribed by a half-million dollars. A chairman's report to the public, issued on 31 December 1956, carried the statement that when the still unpaid pledges had been received, all the remaining bonds issued by the congregation for capital requirements would be redeemed, leaving a small balance for future capital requirements.

There remains to be recorded something about the woman who played such a pivotal role in meeting the challenges of these times – Sister Maura (Estelle McGuire, born in Toronto on 1 July 1900). Sister Maura was fifty years of age when, after six years as secretary-treasurer, she was appointed superintendent in 1950. Her abilities as an executive are clearly revealed in the records of the board of governors and the medical advisory board. These records underline Sister Maura's clear understanding of the complex world of the hospital with all its jurisdictional lines and limits – a world where she assumed her own place with authority, but was at the same time as attentive to seeking proper authorization from the board as she was careful never to infringe upon the prerogatives of the medical staff. With the latter, Sister Maura did not shrink from tabling unpopular issues, nor did she give up easily; she refused to have hospital department heads assume responsibility for matters of discipline which properly belonged to the medical chiefs. With both the board of governors and the medical advisory board she was attentive to legislation, resourceful, prompt, and flexible in addressing problems, and scrupulously careful in accounting for funds received and expended.

Throughout the ambitious expansion and reconstruction projects of her term, Sister Maura prowled the construction sites after the labourers left each day, satisfying herself that the quality of workmanship conformed to the plans and to her own high standards. She used to say, "We can't afford to build cheaply – we would only have to rebuild within a few years if we did." Colleague and friend alike of church leaders, government officials, and business tycoons, Sister Maura could yet say with complete conviction, "The chief aim of a Catholic hospital is the care of the underprivileged."

Indeed, her open-handed charity was well known. It extended from the poor men who stopped at her office door to ask for a sandwich, to the graduating students who found a fleet of taxis waiting to take them to their own doors at the end of a long day; and from the immigrant cloistered nuns whom she would regularly visit with a car packed with provisions, to a prestigious and long-established religious community in straightened circumstances.

When Sister Maura left the hospital field upon her election to the office of superior general in 1956, one prominent hospital official wrote to her, "St Michael's without Sister Maura will seem very strange."[67] In her new office Sister Maura soon negotiated with the provincial government the sale of the existing motherhouse property on Wellesley Street (where the Macdonald Ferguson Block now stands), and directed the construction of the present spacious headquarters of the congregation on Bayview Avenue, Willowdale.

Although Sister Maura was never personally showy, she was widely known as a woman of courage, integrity, justice, and foresight. So it was perhaps not surprising that, when the Order of Canada was established in 1967, she was among the ninety Canadians selected for membership. In the countless congratulatory notes she received, one recurring sentiment was expressed by the writers – "I am so proud; I know of no one more worthy of this honour." A woman of remarkable achievements, Sister Maura would nevertheless say, when speaking of her almost-fatal illness in 1962-63, "I wanted to live, so that my hands would not be so empty!"

7

The Tempo Accelerates

Change was to be the defining characteristic of the years from 1956 to 1966. Although this change was often imperceptible, it nevertheless opened the door for a glimpse of more, and more profound, change yet to come. The decade brought government-sponsored hospital insurance, new or expanded medical and para-medical specialties and hospital services, a shifting of the patterns and personnel for providing patient care, and finally, as in almost every previous decade, a towering new wing to accommodate current needs and future aspirations.

The population swell that followed the Second World War continued into this decade, giving Metropolitan Toronto a population of 1,825,099 by 1966. As the city's downtown core and suburbs both continued to grow, hospitals mushroomed to meet the needs of their citizens – nine hospitals in all, within a nine-year span.[1] Breaking with the earlier pattern of establishing a school of nursing in conjunction with the hospital, some of the new centres rather drew upon the established schools and hospitals – not only for nurses, but also for x-ray and laboratory technicians, medical-record librarians, and, of course, medical staff.[2]

It was during this decade that the presence of Toronto's immigrant peoples became noticeable at St Michael's – both as patients and as staff members. The variety of foreign tongues among patients in the emergency department or on the wards called for a roster of interpreters; the ease with which such a roster was assembled from among the staff was evidence of the dramatic shift that had taken place in the short span of fifteen to twenty years.

Administration and Governance

For most of this decade, Sister Janet Murray's was the steadying hand at the hospital's helm. With an arts degree, teacher's and business-school certificates, and ten years' teaching experience behind her, Sis-

171

ter Janet enrolled in 1953 in the University of Toronto's program in hospital administration – the first of the sisters to undertake university preparation in this field.

During her seven years as administrator and superior (1956-63) Sister Janet collaborated closely with her counterparts at the Toronto General and Toronto Western hospitals on the issues facing them all, many of which were stamped with a large dollar sign. Very much a hands-on administrator (she visited most of the nursing floors on her way to her office each morning, and never left in the evening without going to the emergency department to check how things were there), Sister Janet was deeply involved in all aspects of the hospital's development. After her term at St Michael's, she did valuable work at St Joseph's Hospital, furthering its evolution into a well-rounded community hospital which provided a support system for a host of agencies and programs in the city's west end. Her accomplishments in the two hospitals and her service on numerous boards and committees of the provincial and national hospital associations were acknowledged when York University awarded her an honorary doctorate in 1979, and the Canadian Council of Christians and Jews honoured her with its Human Relations Award in 1983.

A second person who served St Michael's through these and previous years of change was the chairman of the board, John J. Fitzgibbons. The first layman to hold this office at St Michael's, Fitzgibbons aided and advised four successive sister-administrators from 1940 through 1963, a period that spanned the cramped war years and the massive redevelopments and fund-raising projects of Sister Maura's time. President and managing director of Famous Players Theatres, Fitzgibbons had a keen sense of timing and of the public-relations and political aspects of any project needed or undertaken. In 1963, with his plans completed for a move to New York, Fitzgibbons resigned and accepted the honorary chairmanship of the board.

The Early Issues of This Decade

Remuneration of Interns

One of the first issues facing Sister Janet was that of an increasingly vocal and united group of interns who were demanding an improved pay scale.

In October 1956 Drs Brooks and Welsh met with representatives from the other teaching hospitals and recommended that the stipend for junior interns be $500 a year; first-year seniors, $1,000; second-year seniors, $1,400; third-year seniors, $1,800; and residents, also $1,800 – which might be increased to, but not exceed, $3,000.[3]

For the next three years proposals and counter-proposals continued, with hospital administrators maintaining that the money was just not available to make the proposed increases, and the teaching staff warning that the best-qualified interns would be lost to non-teaching hospitals where better salaries were being offered. St Michael's quota of junior interns at the time was thirty-one.

After the introduction of hospital insurance a new pay scale was agreed to, beginning January 1960: a junior intern would receive $1,650, and the senior intern, assistant resident, and resident would advance in $500 steps. Subsequently the university reduced its honorarium to residents from $1,000 to $750; actually, the medical resident's honorarium was reduced to $450 – the difference restored only after repeated protests by Sister Janet.[4]

The First Collective Bargaining Unit

Close on the heels of the interns' demands were those of the hospital's engineers. Negotiations continued throughout 1964, and in January 1965 the board ratified the hospital's first contract with unionized employees – all but five members of the engineering staff would now be members of the Union of Operating Engineers.

The Introduction of Hospital Insurance

In 1956 the provincial government passed the Hospital Services Commission Act and transferred the staff of the public and private hospitals division of the Department of Health to serve under a three-man Ontario Hospital Services Commission appointed by the province.[5] The commission (OHSC) was given wide powers, among them that of administering any system of hospital-care insurance that might be established and determining the amounts to be paid to hospitals for approved services performed for insured patients. The commissioners moved rapidly and within two years were able to announce a plan of hospital insurance, effective 1 January 1959. About the same time it was announced that the federal and provincial governments would now provide about one-third of the cost of public-hospital construction. To oversee the revised capital-grants regulations, the OHSC set up a hospital planning committee to which a hospital's detailed architectural plans and estimates of construction costs must be submitted before final approval of the project for funding.[6]

To avail itself of the benefits of the hospital-insurance plan, the hospital was required to forecast its expenses for the coming year and submit these in detail in an annual budget, for approval by the OHSC. This budget, when approved, became the basis for the per diem rate which the hospital charged its patients and for which it was funded by the Province. The exercise, particularly in the first years of the plan's operation, required untold hours of work. However, while the budget became each department head's annual headache, it also made for more business-like practices as competition for scarce health-care dollars grew ever more keen.

Once hospital insurance was up and running the government of Ontario turned its attention to insurance for medical services. The Medical Services Insurance Act, 1965 made comprehensive medical insurance available to all residents of Ontario, regardless of age, state of health, or financial means. Premiums were modest: $60 a year for single subscribers, and $150 for a family of three or more; the insurance was provided free of charge to most recipients of social assistance. Services of doctors, whether they chose to practice within the plan or to "opt out," were paid at the rate of 90 percent of the Ontario Medical Association fee schedule. OMSIP, as the plan was initially called (but soon came to be referred to as Medicare), was received with mixed sentiments by doctors; they valued the patient-physician relationship and feared third-party interference.

The Role of the Medical Advisory Board

Throughout this decade the membership of the medical advisory board remained unchanged, except for the addition in 1964 of Dr W.E. Hall, president of the medical staff organization. (The efforts to form such an organization, which had fizzled out in 1956, succeeded in 1963 with the election of Dr Hall as president, Dr C. Day as vice-president, Dr B. Bird as secretary, and Dr B. Hamilton-Smith as treasurer.)

Dr Hall was by this time a prominent member of St Michael's staff. After doing his senior internship and medical residency at St Michael's from 1939 to 1941, he served for four years in the RCAF in which he rose to be the officer in charge of the Manning Depot Hospital, Toronto, with the rank of squadron leader. At war's end he was awarded the Alexander McPhedran Research Fellowship in Clinical Medicine, in connection with which he did research in diabetes at the Toronto General Hospital and the Banting Institute. Then, for nineteen busy years as clinician and associate professor in medicine at the University of Toronto, Hall's initial and primary work with diabetes broadened to include the developments within the hospital's metabolic unit, including the artificial kidney. In 1967 Hall resigned from St Michael's to become physician-in-chief at the young Scarborough Centenary Hospital.

A reading of the medical advisory board's minutes throughout this period yields a profile perhaps as much reflective of the individuals on the board as of the group as a whole: serious about their rights and duties, expecting of the board's subcommittees equally serious attention to their delegated duties; somewhat conservative; highly ethical; and with a formality that appears almost quaint by the standards of today.[7]

Among the medical advisory board's functions was that of authorizing purchase of the major (and expensive) pieces of equipment with which the market was suddenly flooded.[8] The board's various committees took on an increasingly active role in those issues that affected patient care. Concerns and suggestions of the nursing department – whose route for communicating its suggestions and concerns had previously been through the administrator to the advisory board – now received a hearing at the committee level, where nursing supervisors were represented. Some enduring patterns thus got their start, including in 1961 the use of the patient Kardex (a compact, portable file containing a card for each patient, with all of that patient's relevant medical data) as a nursing reference, combined doctors' progress notes and order sheet (1964), and metric scales on the surgical units (1965). Innovations were routinely given a trial period on the teaching wards before hospital-wide use.

In 1959, following an accreditation survey, the medical records committee became the medical records and audit committee; the role of the surgical and of the obstetrics and gynaecology committee was similarly extended. These committees assembled data on incomplete charts and other matters and put the information before the chiefs for action, thereby becoming a valuable resource and support for the medical records department.

At the suggestion of the pharmacy and therapeutics committee an intravenous nurse was approved in 1960, attached to the laboratory and blood bank, under the supervision of Dr Gordon Hawks. This nurse was authorized to start intravenous infusions, including blood transfusions, on the private and semi-private patients; the interns continued to have responsibility for the teaching units.

Late to be formed – amazingly late, in view of its future prominence – was the operating room advisory committee (1964). Its role was to consider the purchase and maintenance of increasingly complex equipment, and advise on factors concerning patient care in the operating room and recovery rooms, including safety standards. In connection with the latter, Wolfgang Besser was named "expert advisor" to the committee in 1965; for years he would serve in this capacity to a host of departments and individuals as the electronic age extended its reach into the field of medicine.

One of the busiest of the medical advisory board's committees was the infection committee, which introduced such practices as disposable medicine cups and razors and foot-operated hexachlorophene soap dispensers. Disposable syringes, earlier put "on hold" because of their expense, were also finally authorized. Dr Gordon Hawks, the capable and vigilant director of bacteriology, was commended by the medical advisory board for his part in curtailing post-operative staphylococcus infections.

Unrelated to the work of the infection committee *per se*, but connected with its focus, was an event in 1959: a longstanding practice of serving morning coffee in the operating room (eight gallons of coffee and seventeen quarts of milk in a single morning) ceased abruptly when the coffee machines were spirited away one night by person or persons unknown. Hospital officials did not protest the incident; on the contrary, they suggested that the disappearance of the coffee machines lessened the potential for introducing infection in the operating rooms. The mystery went unsolved.

The Committee for Investigating Patients' Stay in Hospital
The number of long-stay patients remained a continuing concern for the medical advisory board in this decade. The doctors' problems in obtaining beds for their new admissions, despite the hospital's more than 800 adult beds, were compounded by their irritation over the OHSC's calls to explain why certain of their patients were occupying beds beyond the usual length of time.[9] Ever respectful of one another's prerogatives, the admissions and discharge committee sought and received permission from the advisory board to examine the charts of patients brought to their attention. In what seems excessive sensitivity, the board considered whether there would be any legitimate objection to nursing supervisors reminding doctors about their long-stay patients.

Even when additional chronic and convalescent beds finally did become available (for example, Weston, 1961; Hillcrest, 1962; Riverdale, 1963), the concept of transfer for convalescence grew only slowly – partly, perhaps, because the chiefs thought the staff doctor (not the intern, or the nurse) should make the arrangements, and also because a method for follow-up of St Michael's patients by St Michael's doctors took long to be worked out. Dr Welsh himself visited Hillcrest every Sunday morning over a two-year period for this purpose. In 1965 the department of surgery negotiated with Riverdale Hospital to have a certain number of beds under its control, and made arrangements for weekly visits. Beginning in 1966 the movement of long-term patients to nursing homes and convalescent and chronic-care hospitals was greatly facilitated with the inclusion of St Michael's in the Home Care Program, a service administered and financed by the Department of Health. In the following decade, the unique policies, requirements, and restrictions of the various long-term care facilities eventually prompted St Michael's to appoint a full-time discharge planning coordinator.

Appointments to the Medical Staff

Among the eight appointments to the department of medicine during these years, several would have upwards of twenty-five years of distinguished service: Dr H. Fields (cardiology, 1957); Dr E.J. Prokipchuk (gastroenterology, 1963); Dr H. Berry (neurology, 1963); Dr W.T.R. Linton (dermatology, 1964); and Dr L. Casella (cardiology, 1964). In surgery, Dr S. Schatz (1961) joined Dr W.J. Horsey in the division of neurosurgery; that same year Dr W Sapirstein joined Dr C.B. Baker in the division of cardiovascular surgery. In 1961 Dr V. Colapinto joined the division of urology, and Dr W. Kerr the division of general surgery in 1964; both of these would have productive and promising careers cut short by fatal illness. The department of ophthalmology was strengthened by the appointments of Drs M. Shea (1958), W. Hunter (1961), and D. Morin (1965); and the department of otolaryngology by the appointments of Dr Elizabeth McKee (1958), Dr T. Molony (1959), and Dr P. E. Smith (1963). All had had extensive postgraduate training and had earned the fellowship in their respective colleges. Dr G. Arnold Henry, FRCS (Canada), FACS, chief of otolaryngology from 1955 to 1973, records that Dr Molony "quickly made his name in laryngology."[10] Speech therapy became available to the patients of the ear, nose, and throat service, as well as to patients suffering the effects of a stroke, when the first speech therapist, Barbara Moran, was appointed in 1964.

In 1959-60, Dr Brooks and Dr Welsh were promoted to rank of full professor on the university's faculty of medicine, in each case one of only three holding that rank in their respective departments within the faculty. In 1962 St Michael's appointed its first woman resident in medicine, Dr Carol Broadhurst.

After Dr Noonan's resignation as chief of obstetrics and gynaecology in 1959 the university and the hospital failed to agree on the two leading candidates for the position. A compromise was reached whereby the department would be managed by a committee of the staff as a whole, with Dr William Murby as chairman sitting on the medical advisory board and reporting for the department to the board.[11]

In 1962 Dr P. Ryan was appointed director of the outpatient department after the retirement of Dr Hagar Hethrington following twenty-nine years on staff. In his position as director of outpatients and assistant professor at the university, Dr Hethrington had brought the department to a new level of organization and effectiveness.

Lastly, in May 1965 Dr John C. Platt was appointed St Michael's first medical director and a year later Dr C.A. Woolever was appointed physician-in-chief and Dr W.J. Horsey surgeon-in-chief – the latter two being the first geographic full-time heads of departments* at St Michael's. Each would play an important part in the developments of the decade to follow.

New Services, New Departments, New Concepts

The future of the radiotherapy service was discussed from time to time over a period of seven years; the equipment, and the facilities in general, had become inadequate and questions were raised as to whether the service was even necessary when a similar one would be available at the soon-to-be-opened Princess Margaret Hospital. Dr Welsh and Dr Brooks favoured retaining the service and finally the decision was made to make provision for it in the new wing under construction, Dr Shannon to take charge of radiotherapy after Dr Bird had replaced him as chief of radiology.[12]

Orthopedics, as a division of the department of surgery, was established in 1957, with Dr Paul McGoey in charge. It was not envisioned that the service should handle all fractures but would concentrate, rather, on joint fusions, arthroplasty, primary bone tumors, and similar more complicated disease processes.

This new surgical division, along with the neurology and neurosurgical divisions and the rheumatology service, became a heavy

---

*A geographic full-time department head was expected to devote all his/her time to teaching, research, and administration within his/her department, with vastly restricted time for private practice; a salary was provided by the university, while office space and secretarial help was provided by the hospital.

user of the department of physical medicine and rehabilitation. The latter was necessarily equipped with a variety of aids: mechanical-traction machines, whirlpool and wax baths, stationary bicycles, and electrical muscle stimulators.[13] By 1969 this department's staff of fifteen qualified full-time physiotherapists was carrying an annual caseload of 59,000 patient visits, and had become an important training centre with twelve intern physiotherapists and thirty-five students.

The medical advisory board's carefulness to safeguard patient care and the teaching program and to screen out services not requiring the facilities of a large teaching hospital – as well as a certain wariness of newcomers – is suggested by its decisions with regard to general practice, chiropody, and dentistry. When the question of extending admitting privileges to the dentists arose in 1957, the advisory board took the position that dentistry should be under one of the existing departments, for example, ear, nose, and throat, with consultation and supervision by a member of the medical staff; similarly, chiropody should be under the supervision of the orthopedic surgeons. In 1958 the request of the general practitioners to organize a department of general practice was rejected as being too difficult to adapt to the program of a teaching hospital. However, beginning in 1959 one student from the general practitioner's course was accepted every four months and the Clinic Day of 1962 was directed, as in earlier years, towards the general practitioner.

The metabolic investigation unit was an important development in 1962.[14] It was located on 3-D south and, like most new ventures at St Michael's, the initial space and furnishings were extremely modest. However, the staff was of the finest: the advisory board appointed Dr J. Alick Little as director, and recommended Drs D.J. Currie, V. Colapinto, W.E. Hall, and P. Higgins to work with him. At the same time, Dr Little assumed responsibility for setting up St Michael's first artificial kidney, along with Dr V. Colapinto and M. O'Sullivan (head of biochemistry). Peritoneal dialysis had been established earlier, in 1961, using equipment provided by the pharmaceutical companies. Now a dialyzing machine was installed in 201A, and haemodialysis was begun on patients in October 1963 in Toronto's first haemodialysis centre. Within a few months Dr Little, who had served as nephrologist on the team, was selected by the university to serve on the team for lipid investigation; Dr Colapinto attempted the demanding role of nephrologist-urologist-teacher, in addition to his experimentation with kidney transplants in animals, but within a few months the activities of the haemodialysis unit had to be suspended. In 1969, at

Dr Colapinto's initiative the unit was reopened and enlarged (201, 202, and 203A), by which time the dialyzing machines had been improved to complete their run in six hours rather than the previous ten.[15]

To return now to the metabolic unit, in 1964 it was relocated to 6B. Accommodating their work to quarters that were usually temporary, often widely scattered, and always cramped, Dr Little, his staff, and his research fellows would nevertheless, within a very few years, do some important work. Among their earliest studies were those connected with the estimation of serum lipids, lipoproteins, and various enzymes important in lipid and carbohydrate metabolism, including a study of the first Canadian case of hereditary fructose intolerance and the first report in the world of electron-microscopic findings.[16]

Radioisotopes came to St Michael's in 1956 when Dr P. Higgins obtained a licence for their use from the Atomic Energy Commission. Dr Higgins set up a low-level radio-isotope laboratory in two small rooms on 1-D north, and within a very few years the demand for his work grew dramatically, beginning primarily in thyroid studies and expanding to radioactive renograms and blood volumes. By the end of the decade the laboratory had been relocated to more spacious quarters on the ninth floor of the new F-wing, and had obtained a gamma camera (only the second in Canada) for the imaging of organs, and a refrigerated centrifuge. By this time Dr Higgins's own role had expanded from that of combined technician-secretary and physician-in-charge to a division head, with an assistant doctor, a registered nurse, and three technicians under him. A leader in the field since its inception, the laboratory would undergo rapid change in the coming decade, both in the volume of work and in the pattern of demands.[17]

A cardiovascular laboratory was the next major development. While a cardiac division had existed for several years, and heart surgery had been performed at St Michael's since 1954,[18] no haemodynamic studies were done until July 1959 when Drs H. Fields and P. Forbath joined the staff. The cardiac team at that time consisted of Dr C. Baker (surgeon), Dr P. Bailey (cardiac anaesthetist), and Dr D. Moran (acting head of the medical division, which was composed of Drs Fields, P .Forbath, and J.K. Wilson).[19]

While Wilson and Dr Clare Baker both did sporadic heart catheterizations between 1953 and 1958, the procedure was begun on a regular basis only in 1959, primarily by Drs Wilson and Forbath. The work was done in the radiology room, one of the theatres on the operating-room floor which served for both neurological and haemo-dynamic studies.[20] In 1962 Wolfgang Besser was hired as the first full-time electronics technician, and a year later the hospital made what would be the first of many purchases for the cardiovascular laboratory – an elaborate electronic polygraph, financed by a grant from the Atkinson Charitable Foundation, matched by a pledge from a group of staff physicians, and serviced from the beginning by St Michael's own staff. During the hospital's planning years of 1962 to 1965 an area was assigned for haemodynamic investigations and the premises were specifically built for a catheterization laboratory and phono-cardiographic laboratory, complete in every detail. The ninth floor of the new F-wing was occupied for this purpose in 1965.

Accompanying all three developments was the sudden need for and proliferation of specialists within the emerging field of medical technology. Although St Michael's had for more than ten years conducted a twelve-month course for laboratory technologists,[21] the times called for something more. With the establishment of the Toronto Institute of Medical Technology in 1966, there became available a pool of prepared people – medical-laboratory technologists, nuclear-medicine technicians, radiology technicians, respiratory technicians, and cytotechnologists, to name a few – all of whom were welcome additions to St Michael's staff.

With the move into haemodynamic studies, a laboratory for this purpose on the drawing board, and the initiation in 1960 of open-heart surgery utilizing the heart-lung machine,[22] the medical advisory board moved in 1962 to establish a separate division of cardiovascular surgery headed by Dr C.B. Baker. About this time the techniques for resuscitating patients after cardiac arrest were becoming more widely known and practised; intern and nursing staff were trained in the technique, and resuscitation carts with all the necessary drugs and equipment were furnished to key areas.[23]

Then followed a nine-bed intensive care unit on 4D – a temporary move, pending approval by the OHSC for more extensive reconstruction once the new F-wing would be completed. The unit was opened on 3 February 1964, with a five-member medical staff (Drs Horsey, J.K. Wilson, A. Dunn, D.C. Finlayson, and W. Young – a surgeon, a cardiologist, and three anaesthetists). A month later, Sister Mary Zimmerman, administrator, was questioning the low patient numbers and was told that during the unit's first five days there was not a single patient in the hospital requiring mechanical respiratory assistance; the statistics would change dramatically in the next decade.

To service the equipment in this new unit an inhalation therapy department (later called respiratory therapy services) was established in 1965, initially under the supervision of the nursing department with an anaesthetist (Dr J. Jacobs) as consultant. The department expanded with the growth of the cardiovascular and other services – from a staff of five in 1967, primarily occupied in the simple task of replacing medical-gas cylinders, to a staff of nineteen to twenty in 1988. These staff members were capable of assisting in cardiopulmonary resuscitation and support, and of administering aerosol and humidity therapy, as well as other forms of direct patient-care.[24]

The department of pathology, meanwhile, was initiating changes that would, within the next few years, result in a fully rounded centre for service, undergraduate and post-graduate teaching, and research. Dr Roderick Ross had been engaged by Sister Maura in November 1952 to restore department which, after Dr Magner's death, had been reduced to a staff of one, part-time.[25] A graduate of the University of Toronto in 1940, Ross served for more than four years in the Royal Canadian Navy and afterwards began post-graduate studies in pathology – first at McGill University and then at the New York Hospital under George Papanicolaou, the father of exfoliative cytology (study of the scaling off of dead tissue cells).

After a stint at St Mary's Hospital, Montreal, and McGill University, Dr Ross took up his duties at St Michael's. He was soon joined by a former colleague, Dr Terry Van Patter, who took over the subdepartment of cytology, and then Dr Allan Katz, who developed the department's capacity for fluorescent microscopy.

The department took a giant step forward in 1965-66 with the setting up of its subdepartment of electron microscopy. Dr Ross credits his resident at that time, Dr Norton Medline, with being largely instrumental in this development for he selected the type of machine that was purchased and organized the technical aspects connected with its use. Dr Medline subsequently held a staff appointment in pathology from 1967 to 1971. With the addition of Dr Arvind Bhagwat to the staff at about this time, the capacity of the department for carrying out investigative work related to the study of liver biopsies and experimental liver disease was greatly enhanced; much more was yet to come.

Other new services opened during these years included a rheumatology clinic under Dr John Digby (March 1963), and the hard-of-hearing clinic led the way into the computer-assisted future with an IBM data-processing machine. A department of psychology was begun in 1962, and it was further and more formally organized in 1968 under Pius Riffel, PhD.

The possibilities for treatment and cure that accompanied break-throughs in the pharmaceutical industry brought with them the need for constant vigilance, as well as recommendations and policy decisions on the part of the medical advisory board and its committees.[26] As a result, it became the practice for all investigational drugs to be dispensed only through the pharmacy, with appropriate literature. With the literature relative to the new drugs becoming ever more vast and complex, and the problem of adverse drug reactions fast developing into a subject of great concern to all in the hospital field, St Michael's opened in 1965 a drug information centre. Strategically located, adjacent to the medical library and across from the pharmacy, and staffed by an experienced pharmacist, the centre quickly became, and remains, a valuable resource for physicians, nurses, and pharmacists. The person behind this development was Sister Liguori McCarthy, director of pharmacy from 1962 to 1973. After three years as assistant administrator, Sister Liguori left St Michael's in 1976 to become executive director of Providence Hospital and Villa.

Finally, the developments of these years included two for the benefit of the hospital staff: an employees' pension plan, effective 1 January 1958, underwritten by the Canada Life Assurance Company; and an employees' health unit in June 1962, directed by Dr J.N. Reichert with Marie Meehan as head nurse. Established for the purposes of providing pre- and post-employment medical examinations and centralizing the health records of hospital personnel, the unit proved its worth within a few months, picking up several instances of conditions that required immediate attention.[27]

Some initiatives for making the hospital more business-like and facilitating communication within an increasingly complex milieu were an addressograph system of patient identification (1957), a patient-information brochure (1959), and a hospital bulletin (1962) – the last a publication of the medical advisory board which had had only variable success in communicating its decisions. Electronic "bell-boys" were introduced for contacting doctors and certain other staff in 1964, replacing the electric-light-flash system which had been installed in 1938. (St Michael's has never used the audio paging system so widely used in hospitals.) The bell-boys were available only on a rental basis from Bell Canada; the cost-tag attached to their use was deleted by OHSC from its 1964 budget approvals, and again in 1965.[28]

Organizing for the Support and Coordination of Research

In May 1958 St Michael's Hospital Research Society was founded; its by-laws made provision for a scientific advisory committee, a research fund, and a research finances committee. The board of governors appointed two of its members (Dr P.J. Moloney and H. Roesler) to sit on the research finance committee and encouraged board members and their friends to contribute to the research fund.

Donations at first came slowly: for example $5,000 from R.O. Pitman in 1960, through a board initiative. However, early requests for research funds were, likewise, modest by today's standards – for instance, $250.38 from Dr Roderick Ross in 1960 for a study of the ultra structure of the adrenal gland in primary aldosteronism. Requests generally were for funds to cover development of necessary equipment, to supplement salaries of assistants, and to pay for laboratory tests not covered by the OHSC. Two substantial donations were received from the Atkinson Charitable Foundation in 1965, both for expensive equipment: $26,000 for a gamma-scintillation camera for the radioisotope laboratory; and $50,000 for equipment for the hard-of-hearing clinic, to which Dominion Stores also made a generous contribution.[29]

In 1962 the advisory board, acting on Dr Brooks's recommendation, approved the appointment of Dr J. Alick Little as coordinator of research, and the following year St Michael's research committee was formed with Dr Little in the dual role of secretary-coordinator of research, an office he fulfilled until he retired in 1991.

Dr Little was a 1946 graduate in medicine from the University of Toronto. His post-graduate work included a National Research Council Fellowship in the department of biochemistry, University of Toronto, from 1947 to 1949, and a master's degree in biochemistry at the same university in 1950. Little was awarded his FRCP (Canada) in 1952 and was appointed to St Michael's department of medicine in 1954. He served as director of the diabetic clinic from 1954 to 1960, of the lipid clinic from 1966, and of endocrinology, metabolism, and nephrology from 1970 to 1972. Concurrently, Little held teaching appointments in the University of Toronto's faculty of medicine, advancing from associate in medicine to full professor in 1974.

The extent of Dr Little's involvement in research can be gauged from the fact that he was the author or co-author of no less than sixty-five published studies between 1951 and 1980.[30] Of particular significance was his role in the mammoth ten-year clinical trial sponsored by the United States National Institutes of Health and the Ontario Heart Foundation of the effect of a cholesterol-lowering drug on the rate of heart attack, involving 3,806 volunteers selected out of half a million men screened for the project. The study was carried out at eleven centres (ten American and one Canadian); the Canadian centre was a combined Toronto-McMaster university clinic under Little's directorship. In January 1984 the researchers published their results: by lowering blood cholesterol levels by 1 percent, risk of coronary heart disease is reduced by 2 percent.[31]

Impressive as Dr Little's own part was in the studies he was involved in, he was careful to acknowledge all those who supported the primary researcher – the laboratory technicians, dietitians, secretaries, mathematicians, and biostatisticians.[32] Among these was Sister Mary Frederick Sheehan.

Sister Mary Frederick Sheehan was named director of dietetics in 1950, when only twenty-nine years of age, and served in that capacity until her death from cancer at age forty-seven. In those intervening eighteen years, Sister Mary Frederick was prominent in her professional associations and was elected to the presidency at both the provincial and national levels. She lectured in the faculty of food services, University of Toronto, from which she had received her BSc, and was instrumental in developing the integrated internship program for dietitians.

With a scholar's enthusiasm for the clinical research underway all around her at St Michael's, Sister Mary Frederick quickly involved herself and her interns in the work of the clinical investigation unit and established with Dr Little a nutrition counselling service for patients with hyperlipidemia. Like so many similar small beginnings at St Michael's, this initial participation of the dietary department in research has grown: in 1990, the department of dietetics shared in a grant of $120,000 to establish a clinical nutrition and risk factor modification centre which provides individual assessment of risk factors contributing to chronic diseases, such as cardiovascular disease.

Nursing

While enrolment in the school of nursing remained high during these years (335 students in 1956), developments in the larger society, and in particular the rising standards of preparation for other professions, was forcing the nursing profession to examine itself.[33] The profession would eventually change course in a way that would prove revolutionary for nurse preparation and for the hospitals.

A new pattern of nurse preparation was being advocated by influential leaders, one that would develop two groups of nurses: a professional group to be educated in the universities, and a clinical group to be educated under "a well-unified and properly administered system of nursing education," probably of two years' duration.[34]

Naturally, the proposal raised questions about the future of the hospital schools of nursing, for imperative within the new thinking was the autonomy of the school, free from the hospital's control. Dr Helen Mussallem, who had earlier gained national recognition by carrying out a study of hospital schools of nursing for the Canadian Nurses' Association, was by 1963 recommending that all schools of nursing be removed from hospital control and placed within the general educational system of each province of Canada.[35] Indictment of the hospital schools was, at the same time, coming from the United States, where experimentation with community-college education for nurses was being undertaken.[36]

Such recommendations, however well intentioned, left the directors of hospital schools of nursing in a painful and ambiguous position, caught between their professional organization, which subscribed to the proposed change, and their sponsoring hospital, an alternative for which had not yet been developed. Sister de Sales Fitzpatrick steered St Michael's school of nursing through most of the turbulent transition period.

An active and popular alumna of St Michael's school of nursing (1932), Sister de Sales had done several years of private-duty nursing before entering the Sisters of St Joseph. She was an excellent nurse and, after obtaining her bachelor of nursing education degree at St Louis University, was appointed to the school of nursing at St Michael's. There she instructed twenty classes of nurses (a large and a smaller class each calendar year) over a ten-year period. Many would agree that few, if any, excelled Sister de Sales as a teacher of nursing arts at St Michael's. Over a period of twenty years Sister de Sales – fun-loving and creative, with an active intelligence and a well-developed philosophy of nursing –[37] inspired literally hundreds of student nurses to emulate her own high ideals and values; they, in their turn, became "carriers of the culture" that was St Michael's school of nursing.

When Sister de Sales became director of the school of nursing in 1958 she moved quickly to build up the teaching staff, new regulations having come into effect with regard to student supervision on the wards. By 1960 she had recruited a clinical coordinator with a master's degree (Mary Shaver), eight part-time teachers with bachelor of science degrees, and twelve with university certificates. Throughout her tenure Sister de Sales engaged additional well-qualified staff and improved the educational program through better integration of theory and practice and better control of the students' time. A barometer of her success (and further confusing the issue of the school's future) was the attraction the program held for students of excellent potential, and the continued high enrolment – including granddaughters, daughters, and sisters of former graduates.[38]

The hospital's department of nursing service, meanwhile, struggled to adapt to the partial loss of students and to the thinning of its ranks because of nursing opportunities elsewhere.[39] To help fill the gap left by the nursing students' withdrawal, as well as to fulfil the dreams of young women who wanted to nurse but lacked the necessary educational background, Sister de Sales established in 1961 a school for registered nursing assistants with Ann Ford as its first director. Initially this school was headquartered in the old Underwood Building next to the hospital, where the instructors were somewhat uneasy tenants alongside the research animals that also had space there. The school was later moved to the north nurses' residence.

While the registered nursing assistants, both student and graduate, were welcome additions to the hospital's nursing service, requirements of the emerging new specialties (which many nurses saw as attractive alternatives to the traditional nursing wards) sorely strained its resources. Fortunately, well-prepared immigrant nurses from Australia, New Zealand, and the United Kingdom, as well as from the Philippines via the big American medical centres, took up the slack. To assist the newcomers' adjustment, a staff educator was appointed; to create a cohesive working group out of the newcomers and the registered nursing assistants, team nursing was inaugurated;[40] and beleaguered head nurses were sponsored for the extension course in nursing-unit administration offered by the Canadian Hospital Association.

These years saw the beginning of regulated transfer of medical duties from doctors to nurses, many of which surrounded intravenous feeding and intravenous medications. Beginning with the metabolic unit and the artificial kidney, and then continuing with the intensive care unit, nurses were instructed (usually by the doctor in charge) to assume ever more complicated duties. After much consultation with the College of Physicians and Surgeons of Ontario, the first IV team of three nurses was trained – with the cooperation of the anaesthetists and under the aegis of the blood bank – to take blood samples and begin intravenous infusions, including blood transfusions.

Redevelopment and New Construction

With the expansion of the early 1950s just completed, there came relocations and new needs. The old laundry building became the home base of the engineering department and that indispensable corps of carpenters, painters, upholsterers, and surgical instrument repairmen which keeps a hospital looking good and running smoothly. Obstetrics was feeling acutely its obsolescent delivery-room facilities, and pathology was finding that the carrying out of its tests at the Banting Institute was wasteful of staff time. Their turn would come, but only after extensive renovation and enlargement of the radiology department: in the viewing room and film library a Kodak X-omat processing machine was installed to speed development of films, and two gastric rooms were remodelled in late 1957 – all with the assistance of a special government grant for rehabilitation and capital expenditures. At the same time, five new appointments to the radiology staff were made.[41]

But more was needed. After first studying the possibilities of building atop the new laundry building (a two-storey structure with a foundation capable of supporting eight storeys, but with the disadvantage of being detached from the hospital) the board decided on a new wing that would run from the B-wing to Queen Street and then east on Queen to join up with the AS-wing. The Day property east of Victoria Lane, that is, 36-38 Queen Street East was purchased for $150,000; the property west of Victoria Lane, 32-34 Queen Street East, for $115,000; and the Underwood Building for $355,000. Application was made to have Victoria Lane closed and the land conveyed to the congregation.[42]

Sister Janet, in a departure from the past, invited the active involvement of the medical staff in the planning and passed on the briefs from their two planning committees to the architects.[43] In January 1962 she brought to the board of governors a proposal for a $5,426,000 project, together with her plans for financing it, and received the board's approval. Three months later the OHSC approved the plans. The only hurdle remaining was that of converting the proposed site from its current use, parking for the interns' cars. The issue was resolved in a two-step arrangement: City Parking took over the hospital's parking garage and returned 50 percent of the revenue (the staff doctors would be charged $15 a month) to the hospital; the hospital applied this to the rental of new parking sites arranged for the interns by City Parking at Bertie and Queen and Dalhousie and Queen – the intern paying $5 a month for his or her car and the hospital paying the extra $13. There would never be any simple answer to the question of parking for St Michael's people.[44]

With her term at St Michael's about to expire within a few months, Sister Janet was able to report to the board on 21 February 1963 that work on the new construction had begun the day previous: a ten-storey wing, plus basement and subbasement, air-cooled throughout, would house – from the top down – an animal laboratory for the development of techniques in open-heart and neurosurgical procedures; cardiovascular- and radioisotope-investigation units; a central surgical supply department and a handsome conference/reception room; a gynaecological department complete with examining rooms and classrooms; an obstetrical department of five delivery rooms, one Caesarean section room, a recovery room, 100 patient beds, and 120 bassinets; a pulmonary-respiratory investigation unit; two floors of accommodation for interns; a medical-records department and a school for medical-records librarians; an amphitheatre with seating capacity for 150 medical students;[45] an x-ray therapy department; and locker rooms and storerooms. Fronting on Queen Street to which it had access via a curved driveway, the wing had a street-floor lobby which was graceful but left somewhat too shallow by reason of the gift shop that opened onto it. The cost was to be financed by $1,300,000 in government grants, $1,200,000 in hospital funds, and a bond issue covering the balance of $4,000,000.[46]

The building, called the F-wing, was completed 1 October 1964. Post-partum patients were moved from 6-AS and that area was converted for surgical patients. In due time, the interns were moved to their new quarters in the new wing, freeing up 3-AS for medical patients and 2-AS for urology patients. This extended the urology department to occupy the whole of the second level of A, B, and C wings – seventy patient beds in all. Over the whole was Sister St Matthew Reich as supervisor, with capable lieutenants Mary Ramey as head nurse in cysto and Jacqueline Mulcahey as head nurse on the floor.

Sister St Matthew was progressive, scrupulous about surgical and aseptic technique (she had been an operating-room supervisor and had spent time at the Mayo Clinic), and possessed of sound administrative and pedagogic instincts. She was possessed, also, of a sometimes acerbic wit, but was widely esteemed by patients and their families, students, staff, and doctors.

Among the latter was Dr J.L. Thomas Russell, chief of the division of urology from 1950 until 1983. Russell graduated in medicine from the University of Toronto in 1941, and then served in the Royal Canadian Navy in Canada and overseas, eventually becoming the principal medical officer on *HMS York*. After the war he undertook graduate studies under some of Canada's leading surgeons and at some of the major American centres on a travelling fellowship. Russell obtained his FRCS (Canada) in 1949 and, after one year at the Toronto General Hospital, was appointed urologist-in-chief at St Michael's and assistant professor at the University of Toronto. An innovator in surgical techniques in his field, especially in urinary diversion methods and substitute bladders,[47] Russell was at the same time intensely concerned for the comfort and quality of life of his patients. Like Sister St Matthew, Russell was energetic and resourceful in obtaining always the latest and the best for the urology division, and together they worked as a highly successful team for more than twenty years.

The University's Influence on Hospital Planning

Running concurrently with the hospital's planning for the new F-wing were meetings of the joint university-hospital planning committee, which focussed on the university's requirements of St Michael's as an affiliated hospital,[48] and of the university and university-affiliated hospitals committee, which aimed at coordinating the teaching hospitals' operations with the faculty of medicine.[49]

So, with the plaster barely dry on the new wing, St Michael's was plunged into another round of planning for its future as a teaching hospital – this time within a wider circle of decision-makers and within an environment increasingly competitive and increasingly regulated by government. The latter also exercised more and more control of the purse-strings.

A composite of every hospital department's plans for a ten-year period was prepared by a staff planning committee, and in October 1964 Sister Mary Zimmerman, who had replaced Sister Janet as administrator, brought before the board two suggested plans for new construction as an alternative to renovating the existing buildings: a twelve-storey tower, at a cost of $6,978,000, or a sixteen-storey building to replace the A, B, and C wings, at a cost of $8,220,000 – both estimates exclusive of architects' fees, equipment, and furnishings. In January 1965 Senator D'Arcy Leonard, chairman of St Michael's board of directors,* reported to the board that he had met with the

---

*The name "board of directors" replaced "board of governors" in 1963.

premier (John Robarts) and the dean of the university's faculty of medicine (John Hamilton), that the hospital's proposed expansion program was favourably received, and that, although no definite commitment was made by the Province, it was expected that funds would be allocated in the 1966 provincial budget.

This good news was soon overshadowed by the faculty of medicine's announcement, via Dean Hamilton in a presentation to the medical advisory board, of "the new curriculum" for its medical students along with a proposed increase of students to 250 each year – up from 175 – and a necessary enlargement of medical faculty.[50] Dean Hamilton followed this up by a comprehensive letter to Sister Mary, placing before her the implications of "accepting the burden of becoming a clinical school ... within the University."[51]

Briefly, the plan involved the following: St Michael's would become entirely responsible for the curriculum of fifty third-year and fifty fourth-year medical students; an associate dean would be appointed at each clinical school; clinical teaching units must be clearly defined (St Michael's had approximately 450 teaching beds at the time); teaching staff and heads of service would be jointly appointed by the university and the hospital, with the university holding the dominant responsibility in appointment of teaching staff; approximately forty full-time teaching staff would devote all their time, with the exception of two half-days per week of private practice, to teaching, research, and administration – each teacher's salary provided by the university,[52] but with office space provided by the hospital free of rent and a part-time secretary paid by the hospital; the university would accept the responsibility for the allocation of special services, such as chronic dialysis, in order to avoid duplication of expensive equipment and dispersion of specialized personnel (the university acknowledged that this was an encroachment on the sovereignty of the individual hospital); the hospital would be responsible for providing research space, laboratories, and lecture rooms, each capable of accommodating fifty students, and living accommodations for those students required to live in during certain rotations.

It was within a cloud of great uncertainty – vastly expanded resources required for continued participation in undergraduate medical education, and no firm assurance of government funding to provide them – that the board attempted to chart a course. In December 1965 the Herman property on the northeast corner of Queen and Victoria streets was purchased ($387,500) and negotiations for the adjoining

Abrams property at 28-30 Queen Street were begun; a year later this property was acquired for $300,000. In April 1966 the board was told that the OHSC had still made no definite commitment to finance the proposed new building, and that a series of meetings would be held to discuss the university's requirements for the teaching hospitals and the role of these hospitals in the new curriculum. As it developed, St Michael's responsibilities as a teaching hospital would be a major preoccupation of its board of directors, administration, and medical staff for the whole of the coming decade.

Some Final Observations

While unresolved issues of major proportions remained, the decade from 1956 to 1966 had its moments of rejoicing. In April 1959 Dr Brooks was awarded the FRCP (London) and that same year twenty of St Michael's doctors were off to Edinburgh to a joint meeting of the Canadian and British Medical Associations. (The almost-routine annual jaunts to faraway places were still in the future.) A few months later, Dr D. Currie and A. Smialowski were awarded the prestigious Lancet Trophy for their series of articles on medical photography – the first time the award had been made to individuals outside the United Kingdom. In November 1961 Dr Welsh was appointed exchange professor at Middlesex Hospital Medical School, London, England.

On the dark side, with nuclear weapons now stored on Canadian soil and in the wake of the Cuban missile crisis, the hospital clearly established steps to be taken in the event of war or of a disaster (defined as fifty persons requiring immediate medical attention and admission as an inpatient), including a method of triage – the sorting out and classification of casualties to determine priority of needs and proper place of treatment –[53] as well as a plan for total evacuation of the hospital. And there were other worrisome incidents – two cases of impersonation of doctors within a matter of weeks,[54] and an injunction from the Ontario Hospital Association in May 1964 to be on the lookout for cases of suspected child abuse. All of these were signs of what the future might hold for the downtown, big-city hospitals in the closing years of the twentieth century. And on the lighter side, but again consistent with St Michael's history and location, the Christmas crèche that was erected each year in the Bond Street lobby began gradually to lose more and more of its sheep – until one year St Joseph was finally left alone with the infant Jesus.

8

In the Eye of the Hurricane

The years from 1966 to 1976 began with a burst of optimism as Canada hosted Expo 67, and ended on a sober note as the free-spending of the previous few years caught up with the government of Ontario, the institutions it funded, and the professions for whose services it paid.[1] Similarly, in Catholic religious life, the Second Vatican Council illuminated the early part of this period with its quickened hope and promise but was followed within a few years by unrest, confusion, and disappointment for many.

Hospitals continued to spring up in and around Toronto,[2] and the University of Toronto bought Sunnybrook Hospital for $1 from the federal government. Meanwhile, the existing major teaching hospitals were plunging into that world of high technology and extremely specialized services which would become the trademark of the tertiary care centre. A heliport on the roof of the Hospital for Sick Children became available to the downtown teaching hospitals to handle the transfer of patients referred for their special care. This decade saw the beginning of organ transplants, with their attendant legal and ethical issues, and the same issues were at the forefront of the controversy surrounding the decriminalization of abortion. Even one's height and weight became suddenly unfamiliar as the decade brought complete conversion to the metric system of weights and measures.

The growth of hospitals, health-care services, and health professionals made heavy demands on the health-care dollars. As a result, a mind-boggling stream of fact-finding surveys, reports, commissions, and consultants commanded the attention of hospitals and their boards. This was an era when old established traditions suffered erosion: many doctors perceived their professional autonomy and their social and economic privileges to be threatened by universal health insurance (1969),[3] and many nurses felt a little less professional as their members adopted collective bargaining (1974), their ambivalence

193

reflected, perhaps, by the use of this phrase rather than the term "unionization." Finally, these were the years when many nurses discarded the cap, and many the uniform – beginning in the psychiatric units where dangling earrings became commonplace.

In the wake of Vatican II, the congregation opened its first foreign mission – in Guatemala – after Sister Maura had gone herself to assess the need. The hospital's chaplaincy department developed a distinctly ecumenical character; and many of the sisters exchanged the names they had received on reception into the congregation for their baptismal names, a move that brought its own confusion. This confusion was intensified by the exchange of the sisters' traditional religious habit, first for a modified form and later for secular dress. Their numbers held fairly constant, however (between forty-six and fifty-one at the hospital throughout this decade); the big loss would come in the 1980s. Let us try to pick our way through this exciting, disturbing, highly volatile time from the mid-1960s to the mid-1970s.

Governance and Management

The membership of the board of directors remained strong and deeply involved throughout this decade, under the successive chairmen: Senator T. D'Arcy Leonard (1964-69), Robert Davies (1969-75),and A.G.S. Griffin, whose term extended from 1975 to 1985.[4]

The hospital's administrative structure underwent development and redevelopment: in November 1968 Sister Mary's title was changed to executive director; Sister Regina Marie (who later resumed her baptismal name of Sister Margaret McNamara) became assistant executive director, and Dr John Platt continued as medical director. Next, George Morgan joined the team as administrative consultant to both St Michael's and St Joseph's hospitals, and Sister Catherine McDonough became secretary-treasurer. In early 1973, in response to the increasing complexity, a further restructuring was done when six assistant administrators were appointed. Related departments were now grouped under one senior person: administrative services (Sister Catherine McDonough), finance (Larry Thalheimer), hospital services (Errol Pickering), special services (Sister Liguori McCarthy), and patient care (the author). This group, with Rita Halsall, the hospital's competent and gracious public-relations officer, formed the first administrative council, which became an effective forum for joint planning, consultation, and decision-making.

The Medical Advisory Board

This board's membership changed as chiefs of departments changed and new departments were created (family practice, 1970; dentistry, 1975). Faced with the massive reorganization implied in conversion to a semi-autonomous medical school, and despite his still brisk and youthful manner, Dr Edward Brooks asked that his retirement be accepted as of 30 June 1967. (He carried on as acting head of the department of medicine for a further two years until a decision was made as to his successor, and chaired the medical advisory board until the end of 1968.) Dr William Horsey assumed the chairmanship in March 1969, and with wisdom and even-handedness handled the wide range of issues – often controversial – that crowded the board's agenda throughout these years of phenomenal growth and unprecedented difficulty.

During the same period, and extending beyond it, Dr John Platt served as secretary to the advisory board and to many of its senior committees, while serving for much of the time as head of the redevelopment program. Platt had followed his MD and MBA studies (University of Western Ontario) with a program in hospital administration; for the next twenty years, in his capacity as surveyor for the Canadian Council on Hospital Administration, he gained a wealth of knowledge about hospital matters on a national scale, knowledge of which St Michael's and students at the university's school of hygiene, where he held an appointment, became the benefactors. Generously blessed with interpersonal skills, a quick grasp of complex issues, and an encyclopedic memory, Dr Platt was, and remains in 1992, a highly respected member of the administrative team.

A Hospital Under Siege

Without a doubt the central concern of this decade was the place St Michael's would occupy within the bold initiatives contained in the recommendations of two major reports and the subsequent response of governments. The report of the Royal Commission on Health Service in 1964 had revealed an urgent need for more health professionals, while the Gundy Report of 1966 emphasized the need for medical research and for the provision of facilities that would promote research and keep teacher-scientists in Canada. Finally, the Health Resources Fund Act was passed, whereby the federal and provincial governments agreed to provide the substantial capital necessary to build and equip health-sciences buildings and related patient-care, research, and teaching facilities in university-affiliated teaching hospitals. The university had already planned a new curriculum, along with a greatly increased enrolment, and a new basic sciences building would be ready by 1969. What remained to be worked out was the place of the teaching hospitals in the grand design. Thence began a five-year saga marked by unprecedented rancour and mistrust between and among the university and its affiliated hospitals, a time of shifting parameters as government reneged on its promises and powerful vested interests resorted to more than occasional hardball.

St Michael's knew it would have to build if it was to accommodate the future teaching load. So that there would be no interruption of its existing teaching commitments it planned, and received approval for, five additional storeys atop the ten-storey F-wing, with a view to demolishing the A, B, and C wings, all built before 1930. In April 1967 the OHSC expressed a wish that St Michael's would undertake a parallel expansion of the hospital and the school of nursing. Later that year, however, it expressed concern about the building plans, and recommended that no further construction be done until further property had been acquired and a study conducted of the facilities to be located thereon.

This decision requires a short explanation. As early as March 1967 the government had indicated that the university would be responsible for approving all major capital expenditures related to teaching and research programs. In Toronto alone the government had requests amounting to $300 million, each hospital having far-advanced plans of its own for which it was seeking university approval, and without which it could not get government support. Suspecting that there might be unnecessary duplication of teaching areas and research facilities, the government looked to the university to determine the actual requirements.[5]

The university then employed management consultants to survey and make recommendations regarding, broadly, the faculty of medicine and its relationship with the teaching hospitals and with government. The consultants' report was not accepted by the university's joint board of governors and faculty committee, whereupon the faculty of medicine's departmental chairmen produced their own statement of the faculty's needs for staff and beds, and forwarded it to government. It was about this time that St Michael's first learned that the university was recommending that St Michael's redevelopment program be "staged later on" but that "the previous teaching responsibility assigned to St Michael's would continue."[6] It was noted at this time, too, that a high level of suspicion had developed among the teaching staffs of the various teaching hospitals.

In response to the faculty's submission, the three-member senior coordinating committee (SCC) of the OHSC informed the university in November 1968 that the latter must establish some priorities and a suggested schedule for building and redevelopment. Further, the SCC would not extend active treatment beds beyond those already approved (of the major teaching hospitals, Toronto General – 1,317; St Michael's – 894; Toronto Western – 950; Sunnybrook – 637), and until a further report was submitted it would not approve new facilities.

It was at this point, with the collapse of efforts on the part of the university and its teaching hospitals to plan together for the vastly expanded needs for medical education, that the independent planning committee (IPC) was constituted as a result of a resolution of the council of the faculty of medicine. It was to be independent, in that it would not be under the jurisdiction of either the university or the hospitals and would not be an arm of government. It was charged with reporting to the SCC on requirements for teaching and research facilities in the teaching hospitals to the year 1975. Robert Davies of St Michael's board became chairman of this important committee following the death, early in the committee's work, of the original chairman, Senator Wallace McCutcheon. Davies recalled that it was "a time of total war between the University and its teaching hospitals, each separately struggling to maintain its individual personality."[7]

The IPC submitted its report to the SCC in October 1969 – an exhaustive, detailed survey of existing facilities and staff and a projection of what would be needed to support the new curriculum, including teachers, research space, and office space. It drew attention to the very real competition posed by the community hospitals in and around Toronto, and the need to provide adequate office and consulting rooms in the downtown hospitals to provide for the continuous flow of the patients necessary to mount a teaching program. Acknowledging the tensions between and among the "partners" in the medical-education process, and their unwillingness or inability to collaborate in the efforts of 1965-68, it recommended a formal structure to ensure future coordinated planning. As it turned out, this was not to happen until other methods had been tried and had failed.

Meanwhile, St Michael's school of nursing with high hopes had moved on the suggestion of the OHSC and submitted detailed plans for a new facility. A few months later the OHSC announced a freeze on development plans of teaching hospitals, as well as a 5 percent reduction in operating budgets, and suggested that the St Michael's school of nursing convert bedrooms to classrooms and seminar rooms. With government purse-strings thus suddenly tightened, the board considered a two-step plan – to conduct a public campaign for funds, and to borrow, on the strength of the campaign, the money required to finance the needs of the school, necessary research space, the five new floors, and a clinic building on the northeast corner of Queen and Victoria streets. In his meeting with the OHSC in this regard, the board chairman was assured that St Michael's could expect $20 million in Ontario Health Resource Funds (hereafter called OHRDP funds) and another $12 million through capital financial assistance,[8] and would be required to raise $4-5 million on its own.[9] This was encouraging.

In October 1969 the university's school of medicine and affiliated hospitals were assigned $150 million in OHRDP funds and a working committee, established by Dr J. Hamilton, vice-president of the university's health sciences department, was charged with establishing priorities for disbursement. Moving quickly, Robert Davies – who had replaced Senator Leonard as chairman of the board – informed the dean of the faculty of medicine of St Michael's intentions, as described above. Three months later, the chairman of the OHSC informed the board that "there is no way I could indicate that actual construction in your programme could commence in 1970."[10] With plans thus put on hold, and a doubled number of medical students in the new curriculum as of January 1970, the hospital bought a building at 209 Victoria Street to free up hospital space to accommodate the students.

But for Davies and the board, "on hold" did not translate into "no action." Since it would be almost impossible to keep the present hospital in operation during a major renovation project (the possibility of the nurses' residence site becoming available was not yet envisioned), the board began to entertain ideas for a new site altogether. Two architectural firms – Mathers and Haldenby, and John J. Farrugia – were commissioned to prepare plans for a new St Michael's Hospital.[11] Estimates had revealed that by building on a new site millions of dollars could be saved, the time of construction could be reduced by four years, and a more creative product could result.

With a new site in mind, in July 1970 hospital representatives began a series of meetings with members of the congregation of Metropolitan United Church, just across Bond Street on the east, with a view to purchasing that property, appraised at $2.4 million. The proposal for a new site met with a sympathetic response at a meeting with the chairman of the OHSC, but the latter was waiting for the university's position as to priorities in the assignment of OHRDP funds. Officially advised of St Michael's plans, the university's vice-president of health sciences – who appeared to have considerable authority in the matter – said that in his view St Michael's was fourth in priority, after the faculty of dentistry, the Toronto General Hospital, and the Toronto Western Hospital. On 25 September 1970 this official presented to government his guidelines for disbursing OHRDP funds.[12] With St Michael's ranked fourth, it was unlikely that new construction would be authorized before ten years. While the guidelines confirmed the role of St Michael's as an integral part of the teaching function of the faculty of medicine, its doctors feared that they would not be able to attract quality staff; further, if St Michael's refused to take an increased number of students in the present inadequate teaching and patient facilities, its teaching function might be transferred to other teaching hospitals.[13]

Further meetings were held with representatives of Metropolitan United Church, meetings which revealed that the latter was not yet ready to make a definitive decision to give over that venerable and beautiful edifice to the battering ram. In search of an alternative, the board next considered a site known as Market Square, a city block bounded by King, Jarvis, Front, and Church streets, owned by the city since the eighteenth century and then being operated as a parking lot.

After meeting with the mayor and the executive committee of city council about the Market Square property, and prepared to negotiate the purchase of Market Square and the sale of the existing St Michael's site to the city, the hospital's representatives met with the chairman of the OHSC and his officials. This meeting resulted in agreement that St Michael's was needed as a service hospital and as a teaching hospital, and that redevelopment on the present site was out of the question; the hospital was invited to submit its proposal and its plan for financing for presentation to the minister of health. This was done, but just four days later the OHSC wrote that, while St Michael's proposal was worth looking at very closely, it was concerned about the proposed number of beds (840) and the fact that capital financial assistance funding was largely committed for at least the next three years.

Board minutes do not detail the members' reaction to this communication. To the researcher it appears that they had played their cards openly and honestly with all the players in the field. The question becomes, was it really a "level playing field"? It must be kept in mind that the university now owned Sunnybrook and that a special act of the legislature had earlier bonded the Toronto General with the university as a university hospital. By contrast, but by no means inconsequential, Toronto Western and St Michael's had only a formal affiliation.

With the increased number of students already crowding its wards, St Michael's pressed forward with negotiations for Market Square, offering to buy from the city 130,000 square feet, at $22 per square foot. In March 1971 city council agreed that St Michael's might purchase the property, but with the proviso that, if the hospital was unable to proceed with its plans, the city would be given the right of first refusal to lease or to repurchase the Market Square site. So, in the face of its university teaching responsibilities and despite the uncertainty of funding (further letters had been exchanged and a meeting held with the OHSC), the board agreed at a meeting charged with high hopes and high resolve to buy Market Square and to proceed with a fund-raising campaign for a new St Michael's Hospital.

In April 1971 it was agreed, at a meeting called by the deputy minister of health with teaching hospitals and the university, that the University Teaching Hospitals Association (UTHA) would be responsible for planning disbursements of OHRDP funds. (This organization had been formed in December 1970 to ensure coordinated planning, with the ten hospitals and the university as members. Robert Davies was named to represent St Michael's within UTHA.) As we shall see, this would prove to be a pivotal factor in the events that shaped St Michael's future.

Keeping the momentum going, the hospital met with the OHSC to request approval to contract for architects' fees in connection with its application for rezoning of the Market Square site. The written response was favourable but was accompanied by a request that the hospital delay planning until release of an official statement concerning financing of the redevelopment program of the principal teaching hospitals, including St Michael's. On 31 August 1971 the hospital arranged to buy Market Square. Aware that its fund-raising campaign was being actively sabotaged by influential members of other boards, St Michael's board decided to obtain an official statement from the minister of health as to the future of St Michael's for both teaching and research; if unfavourable, strong action would be planned.

Finally, on 16 September 1971 the minister of health and the senior coordinating committee met with representatives of the four primary teaching hospitals and presented a proposal for a Toronto health sciences complex, together with recommendations for capital building projects at each of the four: Toronto General to have 1,000 beds (down from 1,317), at $47 million; Toronto Western, 800 beds (down from 950), at $35 million; St Michael's, 600 beds (down from 894), at $35 million; and Sunnybrook, 600 beds (down from 637), at $26 million.

Although disappointed with the anticipated reduction in bed size, and informed of a role study to be commissioned by the SCC to define in greater detail the role of each of the four primary teaching hospitals in relation to the other hospitals and the community, St Michael's pressed ahead with its plans. The chairman of the corporations division of the fund-raising campaign (Hartland MacDougall) presented the Ministry of Health with a letter he wished to send to potential donors, asking the ministry to verify the projected costs contained in his letter and how they would be paid: a $45-million project, paid for by $35 million in government funds and $6 million in campaign funds, plus the $4 million cost of the Market Square site. After first expressing verbal overall agreement, a senior ministry official called to say that the $35 million was to be the total cost of the project, exclusive of the cost of the land, and the campaign funds were to be included in this figure.

With the architects' projection of $41.6 million for a 600-bed hospital in hand, a meeting was arranged with the premier (William Davis) and the senior SCC official at Archbishop Philip Pocock's office. At this meeting Davies requested that the provincial government make a commitment in writing towards a new St Michael's Hospital on Market Square, for at least $35 million, exclusive of the proceeds of the public campaign and of land costs. The hospital was given to understand that a letter to this effect would be forthcoming. The urgency of St Michael's situation as a teaching hospital was further accentuated by the government's new request for the faculty of medicine to graduate 350 medical students annually, instead of the previously announced increase to 250 students a year.

By this time the campaign had pledges of $3.6 million – despite outright opposition by some board members of some other hospitals[14] – but a firm commitment from government was essential to meeting the $6-million goal. So, with "the letter" referred to above still not received, Davies pressed again for an answer from the SCC official; finally, on 23 November 1971, Davies received the written response – "it is agreed that the eventual redevelopment of St. Michael's will be on the Market Square site."[15] With this assurance, the board formally approved a motion to proceed with the construction of a new 600-bed hospital on Market Square.

The optimism surrounding this decision was short-lived. In February 1972 the authors of the study commissioned by government on the roles of the four primary teaching hospitals presented their preliminary report. They recommended, among other things, that – based on Metropolitan Toronto's demographic data – St Michael's should move from Hospital Planning District #5 (downtown Toronto) to District #4 (northeast Scarborough). The consultants had adopted a preferred ratio of four active treatment beds per 1,000 population, instead of the current 5:1000 – a change that would result in an anticipated bed surplus in downtown Toronto by 1976; they argued that, since St Michael's had already planned to move, it should move right out of the district, thus eliminating the buildup of surplus beds.

In their final report the consultants proposed two alternatives – either a move to Market Square, or to Scarborough – but expressed a preference for Scarborough. There, they suggested, St Michael's could form with Sunnybrook the nucleus of a sixth medical school, associated with York University.[16] (As it turned out, by 1975 another study, the Henderson Report, recommended controlling the number of licensed doctors and limiting the capacity of medical schools – a move that might have left St Michael's high and dry, as far as teaching was concerned, had it moved to Scarborough.)

Within two weeks of receiving this report, hospital representatives began a four-part rebuttal before the SCC and hired a consulting firm (Arthur Andersen and Company) to review the first firm's work. This company brought statisticians and consultants from its New York office who, in their turn, presented some compelling evidence that government should not act on the earlier recommendations. A meeting of St Michael's representatives was quickly arranged with the minister of health before the first report was presented to the legislature.

At this meeting the hospital argued against the move to Scarborough for several reasons: the assumption that medical staff and out-of-town referrals would automatically follow the hospital there was unfounded (in a poll of the medical staff done a few weeks later, 137 out of 165 respondents wanted to stay downtown, regardless of the size of the new hospital);[17] the proposed site was remote, with no public transportation available for even an already-established Scarborough hospital; donors to the fund-raising campaign had given in view of a new hospital at Market Square, and now the uncertainty of the site was causing them considerable apprehension.

The minister of health agreed there was not sufficient evidence to justify moving St Michael's to Scarborough but, owing to a lack of government funds, he would recommend that St Michael's remain on its present site for the present and that the health statistics in relation to the city's growth be reviewed year by year. The deputy minister of health confirmed this recommendation in a letter and suggested that a major review be undertaken during 1976 for a reappraisal of the role and size of St Michael's. But with $2.75 million of borrowed money tied up in Market Square, and income from the parking lot insufficient to cover the interest, no action until 1976 was clearly unacceptable to the board. It decided to try to arrange bridge financing – borrowing sufficient funds to cover all stages of planning up to the beginning of active construction – until such time as provincial revenue would be available; such an arrangement would require a provincial order-in-council.[18] The hospital's request was duly submitted, and was rejected.

The city, meanwhile, had indicated that, in the event that St Michael's did not relocate to Market Square, it (the city) wished to negotiate to buy back the property for use as a parking area.[19]

After further exasperating months of meetings and correspondence, a meeting promised in April 1973 finally took place on 27 August – this time with Premier William Davis and the deputy minister of health, who had participated in the discussions from the start. In a hard-hitting presentation, Davies told the premier that, although ministry officials and members of the SCC had overtly stated that St Michael's was "out of the picture" as far as allocation of funds was concerned, it was resolved to get its fair share of the funds available to the four teaching hospitals, and he was confident of its ability to do so.

Davies outlined the hospital's plans for use of the funds, plans that included a community health clinic on Market Square. If capital funding for this clinic was not approved, and if the government decided that the Market Square site be retained until 1976 (as it had recommended), then government should finance the retention of the site. The premier acknowledged that this was a reasonable position; in addition, the ministry official emphasized that the recommendation concerning the reduction to 600 beds applied, not to the present St Michael's, but to the proposed new hospital.[20]

Four days after this meeting, the deputy minister of health informed Davies that St Michael's would have the same priority as the other three teaching hospitals in the allocation of funds for capital purposes over the next ten years. What had happened to halt and change the direction of events? Two years earlier, as has been noted, government had agreed to allow UTHA to make the decision regarding the allocation of OHRDP funds. A subcommittee of UTHA, under its president, John Law, subsequently assigned a working party composed of the executive directors of the four teaching hospitals, along with the dean of medicine, to come up with a coordinated plan for funding hospital facilities. The subcommittee did its work, Law forwarded it to government, and government accepted the recommendations – an excellent illustration of appropriate delegation, where the decision-making role was finally wrested from the power-brokers and given to those who were most keenly aware of the needs of the members and who would be most affected by the decision.

The Ministry of Health had indicated to UTHA that, if the latter's planning committee agreed that St Michael's receive a "substantial share of the funds, i.e. substantially more than one million dollars, we would regard this as an indication that planning should begin for the development of a modern facility ... to a maximum of 600 beds."[21] Government still seemed fixated on that figure, despite its protests to the contrary. Within the month St Michael's presented to the deputy minister of health and to UTHA a plan for a four-stage redevelopment on the Bond Street site, now made possible because of changes in nursing education which freed up the nurses' residence site for hospital use. UTHA promptly recommended to government that $19,750,000 of OHRDP funds be allocated to St Michael's and a relieved, if somewhat disappointed, Sister Mary informed all connected with St Michael's that the hospital would remain downtown, but not on Market Square as planned. That property was still on the board's hands, however, interest on the money borrowed to purchase it accumulating at the rate of $15,000 a month.

Shortly before a planned meeting with the mayor to discuss the resale of Market Square back to the city, the hospital – without soliciting – was approached by another party with a letter offering $7 million for the property. The mayor was made aware of this offer. Negotiations proceeded with the prospective buyer, and the executed agreement of purchase and sale was submitted to the city clerk and officially recorded by him on 20 March 1974. Under the provisions of the original agreement, the city had thirty days to match or better the offer. A member of St Michael's board met with the mayor and executive committee, and the latter were fully aware of their rights. Then, four days after the expiry of the thirty-day period, the city sent the hospital a letter objecting to the proposed sale.[22]

Responding to a storm of protest from certain council members when the news was out that the property had been sold at a tidy profit, the city attempted to block the sale but the Supreme Court ruled that the owners (the sisters) were not in breach of their original agreement. The city appealed, unsuccessfully, and then launched a third attempt – a judicial review; however, on the day before the motion was to be argued, the city abandoned all proceedings[23] and the site passed to its new owners.

Meanwhile, the Ministry of Health approved, through UTHA, the preparation of master plans for each of the four hospitals. St Michael's plans were facilitated by the availability (unexpected) of the nurses' residence site, as well as the offer made by the Toronto Hydro Electric Commission that the hospital buy steam from that agency, making unnecessary a new boiler-house for the hospital. Soon the battering rams, followed by the bulldozers, were aimed at the old residence, and instead of a new hospital that could have been built in three years at a projected cost of $55 million, a $90-million redevelopment program was launched, phased over an eleven-year period.

Powerfully leading the struggle for St Michael's place in the overall scheme of things in this period was Robert Davies, who had been appointed to the board in April 1968 and elected chairman the following year. Forty-three years of age, he had already earned prominence, respect, and success as a corporation lawyer.[24] While the events recorded above offer a profile of this gifted and remarkable man, his true measure is best appreciated by a reading of the tributes that poured in to the hospital when he died suddenly, of an aneurysm, on 18 April 1975. Among them were the phrases contained in a letter from Michael Barstow, senior architect of the redeveloped St Michael's Hospital: "Vigorous and invigorating ... [all his actions marked by] enthusiasm and devotion ... a considerable source of strength and sound advice ... a good and gracious friend."[25]

The Fund-raising Campaign, and
Some Comments on "Wasted" Efforts

A fund-raising campaign, to which reference was made earlier, was planned in late 1969 and finally launched in early 1971, under A.G.S. Griffin as chairman and S. Paton, W.R. Allen, and J.H. Moore as vice-chairmen; "Bud" McDougald was honorary chairman, and the Hon.

Walter Gordon honorary treasurer. Although plagued from the start by the indecision of government with regard to the future of St Michael's, by mid-1972 pledges and grants of approximately $5 million had been secured. When it became clear that the new St Michael's – to which enthusiastic citizens had pledged or contributed – was not to be, donors were advised of their privilege to withdraw their donations. While some did indeed request that their contributions be returned and their pledges cancelled, others indicated that their cash contributions should be retained and their pledges sustained; between the two extremes, donors selected from a variety of options. One can only guess how many hours of time – time volunteered by busy executives – was spent returning cheques and adjusting donations.

The indecision of government also meant that St Michael's administration spent much time on planning and replanning. And money was spent unnecessarily for the multitude of architects' drawings and for the official studies commissioned in support of St Michael's position. Sister Margaret McNamara (a fine nurse and administrator, with extensive hospital experience, much of it as supervisor in the operating room or in emergency) was in charge of the planning office for much of this time. Sister Mary Zimmerman, of whom more will be written, was executive director. Can it be said that their time and the board's, as well as the money involved, were really wasted? By no means. The costs of not continuing the struggle would have been great, too – so great, indeed, that the hospital had no choice but to act as it did. The minutes of the board of governors and the medical advisory board reveal a unity and resolve and a depth of engagement with the hospital's life and welfare not evident since the struggles of the first decade. This development can be registered only as a gain.

The Commerce Court Venture

Running concurrently with the "big plan" during four of the above years was the hospital's experiment with an outreach clinic in the heart of the business section: conceived as a community service for hundreds of employees in the downtown office buildings and the citizens of the developimg Harbour City on Toronto's waterfront, and staffed by St Michael's doctors, it was expected that such a clinic would also constitute a valuable centre for teaching and referrals. The hospital leased one floor in the new Canadian Imperial Bank of Commerce complex at King and Bay streets and constructed and furnished there laboratories, a pharmacy, radiology facilities, and doctors' offices. Two doctors (G.A. Callahan and J.C. Paupst) initially took charge of the clinic and undertook to recruit the necessary medical staff. It was intended that the doctors would form a partnership in facilities leased to them by St Michael's.

The clinic opened with five doctors in August 1972. It gradually became apparent that, even after changes in management, the centre was going to continue to operate at a loss to the hospital. In November 1974, eleven St Michael's doctors, headed by John McCulloch, expressed a willingness to assume responsibility for the future of the centre. These formed a corporation and in February 1975 assumed control of the "Commerce Court Medical Centre, affiliated with St. Michael's Hospital"; the centre continues to serve the downtown daytime population – as originally planned.

The Last Years of the School of Nursing

Mention has been made of the expressed goal of the nursing profession to have nursing education become independent of hospital control. At St Michael's, a separate eleven-member board of directors was established in March 1967 for the school, under the chairmanship of Mr Justice H.G. Steen. For the subsequent six years this board was to work long and hard for the preservation of St Michael's school of nursing – if not in its past form, at least in a form recognizable by its philosophy and traditions.[26]

In May 1967, the school, in step with the current wisdom, applied to the College of Nurses for conversion to a "2+1" program – two years of integrated theory and practice, followed by one year of internship or clinical experience in depth; approval was granted. In a sharp break with tradition, third-year students were encouraged to live out of residence as a step toward assuming mature responsibilities, married applicants received consideration similar to single ones, and students were permitted to marry during the program.

In September 1970 the first nurse interns – 107 of them – moved into nursing service, paid at a percentage of the graduate-nurse rate. There were concerns, suddenly, about a surplus of nurses across the province. (A year earlier, the school had moved into a straight two-year program, creating a situation of overlapping programs for a time.)

Aware that change was being discussed by those responsible for funding and those charged with approving curricula, the congregation searched for a plan whereby it might preserve a Catholic presence in nursing education in the event that hospital schools were phased out. With its excellent overall facilities, the occasion seemed ripe for uniting its schools of nursing at St Michael's and St Joseph's hospitals into one educational institute, affiliated with all the health agencies of the congregation situated in Toronto.[27]

In January 1971 the government published an important document containing the proposal that nursing programs currently carried on in hospital schools be placed in community colleges.[28] To avoid this, and after exploratory rounds with several degree-granting institutions in the hopes of establishing an affiliation between these and St Michael's and St Joseph's hospital schools of nursing,[29] the congregation proposed an institute of nursing education under congregation auspices.[30] On Christmas Eve 1971 Mother M. Corinne Meraw, superior general, addressed a letter to the chairman of the OHSC asking for a meeting with government officials with respect to integrating the congregation's two schools into such a single educational unit. Government seemed to be waiting for such an idea. Within two weeks representatives from the OHSC, the Ministry of Colleges and Universities, and the College of Nurses met with representatives of the congregation and the two school boards; and with the encouragement of government officials present at this meeting, a formal proposal was sent to the OHSC in April 1972. In the meantime, it had been observed there was lack of agreement at senior levels of government on the 1971 policy document and some second thoughts about the suitability of the community colleges for all diploma nursing programs.[31] A representative from the Ministry of Colleges and Universities encouraged the sisters' boards to pursue the idea of an institute of nursing education which "could provide a model and an alternative for developing nursing education."[32]

The boards of the two schools continued to work on their proposal. Finally, in January 1973 hospital schools of nursing across the province – including St Michael's – received the government's decision with regard to their future, in its "Guidelines for Transition of Nursing Education into Colleges of Applied Arts and Technology." While hope for a separate institute lingered for several months, the congregation finally made the decision to move in the direction of the government document. It is not clear what prompted the decision; the uncertainty as to funding may have been the deciding factor. In the summer of 1973 representatives from all the downtown schools of nursing gathered to hear from government officials the precise fate of their schools. At that meeting, in the new government building on Wellesley Street, on the site of the old motherhouse where the decision had been made eighty-one years earlier to establish St Michael's school of nursing, the sisters (including the writer) received the definitive announcement that St Michael's school of nursing would be no more.[33] Indeed, not only St Michael's but also four other excellent schools of nursing with long and proud traditions ended a chapter of their lives that day; by September 1973 they were no longer autonomous, each being just one "campus" of George Brown College.[34]

Sister Marion Barron, who had replaced Sister de Sales as director of the school of nursing in 1970, had been deeply involved in these developments. She was uniquely qualified for the task: a 1938 graduate of St Michael's school of nursing, Sister Marion had gone on to become the very successful director of St Joseph's school of nursing. There she was, as well, one of the pioneers in establishing the Quo Vadis School of Nursing for older applicants. Sister Marion returned to St Michael's after receiving a MEd from New York's Columbia University, and a PhD from the Catholic University of America, Washington, DC. With this excellent background in nursing education and in higher education, her proven organizational skills, and her personal philosophy of what constituted a mature professional woman, Sister Marion was the logical choice to be first dean of the nursing division of George Brown College.[35] She held the position with distinction during the division's first fragile years, until her retirement in 1979.

Developments within the Medical Departments

As referred to earlier, the university had given advance notice of a greatly increased student enrolment and, consequently, of an increased teaching load for St Michael's staff. Heads of departments, in response, set about building up their staffs and attracting highly qualified doctors. At the same time there was a loss of staff as valued members resigned to become heads of departments or assume senior positions elsewhere.[36]

More and more evident throughout these years was the tendency to bring a team approach to the complex problems of patient investigation and treatment: obstetricians and gynaecologists with endocrinologists; cardiologists with cardiovascular surgeons and anaesthetists; neurologists with neurosurgeons – and all in collaboration with pathologists and/or radiologists possessed of a special interest or expertise in one or other of these fields.[37] Less prominent, but nevertheless beginning, was the non-physician scientist collaborating in the medical specialists' research.

An overview of each department, in random order, will give a picture of these crowded, stimulating, and productive times.

Obstetrics and Gynaecology

The years under review in this chapter span the complete term of Dr C.A. Woolever as chief of obstetrics and gynaecology, 1 July 1966 to mid-1977, years of dynamic growth and activity within the department. Canadian-trained (University of Western Ontario; FRCS [Canada], 1954), Woolever came to St Michael's following six years at the University of Colorado Medical Center where he was deeply involved in research related to progesterone plasma determination. A year into his new appointment, and with a new women's clinic and research area almost ready for occupancy (the nursery on 7A-south was completely remodelled at a cost of $500,000 for this purpose), Woolever brought Dr Rudi Borth on staff as head of this research laboratory. Holder of a PhD in organic chemistry from Zurich, and with extensive experience at the University of Geneva, Borth was uniquely qualified to take over the position. He held it until 1976 with the exception of two years' leave to work for the World Health Organization on that agency's special program of research in human reproduction. From 1971 onwards, Borth was chairman of St Michael's scientific advisory committee.

In addition to the ongoing research on hormones as related to reproduction, Dr Woolever and his research staff applied themselves to the search for improvements on the various rhythm methods of natural family planning[38] and for alternatives to "the Pill" with its possibly dangerous side-effects. In 1976 an "electronic speculum" – the idea was Woolever's, while biomedical engineer Henry Benoit designed the finished model – was produced and received the endorsement of the church. By means of this instrument the exact time of ovulation could be pinpointed, and the necessary time of sexual abstinence reduced from fourteen to four days each month. (Research teams in Israel, Belgium, and Florida had also been working on such a device, but Woolever's team was believed to have outstripped them.) In the meantime, with the addition to the staff of Dr A. Chalvardjian and Dr D. Gerulath, specialists in gynaecological pathology and oncology, respectively, and of B.R. Bhavnani, PhD, research was undertaken on the relationship between hormones and cancer. Their work was recognized and furthered by the establishment in 1971 of the Toronto Trophoblastic Registry, situated at Princess Margaret Hospital but under the direction of Dr Gerulath.

After changes to the Criminal Code of Canada in late 1967, St Michael's formally reaffirmed its position with regard to therapeutic abortion and advised government that it would not be establishing a therapeutics abortion committee as provided for under the code.[39] As new members joined the staff, the medical advisory board formally charged the heads of medical departments to ensure every staff member's loyalty to the philosophy and ethics of the hospital, particularly in the matters of abortion and referral for abortion – neither of which was permissible.[40]

As recommended in the new Medico-Moral Guide of 1970 for Catholic hospitals, St Michael's established a medico-moral committee "to help those in charge form a moral judgement, in a concrete situation, in the name of the hospital."[41] This committee was charged with developing a protocol and reviewing requests for use of the hospital's facilities for tubal ligations – keeping in mind the guide's emphasis on the uniqueness of the person and the family as well as the importance of prudence and personal conscience in human decisions. This committee's work was to be greatly expanded in the coming years as new ethical concerns – for example, those connected with the new technology and the prolongation of life, to mention only two – became ever more pressing.

Always forward-looking, Dr Woolever was a driving force behind the hospital's move to open in 1971 a storefront clinic, staffed by members of obstetrics and gynaecology and of the new family practice department, in the high-density, low-income Broadview and Gerrard area. The Broadview Clinic moved after four years to its present location in the similarly depressed area at 791 Queen Street East. Sister Therese Cleary, whom Dr Woolever had coached in normal deliveries in preparation for her work as part of the first missionary group of sisters sent to Guatemala in 1968, became and remains in 1992 the nursing director of this highly successful community health clinic.

St Michael's had its first set of quadruplets in October 1975, delivered by Dr Anthony Cecutti and his team of eight doctors and six nurses. The four babies – two boys and two girls – left the hospital in good shape a few weeks later, a happy-sad day for head nurse Margaret Riddell and her staff who had seen the babies and their parents through the first few fragile weeks of getting to know one another as a family.

Cardiology and Cardiovascular Surgery

These two services grew rapidly over the twenty-year period following the first mitral commissurotomy at St Michael's in 1953. St

Michael's first open-heart surgery with the assistance of the heart-lung machine was performed in 1960; its first successful valve replacement in 1962; Canada's first successful cardioversion (the restoration of the heart's rhythm by the application of electric shock) by Dr Peter Forbath and Dr John K. Wilson in 1963; and the hospital's first aorta-coronary by-pass operation in 1969 – a procedure that quickly came to constitute the large proportion of open-heart operations at St Michael's. The volume of work – and more significantly, the successful outcome of the work – of these divisions was made possible by two factors: the new cardiovascular laboratories equipped in 1965, and the quality of the staff.

Prominent throughout these years were Dr Clare B. Baker, head of cardiovascular surgery from the first, and Dr John K. Wilson, who became chief of cardiology in the early 1960s. Baker, FRCS (Canada), a well-trained general surgeon with additional experience in thoracic surgery and cardiac surgery in Holland, had joined the staff in 1953. Wilson, a 1948 graduate in medicine from the University of Toronto, received an appointment to St Michael's staff following his receipt of his FRCP (Canada) in 1954. Over a period of thirty years these two men guided developments in the treatment of heart disease at St Michael's. Each assembled a highly qualified staff that reflected the variety of skills necessary in this branch of medicine as well as the multicultural character of post-Second World War Canada.

Among the earliest of the cardiologists was Dr Peter Forbath, a refugee from Hungary following the revolution in that country in 1956 (earlier Forbath had been the first physician in Hungary to do a heart catheterization, working from a description of how it had been done in Baltimore, Maryland). Then followed Dr Harold Fields; Dr Luigi Casella, from Naples, Italy; Dr Allan Selby; Dr. Narasimhan Ranganathan (a world authority on mitral-valve disease), who came from Madras, India; Dr Trevor Robinson, from Jamaica; and finally, Dr Robert Chisholm. Dr Baker's team included, for the first few years, Dr W. Saperstein; and then Dr John Hart and Dr James Yao – whose appointments date from 1967 and 1968. In addition to their large service load, in a society where heart disease ranks first as a cause of death, the cardiologists carried as well a heavy teaching responsibility at both the undergraduate and graduate levels, and were actively involved in research. A separate, fully equipped coronary care unit was established in 1967 under the direction of Dr L. Casella. The location was excellent – the brightest, airiest section of 3-D facing out on Bond Street where a large chestnut tree was almost within touching distance. Here for the first time St Michael's patients and nurses walked on a carpeted floor. The unit remained in this location until 1984.

In the fall of 1968 Dr Wilson presented to the board of directors a protocol for a heart-transplant program at St Michael's and received approval to proceed. Within days the opportunity and the need arose to put the plan into effect. On 17 November 1968 the first heart transplant was carried out at St Michael's: it was also the first successful one in Toronto. The patient, Perrin Johnston, became a medical triumph and a media celebrity as he went on to enjoy more than six years of quite normal life. (Two months after his surgery he took up jogging.) Until his death in May 1975 he was considered to be the world's longest surviving male heart-transplant patient.

Working with Dr Baker and the thirty-three-member transplant team was Dr James Yao, FRCS (Canada), FACS, and fellow of the American College of Chest Physicians. Born in Fubien, China, Yao had been a gold medallist in his class in medicine at the University of the Philippines and just before coming to St Michael's he had done post-graduate study in Toronto and Bristol, England. Parts of his career at St Michael's had a story-book character and yet were totally consistent with the hospital's tradition of reaching out to the needy. In 1971 Yao led a team to the Philippines where they performed fourteen successful operations, at no charge to the patients. A year later Yao, with cardiologist Dr Casella and anaesthetist Dr William Young as well as a resident and an operating-room nurse, flew to Trinidad for an intensive two weeks. The medical team donated its services; a variety of sponsoring agencies assisted with the remaining costs.[42]

Finally, Dr Clare Baker led an eleven-member team behind the iron curtain to operate in Budapest, Hungary, and Zagreb, Yugoslavia, in October 1973; they went to perform and teach open-heart surgery in those countries, at the request of Hungarian doctors who had visited St Michael's. The team included cardiologists Dr John Wilson and Dr Peter Forbath (who spoke Hungarian), anaesthetists Drs D.C. Finlayson and William Young, two residents, and three nurses – among whom were Ann Wetherall, St Michael's first, and very competent, pump perfusionist, and Tricia Root, the equally competent head nurse of the intensive care unit. The hospital donated much of the necessary small equipment and paid the nurses' salaries.

These were exhilarating times, proud times, for all connected with the cardiac service and with the hospital. Yet there was alarm on the part of some as their very success called for an ever-larger share of capital and operating budgets, of space, and of support staff. To prepare the nurses required for the care of patients in a setting increasingly inundated with new technology, Sister Marion engaged in 1973 a well-prepared nurse to develop a critical care program, twenty-one weeks in length. The program was offered for several years at the hospital and was finally transferred to George Brown College. As the decade was coming to a close the hospital installed its first telephone heart-monitoring system, capable of providing long-distance electrocardiograms (ECG) and pacemaker check-ups. Soon the patient with a pacemaker implant – whether he or she lived in Oshawa, Vancouver, or Rome – would be only a phone call away from printing out an ECG for prompt evaluation by one of St Michael's cardiologists. Dr Julian Loudon could never have foreseen the phenomenal developments that followed his introduction of Canada's first electrocardiograph in 1913.

Anaesthesia[43]

Developments in the department of anaesthesia during these years were closely interconnected with those of the cardiac divisions. Dr J.A. Vining, who had headed the department from 1952 to 1968, serving as secretary to the medical advisory board during most of that time, was succeeded by Dr Lucien E. Morris. (Dr Vining died of lung cancer in 1972, at just fifty-seven years of age.)

In his brief two years as anaesthetist-in-chief, Dr Morris was successful in negotiating superior space and facilities for the department, including a laboratory for basic research. There Drs W. Noble, W.W. Stoyka, and J. Obdrzalik carried on work initiated by Dr Morris, mainly in the areas of cardiopulmonary investigation in dogs as well as studies in cerebral perfusion.

In May 1970 Dr A.J. Dunn was appointed anaesthetist-in-chief. Dr Dunn had been appointed to staff sixteen years earlier, the first member of the anaesthetic staff not involved in general practice. He inherited a department vastly different in size, in daily schedule, and in teaching and practice responsibilities from that which he had entered in 1954. The staff had quadrupled (from five to twenty) and the residents had increased from two to ten over a period when bed numbers had actually shrunk by more than 100 beds. Anaesthetists were no longer free to play golf in the afternoon, after an operating-room schedule generally completed by 2 p.m.; now the anaesthetist was the key person in the intensive care unit, coordinating the treatment plans and orders of the attending physicians and surgeons there on a twenty-four-hour basis. The department of anaesthesia was deeply involved, often leading the way, in the advances of Dr Dunn's early years – recovery rooms and day surgery, preoperative assessment, blood-gas measurement, intraoperative monitoring, use of cardioscopes, and attention to ventilation – developments that made the anaesthetist's task analogous, in Dunn's words, to being at the controls of a 747 aircraft.

The staff headed by Dr Dunn in 1970 – Drs F. P. Rossiter, S.T. Zeglan, S.J. O'Rourke, P. Bailey, Z. Bak, A.H. Cole, W.E. Young, A.C. Finlayson, and W.H. Noble – was further strengthened in the next few years by the addition of Drs W.W. Stoyka, A. Kennedy, D. Sinclair, J. Obdrzalik, H. Samulska, D. McKee, and J. Ewen.

Nephrology and the Renal Unit

With its facilities for acute hemodialysis established, St Michael's was in 1965 approached by government to consider a chronic dialysis unit.[44] Three years later the medical advisory board assigned Drs V. Colapinto, A. Little, and the newly appointed Mitchell L. Halperin to the project. By 1969 they had an acute and chronic dialysis program in place, housed in a four-bed unit in the converted 307-D. Dr Michael Johnson, FRCP (Canada), formerly of Women's College Hospital, was appointed St Michael's first nephrologist in 1969; a year later he was joined by Dr Marc Goldstein, FRCP (Canada), who came from the Royal Victoria Hospital, Montreal. These worked in close collaboration with Dr Colapinto, who now turned his attention to kidney transplants, having successfully carried out the procedure on dogs for several years.[45]

Dr Vincent Colapinto, FRCS (Canada), had pursued his interest in this field in Leeds, England, and in several major American centres. In 1971 Dr Colapinto performed seven transplants; thereafter the number increased each year and by the mid-1970s the renal unit was serving its own patients as well as those from the Wellesley and Sunnybrook hospitals. In 1973 the kidney-transplant team was increased by the addition of Drs M. Barkin and L. Toranger, the university having agreed to three kidney-transplant centres (St Michael's, Toronto General, and Toronto Western).[46] Kidney transplantation was not entered into lightly; the medical advisory board gave serious attention to Colapinto's developed protocol, for example: how the neurological death of the donor was to be determined, and by whom; and the procedure to obtain consent for donation of a cadaver organ, including witnesses to the consent.[47]

As the kidney-transplantation program and the publicity surrounding it grew,[48] more staff and more space became necessary. Dr Robert Bear joined the division in 1975; four beds for peritoneal dialysis were assigned on 6-B, in addition to beds for the transplant patients on 6-A, while the hemodialysis continued on 3-DS. The scheduling of these limited facilities, and the provision of skilled nursing care – each in view of the life-and-death nature of the illness – became both a challenge and a source of satisfaction for all on the team.

In addition to his work in kidney transplants, his teaching, and his publications,[49] Colapinto was recognized as a leading urologist across North America and Europe, especially for his pioneering techniques for surgery of the urethra. His brilliant career was cut short tragically by his death in 1985 from hepatitis B, after pricking his gloved finger while suturing the incision of a patient with that disease.

Neurosciences

Chief of the division of neurosurgery during this decade was Dr William J. Horsey, FRCS (Canada), silver medallist in his graduating class in medicine from the University of Toronto in 1944. Mention was made in Chapter 6 of Dr Horsey's early innovative surgery. Throughout the 1960s and 1970s he carried on a heavy clinical practice, one that frequently brought him to the emergency department in the middle of the night. Many of his patients were referrals from across the province with head and spinal-cord injuries. From 1966 Horsey's time was increasingly occupied, as well, in administration and teaching as surgeon-in-chief at St Michael's and professor of surgery at the university. He was, at the same time, neurosurgeon-in-chief until 1977 and head of rehabilitation medicine from 1980 until his resignation in 1985. Alternating each day between the operating room and the boardroom – his mornings spent in that mysterious zone where the neurosurgeon's responsibility for the quality of a human life intersects with the Creator's, his afternoons spent amidst the projects and politics of the university and its member hospitals – this man of principle conducted with intelligence and grace the duties of his multiple offices, loyal to all that St Michael's stood for, throughout a period of forty years.[50]

In the mid-1960s the neurosciences took over the whole of 4-C, forty-one beds in all, including a fully equipped intensive care unit. Long-stay patients frequently made necessary the admission of new patients to the halls, but morale was always high in these unbelievably busy and cramped facilities. In fact, nurses put their names on a wait-ing list for transfer to the demanding but rewarding work of this unit under the capable (and colourful) head nurseship of Mollie Trimnell, and later, Yvonne (Gilbride) Erwin.[51]

With the coming of Dr Alan R. Hudson to St Michael's in 1970 the work of the division of neurosurgery took on a new dimension. After his basic medical studies in his native Cape Town, South Africa, Hud-son had done nine years of post-graduate training in Toronto (much of it under Dr Horsey) and Great Britain, obtaining fellowships in the Royal College of Surgeons of London, Edinburgh, and Canada before ending up at Oxford University. At Oxford he focussed on elecron-microscopy of peripheral nerve regeneration, and his academic men-tor travelled to St Michael's in 1969 to arrange for the space and financing necessary for Hudson to continue his research in this area.[52] During the subsequent years of research on nerve regeneration and transplantation in the hospital's laboratory, Hudson published exten-sively, travelled widely, and received international recognition.[53] He was also deeply involved at St Michael's and the university in med-ical education, eventually becoming chairman of the university 's division of neurosurgery. The climax of his career occurred in 1987 when he and a team of surgeons performed the world's first sciatic-nerve transplant from a human donor, a procedure that had eluded surgeons for more than a century.[54]

Sharing with Dr Horsey the somewhat dilapidated facilities on 4-C was Dr Joseph T. Marotta, neurologist-in-chief from 1956 until 1969; Dr Marotta continued as practising neurologist and professor of neurology after becoming physician-in-chief in April 1969. One example will illustrate the esteem in which the Horsey-Marotta team was held: in 1977 a father and son, both patients of Drs Horsey and Marotta, donated – in gratitude to them and for the care they received on 4-C – one-third of the $300,000 cost of the hospital's ACTA scanner, the first full-body scanner in Canada. Painless for the patient, who could now undergo his or her diagnostic tests on an out-patient basis, the scanner became a valuable non-invasive diagnostic aid much in demand by the other hospitals in Toronto.[55]

Dr Joseph T. Marotta, FRCP (Canada), was neurologist-in-chief at St Michael's from 1956 to 1969. A philosopher of medicine, of medical practice, and of medical education, Marotta was also an eloquent teacher, both by word and example, as well as a clinician deeply inter-ested in his patients' welfare.[56] After graduation in medicine from the University of Toronto in 1949, and a chief residency in medicine at St

Michael's, Marotta did three years of post-graduate study at the Neu-rological Institute of New York, followed by a year in London, Eng-land. He then served for thirteen years as head of neurology, before assuming the larger responsibilities of physician-in-chief at St Michael's and professor of medicine at the University of Toronto. The confidence and esteem in which Marotta was held, and the skill with which he fulfilled his administrative role, can be gauged from the quality of practitioner he was able to attract as he fashioned a depart-ment of medicine fit for the closing decades of the twentieth century.

The Department of Medicine

In preparation for the announced major shift in the medical curricu-lum that would assign to St Michael's the total responsibility for a block of students in their final two years, Dr Marotta set about build-ing a strong and rounded department of medicine, where the major part of the teaching would be done.

The division of cardiology and nephrology, and to a lesser extent nephrology, have been commented on. Dr Trevor Gray, whose work will be covered in greater detail, joined Dr Marotta and Dr Henry Berry in neurology in 1970.

One of the oldest divisions, the chest service, was strengthened in 1968 with the addition of Dr Fred Douglas and the establishment in 1972 of a pulmonary function laboratory and inpatient unit on 4-F, an area seconded from obstetrics. Dr Adrian Anglin's years of service and teaching of chest disease were acknowledged in his promotion to full professor in 1968. After Dr Douglas's sudden and premature death, Dr Peter Thomas was appointed to head the division in 1976.

Haematology, which had earlier been developed by Dr C.J. Bar-dawill and then Dr K. Butler, was bolstered by the addition of Dr Bernadette Garvey in 1968. Dr J.J. Freedman was appointed in 1976 and took charge of the relocated and improved blood bank on 2-DS.

Dr Ralph Warren came in 1968 to the gastroenterology division, headed by Dr E.J. Prokipchuk; a year later an inflammatory bowel dis-ease clinic, also headed by Dr Prokipchuk, was established. Dr Prokipchuk's interest and skill in the treatment of drug abuse was rec-ognized by his appointment in 1970 to treat referrals to St Michael's from the Addiction Research Foundation's crisis intervention centre.

The division of endocrinology and metabolism and the isotope laboratory, all headed by Dr H.P. Higgins, were strengthened by the appointment of Dr William Singer (1970), Dr Randolph Lee (1971), Dr G.S. Wong (1971), and Dr T. A. Bayley (1970).

St Michael's appointed its first oncologist in 1968, Dr J.H. Goldie. In 1972 the medical advisory board approved the establishment of an oncology service, together with an oncology clinic, and a four-bed block of chemotherapy beds on 6-AS. Dr W. Allt, of the Princess Margaret Hospital's staff, was given a cross-appointment at St Michael's as consultant in radiotherapy.

Dermatology, formerly in the charge of Dr Arthur Hudson, was headed by Dr W.T.R. Linton from 1964; in 1973 a second dermatologist, Dr W. Medwisky, was appointed. Allergist Dr M.M. Nedilski was appointed in 1969, followed two years later by Dr A. Leznoff.

The key division of internal medicine acquired well-qualified new staff: Dr Peter Kopplin in 1970, Dr J. Zownir in 1973, Dr R. Snihura in 1975, and Dr K.Y. Lee in 1976. In addition to their duties within the division of internal medicine, Dr Kopplin was director of ambulatory care from 1971, and Dr Zownir was director of emergency.

Dr T.M. Murray, whose important work in calcium metabolism will be referred to later, joined the staff in 1971; Dr S. Gershon, rheumatologist, was appointed in 1973; and finally, out of concern for the transportability of disease in an era of world-wide jet travel, Dr I.W. Fong, a specialist in infectious diseases, was appointed in 1976. The establishment of an international travel clinic, at the initiative of Dr T.A. Patterson of the department of microbiology, was accomplished that same year. These physicians, each highly qualified in his field, were appointed during Dr Marotta's tenure as physician-in-chief; all, with the exception of Dr Goldie, are still with St Michael's in 1992.

The trend to specialization in an era of rapidly expanding knowledge, as illustrated above, left the ranks of general practitioners growing ever thinner. The University of Toronto addressed the issue in 1969 when the faculty of medicine set up a department of family and community medicine, the first such in any Canadian faculty of medicine. With the ribbon-cutting of St Michael's first family practice clinic, in the basement of C-wing on 6 October 1969, there began a phase of medical practice at St Michael's designed to complement and counterbalance the move to specialization and high technology.

Dr Lance Murray Cathcart was named head of the new family practice division, which initially had but five members: Drs B. Hamilton-Smith, R. Nishikawa, M. Scandiffio, R. Welch, and D. MacAuley. Within a year Dr Cathcart had twenty-five doctors, six with university appointments, giving a part of their time to the clinic. In 1973 the family practitioners were given their own block of beds on 5-B. That same year, they opened and staffed a "stat clinic" to examine and treat the large proportion of patients presenting in the emergency department with complaints not of an emergency nature.

While a department of rehabilitation medicine had existed for several years, it was only in 1970 that an eight-bed inpatient area was provided, with physiatrist Dr J. Houston directing the whole operation. Prominent among the patients there were young men who had had neurosurgery after motorcycle or automobile accidents, beginning (often angrily) their long road back under the competent care of head nurse Ane Marie Hansen. The university's stamp of approval was put on Dr Houston's department in 1975 when it was recognized for post-graduate training in this field.

Ophthalmology

When Dr R.G.C. Kelly joined St Michael's as ophthalmologist-in-chief upon his release from the navy in 1946, he embarked on a vigorous program to staff and equip his department in keeping with its status as a university teaching hospital. When he retired in 1972, Dr Kelly was able to say, with justifiable pride and satisfaction, "We have done our fair share of the teaching of medical students and the training of ophthalmologists, who are scattered from coast to coast, and we have equipment second to none in the country."[57]

Indeed, the number of "firsts," both in equipment and in surgical procedures performed, is impressive: the first upright image-indirect ophthalmoscope for vitrectomy in the world; the first retina unit in Canada (1958); the first silicone implant in the sclera in Canada; the first xenon photocoagulation in Canada; the first cryosurgery of retina and cataract in Canada; the first operating microscope in Canada; the first vitrectomy in Canada (1975); and the first argon lazer in Ontario.[58]

Dr Kelly recruited staff with training across the whole field of ophthalmology: Dr O.B. Richarson, 1949-58, ophthalmic pathology; Dr William P. Callahan, 1950; Dr Michael Shea, 1962, retinal surgery; Dr William Hunter, 1964, ophthalmic pathology; Dr Donald Morin, 1968, glaucoma; Dr Gordon Johnston, 1971-73, tissue transplantation.[59]

For three of the above men, lifelong careers at St Michael's began with these appointments. Dr William Callahan (University of Toronto, 1945; Johns Hopkins, Baltimore, 1949-51; FRCS [Canada], 1953), whose deep interest in research dated from his years at Johns Hopkins, became chairman of the Eye Research Institute of Ontario, and he published, while in that position, a comprehensive text on surgery of the eyelids, lacrimal apparatus, and orbit. Dr William S. Hunter

(University of Toronto, 1946; post-graduate study in London, England, and San Francisco; FRCS [Canada] 1964), has dedicated much time and energy to the prevention of blindness (fourteen years as treasurer of the International Association for Prevention of Blindness). From 1966 he has been in charge of the low vision clinic at the CNIB and consultant to that institute, and for nine years he has chaired the contact lens certification committee of the Board of Ophthalmic Dispensers – a remarkable record of public service, and all in addition to his teaching and clinical practice.

Lastly, Dr Michael Shea came in 1958, having completed his undergraduate studies in Galway, with internships in Galway and Dublin, Eire; residencies at Sunnybrook and at the four downtown Toronto hospitals; a year of basic science and research at the University of Toronto; and two years as a fellow at the Massachusetts Eye and Ear Infirmary, Boston. With his FRCS (Canada) awarded, Shea joined St Michael's retina service in 1958, serving at the same time as fellow-in-charge of the eye pathology laboratory at the Banting Institute for two years.

Dr Shea was not long in reaping the rewards of his decade of post-graduate study and research. In late 1964, after three years of experimentation on rabbits, Shea pioneered a procedure for correcting retinal detachment by cryosurgery which involved the use of a specially designed probe and a cooling agent.[60] Thence began a dizzying round of written and oral presentations on this subject: thirty-five publications from 1956 to 1981, as well as a chapter on the subject in a 1968 book on retinal detachment;[61] lectures in Buenos Aires, Johannesburg, Bogota, Zurich, and Nice; and visiting professorships closer to home at Dalhousie University, Halifax, and at Northwestern University, Chicago. Not surprisingly, Shea's patients came from far and wide to his unit and his clinic on 3-B, both of which were supervised by Sister Anne Purcell. Dr Shea succeeded Dr Kelly as head of the department in 1972, and he has ably represented his department and the hospital's interests until the present.

Department of Psychiatry

In 1967 psychiatry was separated from the department of medicine, and in January 1968 Dr William Stauble came from the Clarke Institute to become its full-time geographic head. The mezzanine floor 4M was converted from neurosurgery to well-appointed offices for psychiatrists and their residents, and Stauble set about building up his staff.

Dr Mary McEwan, who became a prominent consultant on women's issues in general, joined the staff in 1968; Dr Cyril Murray and Dr J.M. Divic in 1969; Dr David Sherret in 1970; Drs A. Kindler and J. Salvendy in 1971; and Drs C.T. Rotenberg, Donna E. Stewart, and R. Lamon in 1973. All of the recognized branches of psychiatric therapy were gradually introduced.

Psychological services had been established earlier. As the departments of psychiatry and psychology grew, despite recognition of the latter's autonomy and despite repeated efforts on the part of the medical advisory board to resolve jurisdictional boundary lines, an uneasy relationship between the two persisted for several years, rooted partially in the similarity of training undertaken by their practitioners.[62]

The work of the department of psychiatry was complemented and extended with the establishment in 1969 of the department of social work and the appointment of Les White, who held a master's degree in social work, as director of the department and assistant professor in the school of social work at the University of Toronto. A day treatment unit was established in 1973 on the third floor, D-north; psychiatric inpatient units already occupied the whole of the second and fourth floors of this wing. With the full range of services for the psychiatric patient thus established, it came as no surprise – but stood, nevertheless, to the credit of all involved – that medical students who had taken their psychiatric training in this department ranked first among the seven Toronto teaching hospitals in the LMCC psychiatry examination results for several years, beginning in 1975.[63]

General Surgery

During this and the following decade Dr Donald J. Currie, MSc, FRCS (Edinburgh), FRCS (Canada), FACS, was chief of general surgery and assistant surgeon-in-chief, positions for which he was eminently qualified. He had graduated from the University of Toronto in 1947 and afterwards had done nine years of post-graduate study in Montreal, London, England, and Edinburgh. Then followed a chief residency under Dr Keith Welsh at St Michael's, and further visits to England, Scotland, Germany, and France.

After his initial – and original – research on the effect of potassium deficiency on gastric secretions, and the effect of bile and pancreatic juice on the colon (for his MSc thesis at McGill), Dr Currie continued his study of the alimentary system, publishing numerous articles on his experience with patients and his research on animals. While he carried out many of his own animal studies at the Banting Institute, he served as director of St Michael's animal research laboratory, having been chiefly instrumental in the design of that facility. Currie was instrumental, too, in the establishment in 1965 of the acute care unit for patients requiring intensive care but not respiratory support.

Dr Currie recognized early that medical photography could be a powerful ally in medical education, research, and practice, and he teamed with St Michael's photographer Arthur Smialowski to author no fewer than twenty-one published articles and two books on the subject.[64] He was among the major architects of the new curriculum at the University of Toronto in 1966, and was active in testing medical candidates for both the Medical Council of Canada and the Royal College of Physicians and Surgeons (Canada). In short, his career is a prime example of the complete range of activities of the twentieth-century physician in a university teaching hospital.

Dr Leo J. Mahoney, MS, FRCS (Canada), FACS – who, like Dr Currie had served his residency under Dr Keith Welsh – shared with Dr Currie the same period of St Michael's history. After seven years of post-graduate training in the hospitals of Toronto, Dr Mahoney spent a year as McLaughlin Travelling Fellow in Britain and Sweden, and was appointed staff surgeon at St Michael's and consultant to Princess Margaret Hospital in 1954.

For ten years Mahoney worked with Peter Moloney, PhD, in a search for a method of providing prophylaxis against tetanus in wounded patients. By 1965 they had succeeded in the breakthrough development of human tetanus anti-toxin and toxoid which would provide long-term immunity to tetanus. Dr Mahoney's experience in the use of intra-arterial infusion chemotherapy for head and neck cancer (he had collaborated in the development of a portable pump for injecting the drug)[65] took him on teaching tours to Malaysia and Indonesia in 1969 and 1971.

From 1972 onward Mahoney's attention was increasingly centred on breast cancer in women: its early detection, assessment of the various forms of treatment, and the use of self-examination, mammography, and thermography in diagnoses – making St Michael's the only general surgical service in the Toronto teaching hospitals aggressively studying early breast cancer. Mahoney shared his findings widely in Canada and the United States, and as far afield as Lucerne, Switzerland, and Manchester, England. In 1970 he established his breast cancer detection clinic –a clinic unique in that it is staffed almost entirely by volunteers from the hospital's Women's Auxiliary (of which more will be written), and unique as well for the intelligent, supportive, and courteous attention of these women for whom the saying "the patient comes first" is a motto truly put into practice.[66]

Two others of Dr Welsh's chief residents joined the division of general surgery: Dr John A. MacDonald, FRCS (Canada), after postgraduate work in Chicago; and Dr William Kerr, FRCS (Canada), after study in Bristol, England. Among his accomplishments, MacDonald was a collaborator in the development of the portable infusion pump, which he subsequently used for intra-arterial infusion treatment of hepatic metastases. Kerr was one of two surgeons to introduce transcervical mediastinoscopy to Toronto, and it was he who performed most of these examinations at St Michael's. Both MacDonald and Kerr had promising careers cut short by cancer, at the height of their productivity.

Working closely with Dr Welsh and his "spiritual sons" from the late 1940s through the 1960s was Dorothy Shamess, the knowledgeable and progressive nursing supervisor of the seventy-odd beds for male surgical patients. No ward at St Michael's quite matched Shamess's 2-D (and later 4-D) for its challenges, satisfactions, and not infrequent drama.[67] When 4-D was converted to an acute care unit, the mantle fell on Mary Cassidy, head nurse of that unit, and Noreen Giommi, head nurse on 5-AS, both of whom have made invaluable contributions to the care of St Michael's patients.

Pathology

As mentioned, the department of pathology was augmented in this decade by the appointment of specialists in various areas – neurology, gynaecology, nephrology, and cardiology. In 1971 Dr Ross succeeded in attracting to his department the husband-and-wife team of Dr Kalman Kovacs and Dr Eva Horvath, who came to St Michael's via Montreal where they had worked under the renowned scientist Hans Selye. Within five years their work on diseases of the pituitary gland was widely recognized as being the most advanced in the field. Although their research funding was precarious at times, the hospital supported their efforts: beginning with the Philips 300 electron microscope purchased by the hospital in 1968 (at a cost of $60,000 – and capable of magnifying a piece of organic tissue as much as 570,000 times); a second electron microscope, a Philips 410, at a cost of $340,000; and, because of a frequent breakdown of the 1968 instrument, another Philips 410 in 1985. By that time the Kovacs-Horvath team had published more than one hundred papers and had become the unquestioned world leaders in their field. Dr Kovacs was, at the same time, professor of pathology at the University of Toronto.[68]

Dentistry

In January 1972 the medical advisory board proposed that dental work at St Michael's, at that time limited to extractions, be extended to include restorative work as well as that involving facio-maxillary and mandibular surgery. That same year, Dr V. Direnfeld, qualified in these fields, was appointed to staff. Negotiations with the faculty of dentistry were begun; two modern and fully equipped dental rooms were established; and in 1975 Dr W.J. Fleming was appointed dentist-in-chief of the division which, it was agreed, would remain for a time under the department of surgery.

Major Committees of the Medical Advisory Board

The accomplishments of the various medical departments occurred at a time when the very future of the hospital and its staff was being hotly debated at Queen's Park and elsewhere. Throughout all of this, the medical advisory board's committees soldiered on: in February 1967, the operating-room committee proposed the elimination of the routine shave preparation and the appointment of a shave prep team which would prepare the area by clippers, making unnecessary the 2600 blades and 100 razors requisitioned each week for this purpose; in 1971 all the operating rooms were air-conditioned; and in 1973 the general surgeons began to schedule their cases through block booking (an arrangement whereby a block of time, for example, two whole mornings a week, are reserved for the exclusive use of a particular surgical service). The pharmacy and therapeutic committee supported the extension of clinical pharmacy beyond neurology to urology and the medical wards in 1969; intravenous solutions in glass bottles were replaced by plastic bags in 1971; and the use of paraldehyde was abolished in 1973. The admissions and discharge committee, under the aggressive leadership of orthopaedic surgeon Dr John McCulloch and the Certified Hospital Admission Program (CHAP), reduced St Michael's 13.8 days' average length of stay in 1971 (the longest in the province) to 9.3 days in 1973 (seventh place rather than twenty-first).[69] In 1972 the Sunday admission and discharge of patients began.

The infection control committee extended the provision of stainless-steel isolation carts (modelled after wooden and arborite carts designed ten years earlier by the nurses on 3-DS) in 1970; provided for the installation of a cidematic machine for decontamination of anaesthetic and inhalation therapy equipment in 1975; and secured, in 1973, four beds for reverse isolation for nephrology and hematology patients, in rooms eventually to be provided with a positive-pressure circulation system. However, the committee's proposal in 1972 to supply disposable gloves and syringes throughout the hospital was postponed because of the cost. Dr Gordon Hawk's introduction in 1971 of the hospital's first infection control nurse, Joanne Roy, a 1963 graduate of St Michael's school of nursing, met with considerable resistance on the grounds that it gave a nurse too much authority. But the position has endured, the nurse's authority has widened, and few today would question the resulting benefits to both patients and staff.

Such were some of the signs of changing times. And there were others: in the need to install locks on all medicine cupboards, and to control access to prescription pads as drug addicts began to present the forged signatures of St Michael's staff on prescriptions handed to retail pharmacies; in the need for new policies for consents and for release of information as a myriad of students and new teaching approaches and media (for example, videotaped interviews) invaded the patients' privacy; and in the appearance of young Lawrence of Arabia look-alikes in the operating room, as attempts were made to provide adequate masks and head covering for bearded and long-haired surgeons and surgical trainees.

Medical Research and Medical Education

Throughout these years St Michael's Research Society continued to review for approval those projects for which financial support was requested.[70] In early 1976 Dr Little drew attention to the need for a long-term strategy to support research at St Michael's, since funds through the Medical Research Council of Canada were being drastically reduced. The future seemed brighter when later that year UTHA announced that provincial lottery funds were to be made available, each hospital submitting its research requirements to the University of Toronto research committee.[71]

Frequent reference has been made to the new curriculum and to the recruitment of teaching staff to handle it. The full force of the change came in 1970: the number of medical students doubled, from thirty-six in the fall semester of 1969 to seventy-two for the winter semester of 1970; and then in June 1970 St Michael's received forty junior interns enrolled in one of the four types of internships offered (rotating, straight, mixed, or family practice)[72] along with thirty clinical clerks. Within the year Dr Selby, coordinator at St Michael's for period II of the undergraduate curriculum, reported to the medical advisory board that staff and facilities were "strained to the utmost" and there was great "uneasiness and unhappiness" about the university's plan to increase its enrolment even further; Dr Alan Hudson brought to the medical advisory board a report of the low morale among the clinical clerks who felt that they were not getting adequate teaching;[73] the intern program, too, came in for its share of criticism – clearly, St Michael's doctors had not foreseen the changes, or had not responded quickly enough or vigorously enough to them. Accordingly, Dr A. Leznoff was now delegated to propose an improved intern program, and Dr A. Hudson to arrange for a forward look into both the undergraduate and the graduate programs.[74]

The appointment of an associate dean at St Michael's, frequently discussed,[75] appears not to have been made; in November 1976 Dr Norman Struthers was appointed educational coordinator for the new curriculum which would be fully instituted in 1977.[76] A measure of the success of this appointment, and of the steps taken above, was evident in the 1977 LMCC examination results. A justifiably proud Dr Hudson was then able to announce that St Michael's had stood first overall in the Toronto hospitals in both the 1976 and 1977 LMCC examinations.

The Department Of Nursing

Several of the nurses prominent during these years have been mentioned. The director of nursing for much of this decade was Elizabeth (Courage) Mange – consistently just in her treatment of staff, and unfailingly vigilant for the care and safety of patients in an era when the nurse's role underwent rapid expansion. Her years spanned that difficult period when changes in nursing education wreaked havoc with staffing plans, as the hospital (and, indeed the province) plunged from a surplus of nurses in 1970 as a result of the nurse intern program, to a severe shortage just four years later – all at a time when dynamic developments within the medical departments made heavy demands for more, and more widely prepared, nurses. Gradually nurses, particularly in the critical-care areas, took on duties unthought of in earlier times, ranging from the simple removal of sutures on the wards all the way to the defibrillation of patients in the coronary care unit.

The nurse practitioner, authorized, among other things, to take histories, do hemoglobins, and carry out pelvic examinations – in short, the "work-up" of some patients – was introduced at Broadview

Clinic in 1971 with the powerful endorsement of Dr Woolever, chief of obstetrics and gynaecology. In 1973 the university's school of nursing requested authorization for its students to carry out research studies at St Michael's in connection with their masters' theses. The university-hospital agreement was amended to accommodate these graduate students, who became the pool from which the hospital recruited its first clinical nurse specialists.

In 1974 nurses at St Michael's along with forty-two other hospitals in the province hammered out in joint bargaining sessions on a provincial basis their first union contract, which covered assistant head nurses, registered nurses, and graduate nurses. The settlement reached increased the 1974 budget at St Michael's by a whopping 14.1 percent, or $2,341,000. The nurse-administrator's work would be henceforth more complex, its every move having to be reviewed in the light of the contract. Claudette Brunelle, associate director of nursing at the time of the first contract, quickly became an expert in handling the concerns of both management and staff, and has tirelessly devoted herself to this, and to other personnel matters, right up to the present.

New and/or Expanded Departments

Like the medical advisory board, the hospital administration refused to succumb to paralysis while the hospital's future was being debated, even though from 1971 on authorization from the OHSC was required for any new programs or services.

The establishment of a social work department has been mentioned. (St Michael's had long had a group of public-health nurses, as well as active and innovative volunteers doing what social workers were doing in many hospitals.) By 1973 Les White had assembled a staff of ten well-qualified social workers and was providing service to all the major clinical departments, in addition to receiving social-work students from the University of Toronto and Carleton University, Ottawa.

In 1972 the hospital's medical art department was established under a qualified medical artist (Sister Anne Marie Black), and charged with the responsibility of preparing visual material for teaching and research purposes. In 1975 Sister Camilla Young, a retired high school teacher and librarian, began the prodigious task of organizing the accumulated records of more than eighty years into the hospital's first archives department, an assignment that she carried forward with precision and taste over a fourteen-year period.

The chaplaincy department, working out of enlarged facilities on 3-B, grew steadily throughout the 1970s under its coordinating chaplain, Father Alan J. Tipping, and associate chaplain, Father Charles Prance, both of whom had had formal preparation in clinical pastoral education in Boston. Chaplains of other faiths (Anglican, Baptist, Lutheran, United, and Buddhist) visited regularly, giving the department's ministry a distinctly ecumenical character. In addition to its responsibility to patients and, to a lesser extent, staff, the department offered from 1970 supervised pastoral education to students from the Toronto School of Theology.

To provide better care for the acute alcoholic, a twenty-bed detoxification centre for men was established in 1973 in a house on Adelaide Street purchased by the sisters for this purpose. Sister Anne Marie Carey was appointed director. An appreciative chief of police served on the management committee; his police officers would now have a long-needed alternative to the police cells for the acutely intoxicated man.

And finally, with so many of its patients' diagnostic and survival needs dependent upon electric-powered equipment, the hospital established in 1976 its second diesel generator – a 600-kilowatt unit to supply emergency power to those units not covered by the 400-kilowatt generator installed in 1965, which supplied only such vital areas as the operating rooms, critical care, and the switchboard. Al O'Brien (assistant chief engineer at the time, later chief engineer) was able to report that, in the event of power failure in the downtown area, the two sleeping giants would be automatically aroused and within eight to thirteen seconds would be sending emergency power to essential areas.

Funding for Operating Costs

From 1969 onwards St Michael's, like all the hospitals in the province, was increasingly preoccupied with its operating budget. Prodigious efforts were made each year to bring costs within approved levels. They were followed by appeals for additional funds, followed still later by all or partial makeup by the OHSC, and then the cycle began all over again. Never were staffing levels and service loads so meticulously documented at St Michael's, all under the watchful eye of the assistant administrator of finance, Larry Thalheimer.

Spiralling operating costs were reflected in the standard ward per diem rates authorized by the OHSC (later the Ministry of Health), which rose from $79 in 1971 to $102.30 in 1974. In response to that year's Henderson report the ministry began to hint at controlling the number of beds and the number of doctors in the province. Next the plea – in the Mustard report of 1974 – was for the "rationalization" embodied in coordinated care, a concept strongly endorsed by UTHA, and for the elimination of duplication of facilities.

In 1976, in the wake of the federal government's Anti-Inflation Act, the Ministry of Health instructed St Michael's to chop a full $1 million from its budget base, the constraints to take the form of bed closures and staff reductions; nothing significant was to be done, however, without prior ministry approval. With all possible reductions made, as suggested, the period under review ended with a projected half-million dollars' overrun for 1976-77.

So ends this account of the tumultuous 1966-76 decade – one which demanded that those in administration be willing and able to walk on water. St Michael's was fortunate to have in Sister Mary Zimmerman just such a person.

9

Caregivers under the Knife

War-bride and war-widow, Sister Mary (Lannan) Zimmerman had entered the congregation in 1948. After several years' experience as director of admitting at St Michael's, she completed her preparation for hospital administration, serving for part of that time as executive secretary to Sister Maura, who was by then superior general of the congregation. In 1963 Sister Mary became the administrator of St Michael's and religious superior of the hospital's community, which at that time numbered fifty-six sisters. Five years later her responsibility was reduced to that of administrator only.

Administrator only – but of a 900-bed teaching hospital entering upon a period of development that would catapult it into the front ranks of tertiary care.* Throughout the decade just reviewed and the one to be explored, Sister Mary guided St Michael's deftly through the shoals and narrows of many a treacherous sea. Although she was no doubt assisted by the experience gained in her outside contacts (fellowship in the American College of Hospital Administrators, 1973; associate professor, faculty of medicine, University of Toronto, 1977; board of directors, Ontario Hydro, 1977),[1] Sister Mary's success as chief executive officer at St Michael's probably lay more in the personal attributes she brought to the position: among them, an ability to work with and through all kinds of people; an openness to new ideas, initiatives, and opportunities; an unerring sense of the public-relations dimension of every decision and event; a resiliency in the wake of setbacks; and a capacity to weather difficult times.

Sister Mary was fortunate in the man elected to take the place left vacant by the sudden death of Robert Davies in 1975. With five years' experience on the board, during which time he had chaired the very successful building campaign for the proposed redevelopment of St

---

*Tertiary care has been defined as consultative care of a more specialized nature in a centre that accepts referrals from a wide area, often both national and international in scope.

Michael's Hospital, Anthony G.S. Griffin was unanimously elected chairman of the board of directors in October 1975.

Prominent in the business community (he was chairman of Home Oil Company at the time of his election), Griffin has been referred to as "one of the Establishment's more thoughtful elder statesmen."[2] The qualities of the thoughtful statesman were abundantly evident in his annual messages to staff, published in the hospital's newsletter[3] and in his communications and negotiations with government and university. A keen observer of the political, economic, and social scene, Griffin repeatedly called St Michael's people to a realization of their individual and institutional responsibility towards the public-health system of which they were all the beneficiaries. Board documents during his tenure reveal a man of wide business experience and skill as well as deep personal integrity. They also show him to be a consummate diplomat in the best sense of the word.

With a building program in progress and a campaign for funds on the horizon, the board was further strengthened at this time by the election of several new members:[4] Lawrence Hynes (1977); David Barr (1979); Bishop Leonard Wall, representing Gerald Emmett Cardinal Carter (1980); Justice Charles Dubin and David Braide (both re-elected in 1981); Alan Dilworth (1981); and Paul H. O'Donoghue and Dr Charles Hollenberg (1983). Dr A. Anglin and Dr William Horsey were elected honorary board members in 1981 and 1982 respectively.

Beginning in 1980, a presentation from a medical or hospital department was an agenda item at each meeting; the uniqueness and richness of the individual departments was thus demonstrated, and did much to enhance board members' understanding of the complex undertaking which they directed. In January 1981, with Ontario's economy slipping into a recession, a permanent budget and finance committee of the board was established to provide support and direction to the hospital's hard-pressed director of finance, Larry Thalheimer.

The Social and Political Context

In the health field the decade 1975-85 was characterized, perhaps most of all, by a preoccupation with funding. The Ontario government's concerns around this issue led to the formation of district health councils (DHCs) and area planning boards with extensive powers, and to efforts to control the number and kinds of physicians as well as the amounts physicians billed government and individuals for their services. This was the decade that brought, in 1980, the first strike by interns.[5] It also witnessed, again in 1980, an unprecedented protest staged at Queen's Park by physicians unwilling to accept a government crack-down on extra-billing and, in 1982, job action by the members of the Ontario Medical Association, which had never fully supported universal health-care legislation.[6] From 1981, chiefs of departments were required by the university to undergo every five years a review of their departments by a committee of board members, university nominees, and their medical peers. It was a decade rocked and shocked by continued breakthroughs in new technology and new drugs, and by the attendant costs which threatened to outstrip resources. The decade also brought changing patterns and volumes at both extremes of patient care – tertiary care was carried to new levels of complexity and competence, while primary and ambulatory care received a renewed emphasis. There was a mounting public demand for health services at each level, and a growing realization of an aging population[7] – all in an increasingly pluralistic society.[8] And there were new concerns about old problems – the effects of smoking[9] and noise pollution, as well as the age-old issue of refugees and their health-care requirements. It is within this framework that the life and growth of St Michael's Hospital will be examined throughout the last half of Sister Mary's tenure – and indeed during the stewardship of the sisters in general, whose numbers diminished markedly during these years.

Government Initiatives and St Michael's

Although the struggle for capital funds to begin implementation of the hospital's redevelopment plans had been won, it soon became apparent that the uncertainty of funding would be the major obstacle to progress in the coming decade.

The Ontario government drew upon recommendations from a number of commissioned studies in an effort to impose some order and cost effectiveness on a health-care system growing out of control, and for which government was the chief financier. Of particular significance was the Mustard report of 1974, which had proposed a number of district health councils across the province, each with wide responsibility for planning in its district and for making recommendations to government concerning district-level programs, manpower, and facilities. As well, the Mustard report recommended area health services management boards under which "the activities of all institutions throughout a district must be coordinated within the framework of the district plan …. "[10] These recommendations were viewed with some alarm by hospitals accustomed to considerable planning autonomy; Catholic hospitals were concerned that they would be pressured to integrate their services with institutions that did not share their philosophy.

In addition to this proposal for overall planning, government drew from studies focussed on specific issues. Of these, the influential Henderson report of 1974 recommended controlling the number of licensed doctors and the number and type of training posts as well as curtailing plans to expand the capacity of the medical schools.[11]

Within a year of its receipt, the Ministry of Health moved to implement the recommendations of the Mustard report. UTHA, fearing that government might unilaterally make decisions in the absence of a district health council and recognizing, as well, that government was serious about establishing an integrated health system, proposed to its members a standing committee within UTHA which would assume many of the responsibilities that DHCs elsewhere would carry out: review requests for new programs; establish priorities; examine existing services; and develop plans for rationalization.[12] Two years later, in 1976, there being still no DHC in Metropolitan Toronto, the ministry proposed an expanded role in this regard for UTHA and the Hospital Council of Metropolitan Toronto. In 1981 these two organizations merged, taking the name of the latter, and became the DHC for Metropolitan Toronto; henceforth any new programs established by St Michael's would receive ministry funding approval only upon the recommendation of the new DHC.

Building Redevelopment: Phase I, Stage A

The hospital moved quickly to harness the energy and enthusiasm generated by the approval to launch its redevelopment. Its first step was the demolition of the nurses' residence to make room for the new construction. Unfortunately, an unexpected problem arose: the contractors found huge masses of concrete supporting the building below ground level where an earlier creek had wandered through. This cost heavily – a price tag of $94,500 for demolition of a building erected earlier at the cost of $292,277.[13]

On 14 December 1978 the Ministry of Health issued a press release detailing approval of a $30-million redevelopment for St Michael's Hospital – the first two stages of a four-stage project. The minister was quoted as stating that the new St Lawrence neighbourhood alone (projected population, 10,000) justified rebuilding the hospital down-town.[14] The hospital simultaneously issued its press release: to stay within the $25.8 million available, the latter part of phase I would be shelled in, with the interior only partially completed[15]– the board having approved the planning office's recommendations for complet-ing only the operating-room level of the second stage of develop-ment.[16] That same day, guests were piped to the site for ground-breaking ceremonies, and the still-incredulous chairman of the medi-cal advisory board fulfilled an earlier pledge to provide his members with champagne to toast this new chapter of St Michael's history.

Walls came down (the boiler plant) and others went up, over a period of four years, all under the watchful eye of Graham Constan-tine, director of planning, working with Sister Catherine McDonough and Dr Platt. These three consulted widely with the heads of services to be housed in the new facilities, arbitrated among their competing plans, and enjoyed their confidence to the full. All – planners, archi-tects, and users – learned much in the process. For example, changes made in orders for diagnostic imaging (radiology) alone amounted to $750,000 because of rapid developments in x-ray technology since the start of the project, an experience which prompted the board to direct that the selection of equipment would be postponed in stage B to assure true "state-of-the-art" installations.[17]

The resulting eleven-storey building, the new C-wing, was erected on the corner of Shuter and Victoria streets; the architects were Math-ers and Haldenby and John J. Farrugia, and the contractor was Ellis-Don. The three upper floors housed the neurosciences (including a thirteen-bed intensive care unit), otolaryngology, and ophthalmology – ninety-nine patient beds in all, each of the three having its ambula-tory-care clinic adjacent to its inpatient area; then, moving down-wards, the cystoscopy rooms, a twenty-one-bed day-surgery unit, and recovery rooms; ambulatory care and family practice; diagnostic imaging; pathology, biochemistry, and microbiology laboratories; emergency, with a three-bay ambulance entrance; and the two below-street levels – a mezzanine housing the receiving room and docks, and the engineering/maintenance complex. The sixth floor, just beneath the three inpatient floors, was reserved for the main kitchen, complete with new carbon-dioxide fire extinguishers and offices for dietary administration.

The building was funded by the province; furnishings and equip-ment at a cost of $7.1 million were paid for by the sisters and with private donations. Air-conditioned throughout, and with four high-speed elevators and three service elevators, the new facility added immeasurably to the comfort and efficiency of operations, while the pleasing decor and furnishings gave a tremendous boost to staff pride and morale. While the full effect and effectiveness of the new building would be felt only with the completion of the planned stage B, the official opening on 11 April 1983 was a day of rejoicing. As it turned out, stage B would be long delayed.[18]

Throughout the four years of the new construction project, a number of other physical improvements were made, including piped medical gases throughout the whole hospital, a move of the interns to the north nurses' residence, and a renovation of the interns' former quarters to a thirty-four-bed cardiology unit and a similar cardiovascular surgery inpatient unit (2-F and 3-F). The last remaining public ward (3-DS) was closed and its patients moved to two- and four-bed rooms on 7-B. A new SL-I (stored logic) advanced computerized telephone system replaced the centrex system, necessitating the threading of miles of cable throughout both the old and new buildings – expensive to install, but promising to save the hospital $1 million over a ten-year period. And some proposed projects were deferred. In 1982 Dr Platt proposed to the board and the medical advisory committee a professional office-building, eight floors in all, above the laundry at a cost of $9 million. While the medical advisory committee agreed in principle, members wanted more data as to financial implications. Finally, remembering the Commerce Court experience, the hospital made the decision to shift attention instead to demolition of the old C-wing and planning for stage B.[19]

Although the old C-wing, built in the late 1920s, was demolished in 1984, a part of it survives. A balustrade (window and balcony) that had stood at level two over the original entrance on Victoria Street in the middle of the building was salvaged by the planning department; after the stones of the balustrade had been sand-blasted, they were installed piece by piece in the Bond Street lobby to frame the plaque unveiled by Queen Elizabeth II on her visit to the hospital on 2 October 1984.[20]

Lastly, among the major renovation projects of this decade were those concerning reallocation of areas which the sisters, at their own expense, had provided for themselves when the E-wing was built in 1937 and their numbers were greater. The first to go was their community room on 5-E, a large bright room with well-polished parquet floor, facing Bond Street, which became in 1979 a spacious patient library. In 1982 a large part of their dining-room and all of their visitors' dining-room and large reception room were taken for hospital use. Two years later, all of their seventh floor (twenty-five rooms) was given over to provide the clinical, research, and administrative accommodations for an expanding division of cardiology. At a massive cost,[21] the sisters' rooms on 7-E, together with some patient rooms on 7-A and B, were converted to an eight-bed CCU (coronary care unit); a four-bed step-down unit (for patients who did not require all that was available in the CCU, but were not yet ready for transfer to a general patient unit); a pharmacology research laboratory; relocated ECG, echocardiograph, nuclear cardiology, and pacemaker facilities; seven doctors' offices; and secretarial and other related support services.

A Note about the Sisters' Presence

Mention was made earlier of the Second Vatican Council and the changes it inspired. As religious congregations responded to the council's call for renewal of religious life during the difficult and challenging period of transition to a post-conciliar church, numerous members left their congregations to continue their life and service in a secular context. The Sisters of St Joseph, too, lost many members – most, but not all of them, young sisters – in the years immediately following the council. With the council there came a new freedom for sisters to choose, in dialogue with religious superiors, fields of ministry which they judged better suited to their interest and gifts. As a result some sisters, while remaining in religious life, left the hospital field entirely. Many of these continued to serve the church in a variety of ministries: some in pastoral care in the parishes; some directly with the poor in and around Toronto, in western Canada, and even the Third World; and later a few chose to work among Toronto's immigrant and refugee peoples. Some of those who continued to serve at St Michael's preferred to live elsewhere in a less institutionalized setting. With all of these influences at work, the number of sisters living at St Michael's fell from fifty-six in 1975 to fifteen in 1985.[22]

Medical Departments: Issues and Developments

Cardiology and Cardiovascular Surgery

These divisions moved ahead aggressively, and in doing so put a heavy strain on the operating room and the intensive care unit as well as on the cardiovascular laboratory. The strain on the budget was similarly intense. One example is the lithium pacemaker, introduced around 1978, costing from $1200 to $1900 each; as the cost for these for inpatients was a hospital cost, some referring hospitals – in an effort to avoid cost to themselves – exerted pressure to have their patients admitted to St Michael's, rather than send them as outpatients.[23]

To relieve the strain on the intensive care unit, two additional ventilated spaces were provided in the adjoining ACU (acute care unit, for patients requiring extra nursing care, but not respiratory assistance) in 1980. Throughout this difficult time, Dr William Noble, director of the intensive care unit, took the lead in monitoring and safeguarding patient care, supporting the nursing staff, and negotiating the scheduling of cases with the surgeons.

In 1980 the hospital, acting upon a 1977 recommendation of an in-house cardiovascular review committee, provided a second catheterization laboratory fitted with the latest and best equipment.[24] (Two earlier external studies had recommended that St Michael's volumes should be increased to 500 open-heart surgical procedures and 1000 catheterizations annually.) The 1977 recommendations had pegged the numbers at 1000 catheterizations and 600 open-heart cases annually; by 1980 the same committee was recommending 1500 to 1600 catheterizations and 750 open-heart procedures annually, but the medical advisory board decided that the hospital had neither the physical nor the financial resources to handle such a volume; besides, other surgeons viewed with some alarm the unrelenting growth of this service.[25]

In 1981 the transluminal coronary angioplasty was introduced, a joint venture with the university and the Toronto General and Toronto Western hospitals. While the new procedure promised to be less expensive than the A-C by-pass, Dr Forbath (who was in the forefront of all the new developments in the cardiac laboratories) projected that within two years the hospital would be in critical need of still more laboratory space as well as new angiography equipment.[26] In the midst of this new development, coming after those just described, the cardiovascular surgeons received a jolt – their resident numbers would be cut by one. This was an attempt on the part of the Ministry of Health to impose some limits on expensive programs.

Dr John K. Wilson, as chief of cardiology, had guided his division to levels of patient care and diagnostic investigation undreamed of when he joined St Michael's staff on completion of his training, which by now had been supplemented by fellowship in the American College of Physicians (1966). All the benefits of a continually improving technology were put to use – cardioversion, heart-transplant techniques, echocardiography, angioplasty, stress testing, and the like. During his term Wilson assembled a highly qualified staff, including – besides those already mentioned – Drs R. Chisholm (1976), Michael Freeman (1980), T.R. Hale (1981), and Robert Howard (1981). As associate professor of medicine Wilson had introduced literally hundreds of undergraduate and dozens of post-graduate medical students to the wonders of this field, and was, as well, highly supportive of the nurses and the various technical groups associated with the cardiac service; this was a service nurses asked to go to. In 1981 Pope John Paul II conferred on Wilson the honour of knight commander of the Order of St Sylvester. In 1983 Wilson stepped down as chief and resumed a staff position; Dr Clare Baker resigned as chief of cardiovascular surgery at the same time. The new chiefs, Dr Paul Armstrong and Dr Tomas Salerno, would build upon the strong foundations already in place; the cardiology division's research potential had already been strengthened by the recent addition of Dr Michael Freeman and Dr Robert Howard.

Plastic Surgery[27]

Cardiac services was by no means the only area of growth during these years. Microvascular surgical techniques underwent vast improvement, enabling a team of St Michael's surgeons to perform in 1976 a muscle transplantation – the first in North America. Through the work of this same team (Drs Ralph Manktelow, Nancy McKee, and R.M. Zuker), St Michael's became established as the finger and hand transplantation centre for the Toronto area, Dr Manktelow having gone to Shanghai in 1977 to learn from Chinese surgeons there. When Manktelow was appointed head of plastic surgery at Toronto General in 1979, Dr McDougall preserved the range and depth of his division by the recruitment of Dr James Mahoney (1980) and Dr Susan McKinnon 1982).

Neurosurgery

St Michael's had one of the busiest neurosurgical units in the city during these years, under Dr Alan Hudson, professor and chairman of the neurosurgery department at the University of Toronto from 1979. Much of the emphasis within the division was on management of peripheral nerve injuries, a team effort under Dr Hudson, Dr McDougall (plastics), Dr James Waddell (orthopaedics), and Dr Henry Berry (clinical neurology and electrophysiology).[28] Increasingly the division collaborated in widely based and carefully designed studies directed from other cities and/or institutions. For example,

Dr W.S. Tucker, who joined the staff in 1976, directed the Toronto branch of a world-wide National Institutes of Health study on the timing of aneurysm surgery, organized from Iowa. Within the hospital there was close collaboration with orthopaedics for management of spinal problems, and with Dr Norman Struthers (urology) for management of patients with paralytic bladders.

In 1982 Dr Paul Muller, who had earlier served his residency at St Michael's, returned to the hospital from a University of Calgary appointment; he received from the University of Toronto a mandate to develop and direct a university-wide, multi-disciplinary brain-tumour group – including neurologists, radiologists, chemotherapists, and statisticians. There was already considerable expertise at St Michael's in the areas of neuropathology, neuroanaesthesia, and neuroradiology, and although Dr Hudson judged the operating room and its equipment at St Michael's inadequate for international-level work, he saw an opportunity in stages A and B of the new construction for the hospital to become one of the major neurosurgical units in North America. This was not to be; Dr Hudson was appointed professor and chairman of surgery in the university's faculty of medicine in 1989 and accordingly transferred to the Toronto General Hospital. Earlier Dr Muller had taken over as chief of neurosurgery at St Michael's, university regulations having precluded Dr Hudson holding simultaneously the dual position of chief and chairman of the division.

Orthopaedic Surgery

In 1980 Dr James Waddell (University of Alberta, 1967, FRCP [Canada]) succeeded Dr John Evans as chief of this division. That same year, Dr Thomas Robinson Sullivan was given a staff appointment and quickly leapt into prominence with the establishment of a bone bank and an orthopaedic-research program. Dr Sullivan's special interest was in bone-tumour surgery, with prosthetic and allograft replacement. He performed the first whole-bone transplant at St Michael's in July 1981. In March 1982 Sullivan ("Robin") met with a sudden untimely death by accident. Dr Waddell continued the clinical aspect of Sullivan's work for a time, while Dr Ray Sherman, a basic science research fellow, carried on the work of the research laboratory. In 1984 – after seeing his division further depleted by the departure to the United States of Dr John McCulloch – Waddell recruited Dr Robin Richards, whose interest lay in micro-vascular surgery and hand and upper-limb reconstructive surgery. With the

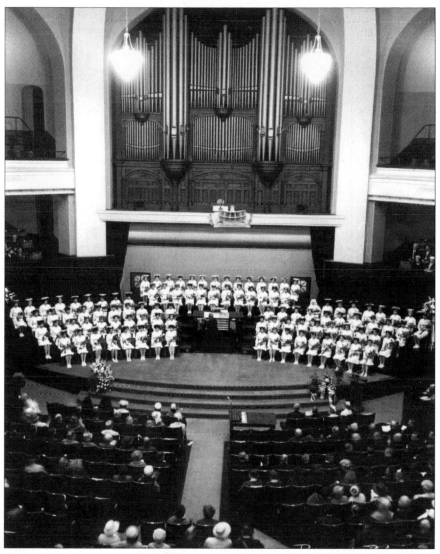

The golden years of the school of nursing – 101 nurses at their graduation at the University of Toronto's Convocation Hall, 1964.

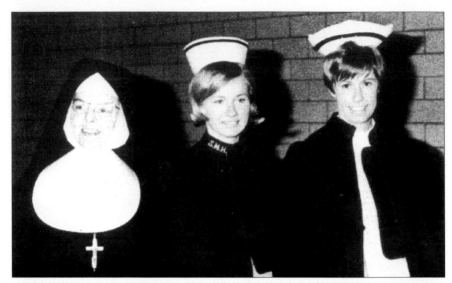

Sister de Sales Fitzpatrick, director of St Michael's school of nursing from 1958 to 1970, with two of the faculty.

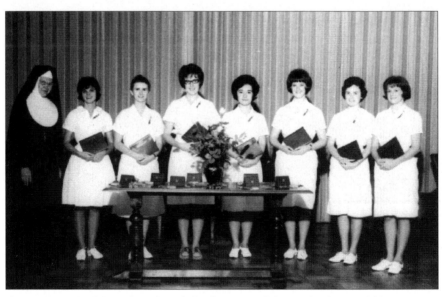

Sister Mary Paul Biss, founder of the first school for medical-record librarians in Canada in 1936, with a class of her graduates, *c*. 1960.

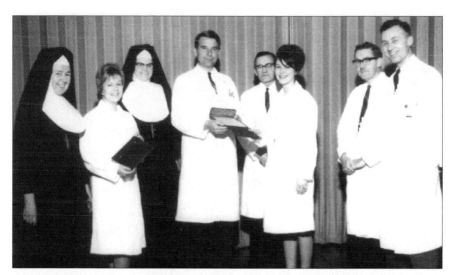

Graduation of medical-laboratory technicians, with their teachers, who were also heads of their divisions, left to right: Dr Roderick Ross (pathology), Dr Charles J. Bardawill (haematology), Michael O'Sullivan (biochemistry), and Dr Gordon Hawks (bacteriology), along with Sister Mary James McMahon, assistant administrator of the hospital, and Sister Michael Edward Allen, laboratory supervisor.

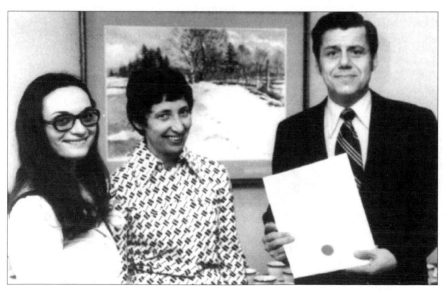

A pharmacy resident receives her diploma from Dr John Platt, associate executive director, medical (1965-92), and Mrs Martha Andrasko (centre), director of pharmacy (1973-85).

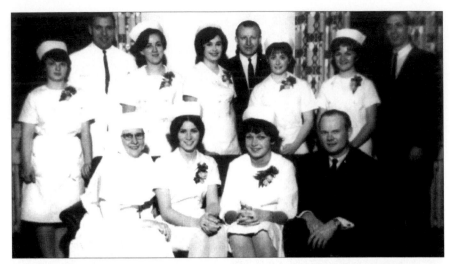

X-ray technologists on graduation day, with Sister Eucheria Smith, supervisor; Dr Bruce Bird, radiologist-in-chief, in the front row, and Drs J. Heslin, J. Sungailia, and Norman Patt in the back row, *c.* 1965.

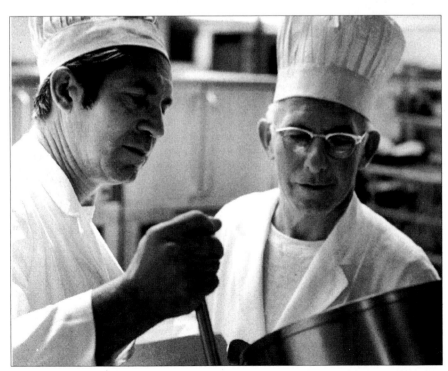

Harold Robinson, shown here on the right, with chef Charles Tagone, was food manager at the hospital for forty years (late 1930s to late 1970s), a period that spanned the hospital's growth to 900 beds.

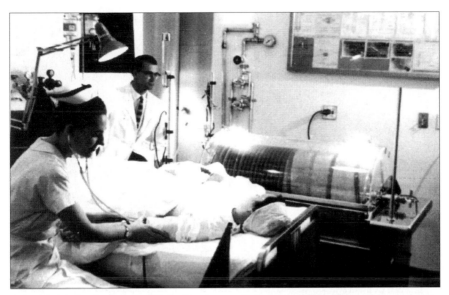

When St Michael's first established its haemodialysis centre in 1963 it chose one of its best medical nurses, Grace Duncan, shown here with an unidentified doctor, to learn the procedure.

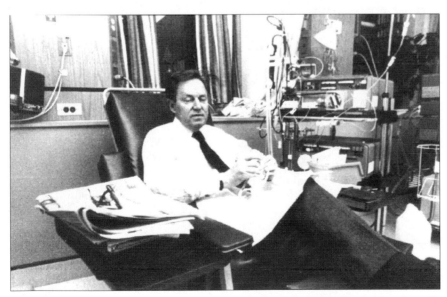

In 1992 highly motivated patients handle the treatment themselves under the self-care program offered in the hospital's renal unit.

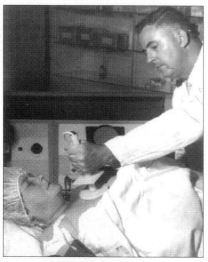

Dr John K. Wilson, chief of cardiology from 1969 to 1984, performed, with Dr Peter Forbath, Canada's first successful cardioversion to restore the heart's rhythm by means of electric shock (1963).

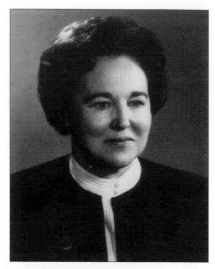

Sister Mary Zimmerman, executive director of St Michael's during the dynamic period from 1963 to 1985.

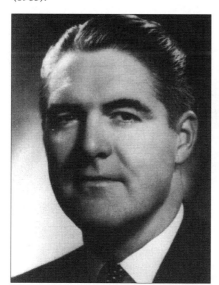

Robert A. Davies, who, as chairman of the board of directors from 1969 to 1975, powerfully represented the hospital's interests during these critical years of competition for the necessary building approvals and grants.

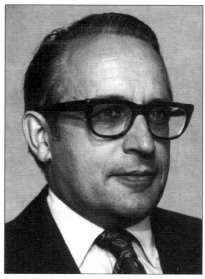

Dr William J. Horsey, neurosurgeon, chief of surgery, and chairman of the medical advisory board/committee during the period of vigorous growth from 1969 to 1984.

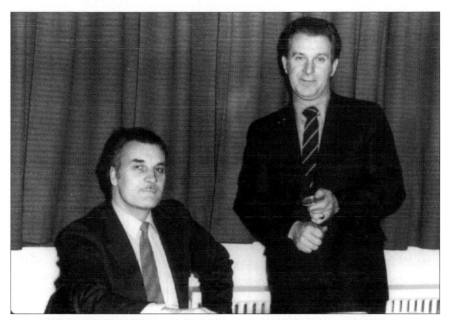

Chief engineer Harry Cunningham, seated, with his successor, Alan O'Brien, *c* 1970.

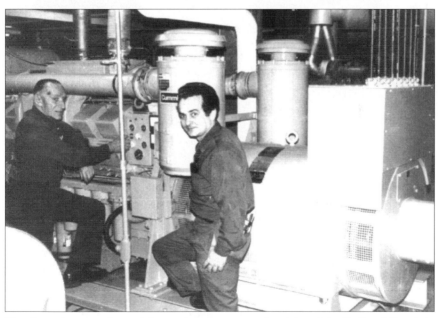

Two long-time members of the engineering team, electricians John Roff and Dominic Amelio, check out the 600-kilowatt diesel generator installed in 1976.

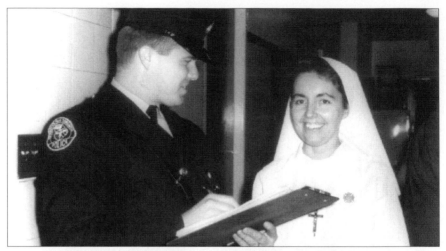

Because of its location in downtown Toronto, St Michael's has always had the police in and out of its emergency ward, investigating the injuries resulting from incidents on the streets or in the homes or lodgings roundabout. Here emergency supervisor Sister Mary Gordon (Rosemary McGinn) assists in the investigation, *c.* 1969.

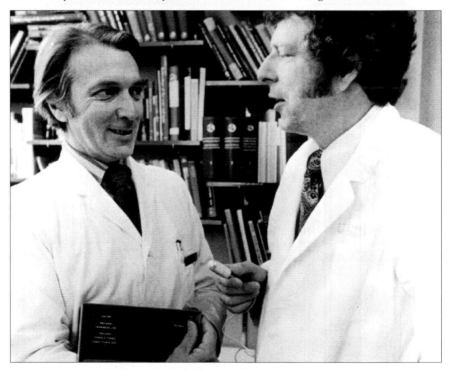

Dr C.A. Woolever, chief of obstetrics and gynaecology from 1964 to 1977, with Henry Benoit (right), and the electronic speculum (an aid in natural family planning) of which they were co-designers in 1976.

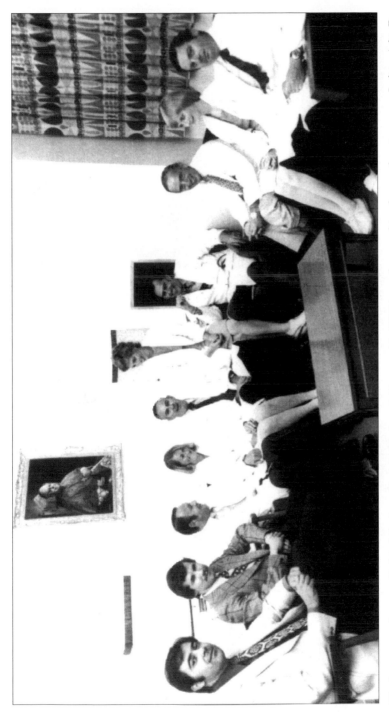

The heart team that went behind the Iron Curtain (Budapest, Hungary) in 1973 to perform and teach open-heart surgery. Left to right: Dr Tom Hanny, Dr Terry Theman (resident), Dr Clare Baker (chief, cardiovascular surgery), Tricia Root (ICU head nurse), Dr John K. Wilson (chief, cardiology), Anne Wetheral (pump perfusionist), Dr Donald Finlayson (anaesthetist), Dr Peter Forbath (specialist in heart catheterization), Sherry Ridgeway (operating-room nurse), and Dr William Young (anaesthetist).

249

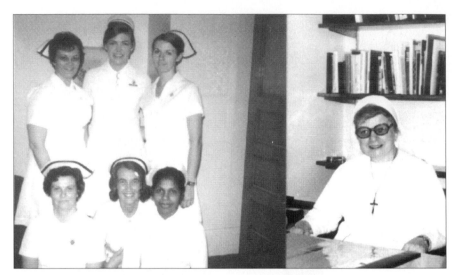

First graduating class of the twenty-one-week course in critical-care nursing, established in 1973 by Sister Marion Barron, director of the school of nursing, shown here on the right. Hospital head nurses Noreen Giommi (left in back row), and Mary Cassidy and Joan Foy (left and centre, front row), were among the graduates.

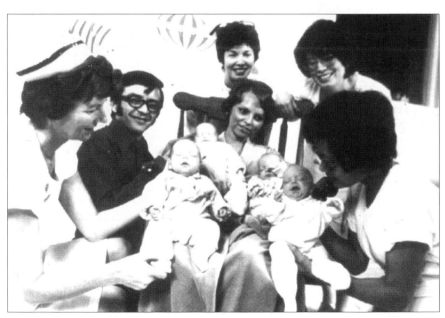

St Michael's first set of quadruplets, delivered by Dr Anthony Cecutti in 1975, shown here with their proud parents and nurses. Nursery head nurse Margaret Riddell is on the left, and nursing coordinator Charlene Shevlen is directly behind the mother.

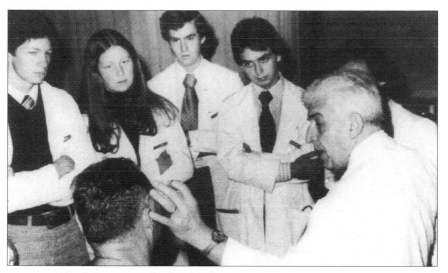

Dr Joseph T. Marotta, neurologist-in-chief from 1956 to 1969, and physician-in-chief from 1969 to 1979, with a group of very serious undergraduate medical students.

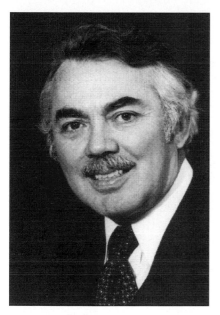

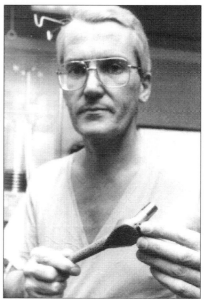

Dr Patrick Higgins, pioneer in the use of radioisotopes, long-time head of the radioisotope laboratory and of the division of endocrinology and metabolism, and physician-in-chief from 1979-89.

Dr James Waddell, chief of orthopaedics from 1980 to 1989, chief of surgery and chairman of the medical advisory committee from 1984 to 1989, shown with the St Michael's hip prosthesis which he designed.

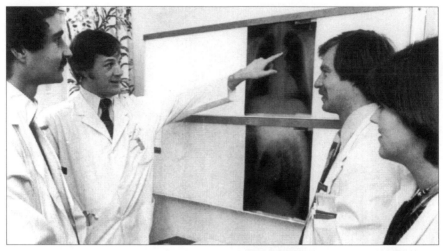

Dr Peter Kopplin, head of the division of internal medicine and director of ambulatory care (1971 –   ), instructing medical residents.

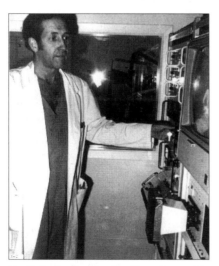

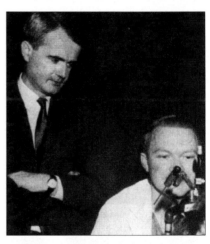

Dr Michael Shea, chief of ophthalmology from 1972 to 1992, supervising a resident in the use of the fixation light of the slit lamp.

Radiologist Dr Charles Gonsalves with the first scanner in Canada capable of producing cross-sectional pictures of the entire human body. Called the ACTA scanner, it was installed at St Michael's in December 1975.

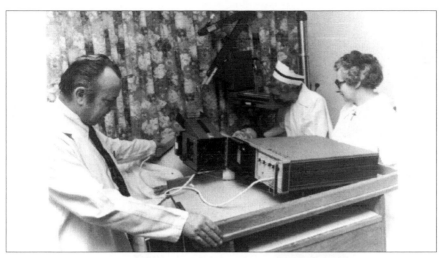

Dr Patrick F. Beirne, staff obstetrician from 1953 and chief of obstetrics from 1977 to 1983, checking a patient by means of the sonar monitor (ultra-sound) which he introduced to St Michael's. With Dr Beirne are nurses Ellen Cassidy and Sister Margaret Ann Hazelton, *c.* 1983.

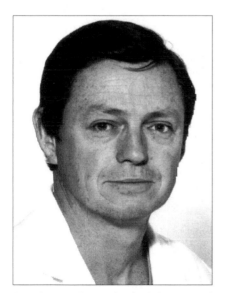

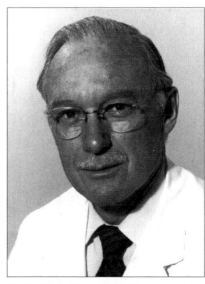

Dr Alan Hudson, chief of division of neurosurgery 1977 to 1979, then professor and chairman of neurosurgery at the University of Toronto from 1979 until 1989, at which time he left St Michael's to become chairman of surgery at the university and chief of surgery, Toronto Hospital.

Dr J. Alick Little, first director of the metabolic-investigation unit, coordinator of research and secretary of St Michael's Research Society from its inception in 1963 to 1991.

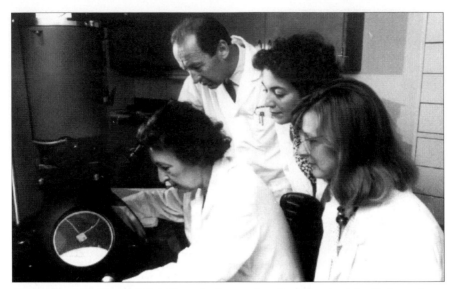

Drs Kalman Kovacs and Eva Horvath, internationally recognized for their work on the nature, function, and classification of tumours of the pituitary gland, shown at the electron microscope, with Dr Sylvia Asa and an unidentified physician in the foreground on the right.

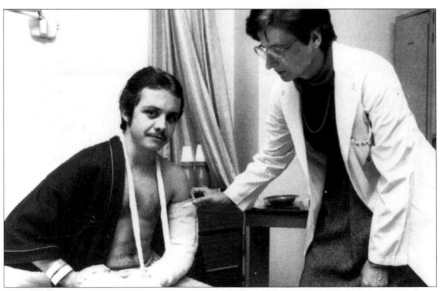

Dr Bernadette Garvey, prominent in the research of the American National Institutes of Health, who founded the centre for adult haemophiliacs at St Michael's in 1982 while serving as well as chief of the division of haematology. Dr Garvey has chaired the Ontario Advisory Committee on AIDS since 1984, and was the first woman to chair St Michael's medical advisory committee (1989-91).

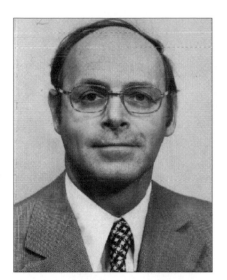

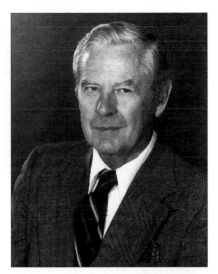

Dr T.D.R. (David) Briant, ophthalmologist-in-chief (1973 –   ) and chairman of medical advisory committee (1991 –   ).

Walter Johnson, PhD, who developed the hospital's vestibular testing facility. A qualified pilot himself, Dr Johnson has long been associated with the NASA aerospace program and has served on the Nobel Prize Selection Committee in medicine and physiology.

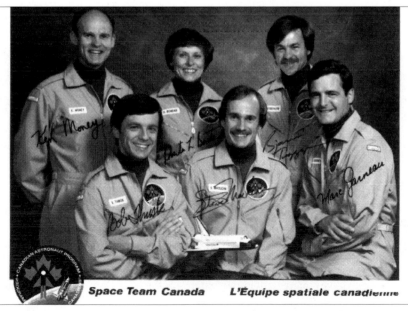

Space Team Canada   L'Équipe spatiale canadienne

Research for a Space Age: Canada's astronauts, all of whom have undergone pre-and post-flight testing in St Michael's vestibular laboratory; their autographed photograph was presented to Queen Elizabeth II when she visited St Michael's in 1984.

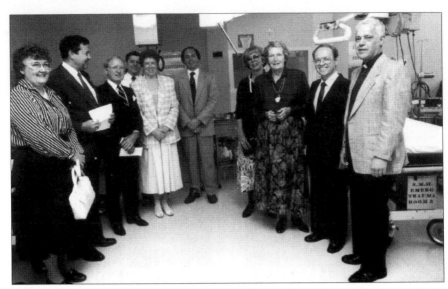

The Wallace B. Chalmers Trauma Unit opened at St Michael's in 1988. Left to right: Patricia McGee, from the Ministry of Health, Dr Martin Barkin, deputy minister of health; Patrick Keenan, board chairman; Dr John Platt; Sister Christine Gaudet, president; Dr Thomas Estall, director of emergency; Clarice Chalmers, generous benefactor of the trama service; Joan Chalmers; Dr William Tucker, head of trauma service; Father Charles Prance, chaplain-in-chief.

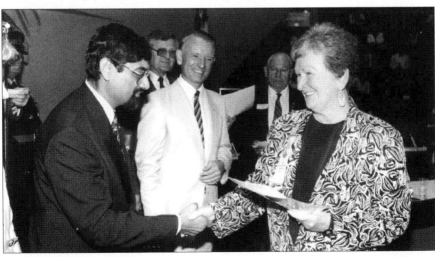

Marie McKeag, former president of St Michael's hospital auxiliary, and a volunteer for twenty-five years, shown receiving Canada's Birthday Achievement Award at Toronto City Hall 15 July 1991. Other hospital volunteers to receive awards were Eileen Murray, Margaret Shumata, Kitty Crofton, and Isabel McLean.

recruitment of Dr Ensor Transfeldt late in 1984, the division was up to strength again – its space needs met by a forty-one-bed unit at St Michael's, plus forty-four convalescent and a share of twenty amputee beds at Riverdale Hospital, as well as a few other beds at Hillcrest and Providence hospitals. In these years Piera Cardella, a St Joseph's (Toronto) graduate, capably provided the nursing leadership for the division.

Urology

Dr J.L.T. Russell remained chief of this three-man division until late 1982, continuing to be recognized as Toronto's foremost instructor of transurethral surgery; he was also active in securing research funds for the division. Dr Norman Struthers's interest was in the dynamics of both the upper and lower urinary tract, for the study of which he arranged the establishment of a urodynamics laboratory. He cooperated closely with the neurosurgeons in management of the traumatic neurogenic bladder and with the neurologists who were treating multiple sclerosis patients with neurological bladder problems.

Dr V. Colapinto's special interest, in addition to kidney transplantation, was in the male lower urinary tract, especially the anatomy and physiology of the urethral sphincters. As a result of his and Dr Struthers's work, St Michael's became a national referral centre for urethral diseases, particulary trauma and stricture. Weekly urology rounds were regularly attended by urologists from the non-teaching Toronto hospitals, and difficult urethral problems were referred from the other Toronto teaching hospitals.

In February 1985 Dr Colapinto took over as chief, envisioning a future when, with the facilities almost completed, St Michael's would be in a position to become the major centre for research and management of lower urinary tract diseases. He did not live to explore fully the possibilities of the new unit he had helped to plan.

General Surgery

Two new general surgeons joined the staff during these years: first, Dr Nicholas Colapinto, FRCS (Canada) – brother of Dr Vincent Colapinto – who had studied immunopotentiating agents at Harrow, England, under Sir Peter Medawar in 1974; and shortly afterwards, Dr Dennis Jirsch, FRCS (Canada), who had had extensive research experience at the University of Alberta. Dr Colapinto developed, with Dr R. MacKenzie of Wellesley Hospital, a technique for liver transplantation in humans, having done extensive experimentation with pig-liver transplants. In addition to developing some new techniques for old problems (liver abscess, thyroidism, inguinal hernia repair), Dr Colapinto became one of the few surgeons at the university to study the surgical care of the morbidly obese. Dr Jirsch studied, within a broad range of research interests, the complications of the immunosuppressed patient and, as well, the etiological agent and the surgical management of Crohn's disease, working closely with the physicians of the inflammatory bowel disease unit.

After sixteen years in the position, Dr Currie stepped down as chief of general surgery in 1984. His division had been recently strengthened by the addition of a thoracic surgeon, Dr Alex Patterson – Dr Horsey's last appointment before resigning as surgeon-in-chief in June 1984. Dr James Waddell became the new chief of surgery.

Members of the department of diagnostic imaging were deeply involved with developments in several of the above divisions – among them, Drs Charles Gonsalves and M.C. Chui, working with the neurosurgeons; Dr Ronald McCallum, in studies of the lower urinary tract with Dr Struthers; and Dr Norman Patt in cardiological research (especially echocardiography, and non-invasive procedures) and peripheral vascular disease.

The Department of Medicine

After thirty years at St Michael's, Dr J.T. Marotta left in 1979 to pursue his research interest in epilepsy at the Wellesley Hospital. His involvement with St Michael's was resumed a few years later in his capacity at the university as associate dean, institutional affairs, faculty of medicine, and as member of St Michael's board of directors. Dr Hubert Patrick McLoughlin Higgins, FRCP (Canada), FACP, succeeded Dr Marotta as physician-in-chief and professor, University of Toronto. After serving for three years in the Canadian Army in the United Kingdom and continental Europe, Higgins had obtained his medical degree at the University of Toronto in 1950. Following residencies and research appointments at St Michael's, Sunnybrook, and the Banting Institute, he studied for a year in London, England, on a McLaughlin travelling fellowship and returned to St Michael's in 1956 to concentrate in endocrinology and metabolism, becoming chief of that division in 1970. In the meantime he had done pioneering work in radioactive isotopes, serving as director of the radioactive isotope laboratory from 1956 to 1976; he also published extensively in his two broad fields of interest throughout these years.[29] Higgins resigned his active staff appointment at St Michael's in 1976 to accept the appointment of physician-in-chief at St Joseph's Hospital, Toronto. It was from here that he came to take up his new chief's duties at St Michael's in 1979, in which position he served until relinquishing it to Dr Joseph J. Connon in July 1989.

The division of respirology was in need of attention following the sudden death in 1978 of Dr Frederick G. Douglas, founder and director of the pulmonary function laboratory. Dr Peter Thomas, MBBS, MPCP, who had been on staff since February 1976, was made acting head in April 1980, and Dr Victor Hoffstein joined staff that same year.

The 1979 appointment to the division of dermatology of Dr James Nethercott became the catalyst for the development of a related new department, which will be discussed presently. Dr Paul Adams was appointed to the staff in 1980 and Dr H. Jacubovics in 1984.

With the departure of Dr Marotta, Dr Trevor Gray became head of neurology in 1980, and the division was strengthened by one further appointment, Dr N. Bayer, also in 1980.

In 1980 a new division of internal medicine was formed, under Dr Peter Kopplin as head, with Drs K.Y. Lee, R. Snikura, J. Zownir, G. Wong, and Robert Josse, the last holding a cross-appointment in endocrinology. The division of endocrinology lost Dr R. Lee in 1982 but gained Dr D. Jenkins in 1983. Dr William Singer became chief in 1983, freeing up Dr Tim Murray to devote more time to research.

In haematology, Dr J.J. Freedman (1976) and Dr J. Teitel (1981) joined Dr K. Butler and Dr M. Bernadette Garvey, who became chief of the division in 1982. Dr Robert Myers, appointed in September 1978, was the lone oncologist, Dr Goldie having resigned in 1976. Dr Rachel Shupak was appointed to rheumatology in 1981. The division of nephrology gained one new member, Dr Edward Cole, in 1984 when administration within the division was shared, Dr Michael Johnson and Dr Marc Goldstein becoming directors of peritoneal dialysis and haemodialysis respectively.

Large in numbers compared with the other medical departments, the department of medicine was similarly large in its research output. In 1981-82 St Michael's stood third among the eleven teaching hospitals of Toronto in allocation of research monies funded – $771,221.[30]

In 1979 St Michael's established, in the former north nurses' residence, a basic-science laboratory dedicated to the memory of John D. McDougald who had chaired the hospital's 1955 campaign for funds. To this Drs Timothy Murray and Mitchell Halperin moved their projects from the medical sciences building; a second laboratory established at this time was the hormone assay (thyroid, pituitary, and sex) laboratory under the direction of Dr William Singer.

Dr Mitchell Halperin – 1973 winner of the gold medal from the Royal College for his work in basic energy metabolism, and of the prestigious Gugenheim fellowship for his work on the action of insulin in 1982-83, which took him to Yale University for a year of research – contributed heavily to the developments within the division of nephrology. Here the work of the team of Halperin, Marc Goldstein, and Robert Bear on electrolyte disturbance earned them a world reputation.[31] This work, and the clinical application of it, particularly by Dr Bear as director of the division, was widely published.[32] In 1985 Drs Goldstein and Bear made a significant contribution to the treatment of chronic glomerulonephritis, the most common cause of kidney failure. The kidney-transplant program reached the 400 mark in 1986, with a success rate of more than 90 percent; that year the division was proud to publish in its report a photograph of one of its patients back at work one month following a kidney transplant – after eleven years of chronic dialysis.[33]

Dr Tim Murray's initial research at St Michael's was into the function of parathyroid hormone in bone tissue, and the control mechanisms in calcium metabolism. In 1980 he collaborated with Dr Robert Josse of the division of endocrinology in establishing a metabolic bone clinic, concerned largely with treatment of osteoporosis and, more significantly, a search for its cause.

In the field of haematology, Dr Bernadette Garvey received international recognition when in 1979 the American National Institutes of Health named her as chair of one of its major research-review committees, with the responsibility for recommending research grants of more than $200 million.[34] At home, she secured a substantial grant to carry out, in collaboration with Dr J. Freedman, a study of platelet cross-matching with a view to improving the prospects of patients with bleeding tendencies.[35]

And there was other research going on, including Drs Kovaks' and Horvath's collaboration with Dr Tim Murray in their continuing study of pituitary disease; Dr Clifford Ottaway's promising work on immunology of the gut, in connection with the work of the inflammatory disease clinic; and Dr Little's ongoing analysis of cardiovascular disease risk factors. While it is the department of medicine that is being reviewed at this point, research – an essential element, in Dr Marotta's words, underlying "the true vitality of the teaching hospital"[36] – was being carried out in a number of other areas: among them, Dr Walter Johnson's continuing study of vestibular disorders, and the research of Canadian astronaut Dr Kenneth Money, with Drs Johnson and Briant; the program of animal and human research in the pathophysiology of respiratory and circulatory problems during post-operative care, under the direction of Dr William Noble of the department of anaesthesia; and, in obstetrics and gynaecology, the work of the department's endocrine laboratory on sex hormones, as well as Dr Gerulath's studies in chemotherapy.

In 1982-83 the university administered grants in excess of $1.5 million for St Michael's researchers, and the hospital's Research Society administered a further $780,000; even so, with space at such a premium at St Michael's the medical staff was concerned that the building projects underway for research at the other university teaching hospitals would make it difficult to attract to St Michael's the staff needed to bring it a step farther among the academic institutions.[37]

The decade 1975-85 closed with the acceptance of St Michael's as one of two Toronto centres for the national study of screening for breast cancer in women, to be carried out in ten screening centres across Canada. Dr Leo Mahoney directed the St Michael's branch of the study, funded by the Cancer Institute of Canada.

Obstetrics and Gynaecology

Dr Patrick Beirne became chief of this department in 1977 following Dr Woolever's resignation to pursue his research interests at McMaster University in Hamilton. Dr Beirne was no newcomer to St Michael's. A native of Galway, Ireland, and a 1946 graduate in medicine from that country's National University, Beirne arrived in Canada in 1948 and, as he himself relates, walked to St Michael's from Toronto's Union Station, carrying his suitcase. After four years as intern and resident at St Michael's, he did post-graduate work at the New York Hospital and the Cornell Medical School, and obtained his FRCS (Canada) in 1953. Thereafter Beirne spent his entire professional career at St Michael's, through the ranks of staffman and assistant professor all the way to chief of the department and professor, University of Toronto.

Early in his career Dr Beirne wrote of "the beauty and even holiness of childbirth," of "the privilege of attending women in childbirth," and the importance of "training the mothers of tomorrow … for it is from them that emanates, unseen and unheard, the greatest single force behind peace and prosperity of a nation."[38] These were no empty words for Dr Beirne, but principles that guided his teaching and practice of obstetrics over a forty-year period.

Dr Beirne is believed to be the first obstetrician in Canada to have employed ultrasound techniques to see and treat a human embryo, and he used the experience so gained in his strong support of the pro-life movement,[39] of which he was a pioneer.

While the number of deliveries at St Michael's decreased by 50 percent over the years of Dr Beirne's practice – following the general decline in the national birthrate – Beirne made a very significant contribution to a side of the medical students' training that had hitherto been neglected: he was primarily responsible for engaging Abbyann Lynch, PhD, of the faculty of philosophy, University of St Michael's College, to lead a series of seminars on ethical problems for the department. Conducted for several years, the seminars were compulsory for the residents, interns, and clinical clerks in the department, and were at the time the only formal exposure to the ethical dimensions of patient care which they received during their medical education.[40]

Dr Beirne built upon the strong staff left by Dr Woolever, among whose last appointments was Dr Christine Derzko, who in 1976 became the first woman with an appointment to active staff in the department. Dr Beirne's appointments included Drs Titus Owolabi, D.V. Haraszthy, Michael Ing, and Louis Burgener; and during his tenure he accepted the resignations of three stalwarts of the department, Drs E. Stuart MacDonald, Gerald Solmes, and James Sorbara, all of whom had shared with him almost his whole career at St Michael's. Dr John Harper, long-time clinician/teacher and contemporary of all of these men, continued on active staff until 1991.

In 1983 Dr Beirne resigned, and Dr Constant Nucci, BA, MD, FRCS (Canada), FCOG, came from Montreal to be chief of the department. That same year Dr Rudi Borth resigned as director of the department's research laboratory, and Gregory Louis, PhD, assumed the position.

Anaesthesia

These were busy years for the department of anaesthesia, under Dr Arthur Dunn as chief until 1981, followed by Dr William Noble. To provide the round-the-clock service necessary for the increased volumes in the thirteen operating rooms, as well as the delivery rooms, cystoscopy, radiology, and the intensive care unit, staff was repeatedly increased, the appointments including Drs Robert Byrick, G. Goldenson, and G.M.G. Sanchez in 1977; Drs A.O. Davies and P. Cole in 1978; D. Bell in 1979; D. McKnight and Keith Rose in 1980; and G.B. Buczko in 1984. Anaesthesia was responsible for supervision of the respiratory therapy department, the quality of which was recognized in 1984 with the award of full three-year accreditation. As mentioned, the department of anaesthesia had an active research program in its own laboratory, unique among anaesthetic departments in the city, and an extensive commitment to the teaching of undergraduate and postgraduate medical students as well as critical care nurses and respiratory technicians. Dr Dunn's contributions to anaesthesia were recognized when he was awarded the Canadian Anaesthetists' Society medal for meritorious service at that body's annual meeting in 1981.

Psychiatry

Dr William Stauble guided the developments of this department until 1983. Remarkable among the appointments to his growing staff during these years was the number of women: Dr Donna Stewart was joined by Drs Farideh deBosset in 1977, Mary Lillie in 1981, and Ophelia MacDonald in 1984. Group psychotherapy was much emphasized on the inpatient units; the outpatient services were directed by Dr John T. Salvendy. Staff psychiatrists were active in the Association of Psychiatric Outpatient Centres of America, an international organization with membership from Canada, the United States, and Mexico, of which Dr David Divic and later Dr Salvendy served terms as president. A few staff psychiatrists were active in clinical research, Dr Salvendy and Dr Klaus Kuch both presenting papers at the annual meeting of the above association in Toronto in 1980. When Dr Stauble stepped aside as chief in 1983, Dr Donna Stewart – highly respected by medical, nursing, and social-work colleagues – acted as chief until the appointment of Dr Isaac Sakinofsky in the spring of 1984.

Ophthalmology and Otolaryngology

These departments moved into the decade 1975-85 under their respective chiefs, Dr Michael Shea and Dr David Briant. Both departments acquired markedly upgraded facilities with their move into the new C-wing, in the planning of which both men had been deeply involved. The department of ophthalmology, which was extensively reviewed earlier, added Dr M.D. Christianson to its members in 1980, and Dr Michael Howcroft in 1981.

During this decade Dr Briant did important studies on patients with recurrent laryngeal nerve injuries. Among the new appointments to the staff were Dr C. MacArthur (1977), Dr D. Rotenberg (1980), and Dr J.M. Willett (1983) Two non-medical members were also added, with allied health care staff appointments: in 1980, Kenneth Money, PhD; and in 1977 Lois Singer, who quickly gained recognition as the department's senior speech pathologist. Singer's research into the application of micro-computers in aphasic therapy was recognized in 1985 when the Speech Foundation of Ontario established the Lois Singer Research Fund in recognition of, and to assist in, this important line of research.

Radiology and Laboratories

Although radiology underwent a name-change in 1982, becoming the department of diagnostic imaging, its activities continued to be directed by Dr Bruce Bird, who was, as well, deeply involved in the expanded, expensive plans for the department in the new C-wing. Members of his department were heavily engaged in the advances of all the medical departments within the hospital. Early in this decade the department lost Sister Eucheria (who later resumed her baptismal name of Sister Rita Mary Smith). Sister Eucheria, a registered nurse, had studied x-ray technology under Dr Shannon and Sister Carmella, passed the qualifying examinations, and served for several years in the department before being appointed to Comox, British Columbia, for four years. Upon her return from there in 1958 Sister Eucheria assumed the non-medical administrative and teaching responsibilities of the department. She shared with staff and students not only her technological expertise but also her own philosophy of patient care – particularly her deep respect for the feelings and the dignity of each patient. When she resigned in 1973 to become director of nursing of the Clinical Institute, Addiction Research Foundation, the same caring, competent attention to patients was continued under chief technologist Lynn Mongeau. St Michael's course in x-ray technology, which had been offered since the 1940s, became the nucleus of a three-year pilot project between 1967 and 1970: students, with their teachers, came from three hospitals (Toronto Western, the Hospital for Sick Children, and the Wellesley) to do their training at St Michael's. Following this experiment it was but a short step to relocate the course to the new Toronto Institute of Medical Technology in 1972 – a move furthered by the prevailing philosophy of removing education out of service institutions and into educational ones.

The laboratories were directed by Dr Robert Lee Patten (McGill University, MDCM, 1962; residencies at Montreal General Hospital, 1962-70; FRCP and FRCS [internal medicine], 1969; FRCP and FRCS [Medical Biochemistry], 1970). As clinical biochemist-in-chief and associate professor at the University of Toronto from 1974, Patten was superbly qualified to collaborate in the research and its clinical applications being undertaken at this time. Roderick Ross, pathologist-in-chief, and vice-chairman of the medical advisory board for several years, resigned in 1980; Dr David Murray, MB, ChB, MRC (Path.), a Glasgow man, came from the Montreal General Hospital and McGill University to head the department. Also in 1980, Dr Norman Hinton, FRCP (Canada), past-chairman of microbiology at the University of Toronto, came to fill the position left vacant a year earlier by the resignation of Dr Gordon Hawks, microbiologist-in-chief.

Patient Care Evaluation Committee

The surveyors from the Canadian Council on Hospital Accreditation (CCHA) had jolted the medical staff when it handed down in 1978 a provisional one-year accreditation, recommending that the medical staff study its committee structure, record keeping, and clinical audit.[41] The main point at issue was the current system for the evaluation of medical care (retrospective medical audit and clinical appraisal), which the CCHA considered no longer adequate. The medical staff had belatedly begun a response[42] to the CCHA's strong endorsement of the method of "criterion audit"[43] but had made little progress by the time of the accreditation survey.

Now the medical staff disbanded its existing departmental record and audit committee and formed one patient care evaluation committee under the chairmanship of Dr Leo Mahoney, and though severely hampered by the lack of appropriate computer assistance, set about applying the recommended methodology. Within the year Dr Mahoney reported to the medical advisory board that the new system had merit – it uncovered deficiencies in the audits of some disease conditions and established the value of certain procedures.[44] The method revealed, as well, the occasional tendency to over-prescribe,[45] particularly on the part of the interns.

In October 1979 the CCHA acknowledged the tremendous efforts underway and awarded a two-year accreditation;[46] in 1981, and again in 1984, full three-year accreditation status was granted. In 1984 the department of dentistry, in a separate survey (its first), received full three-year accreditation.

Patient Care Services

The programs begun or expanded during these years are remarkable, not so much for their number as for their uniqueness and their cost.

Among the six clinics to be mentioned in this connection is the inflammatory bowel disease clinic, pioneered by Dr E.J. Prokipchuk in 1969. Prokipchuk had served as fellow in gastroenterology at Johns Hopkins Hospital, Baltimore, obtained his FRCP (Canada) in 1960, and was appointed to the division of gastroenterology at St Michael's in 1963, becoming chief in 1968. Because of the additional research within the division after Dr Clifford Ottaway's appointment in 1977, the physical facilities were enlarged to take in a row of rooms on the 3B-F corridor.

The family life clinic, begun by Dr Woolever in 1974 with a focus on fertility awareness and responsible parenthood, was expanded and revitalized with the appointment in 1977 of Sister June Dwyer, fresh from her years at Lakehead University, where she earned a BScN, a BA in Psychology, and the dean's medal.

A peripheral nerve injury clinic was established in 1980 under an interdepartmental/divisional team of Drs Alan Hudson, Peter McDougall, James Waddell, and Henry Berry. A sports medicine clinic, staffed by the department of family practice in cooperation with orthopaedics and rehabilitation medicine, was established in 1981. A pain clinic, in which the department of anaesthesia was heavily involved, was begun in 1983. Finally, a multiple sclerosis clinic and an occupational disease clinic were important new initiatives.

In addition, there were the new units, centres, or services: the oncology day care unit and the metabolic day care unit in 1979 – occupying the same physical facilities on alternate days, on 2-D south, linked to their parent facilities on 6-AS and 6-B via rotation of staff through the new units from the inpatient areas. Here the cancer patient, who might spend the better part of a day receiving a blood transfusion, or the new diabetic patient spending hours learning about his/her disease and its management, would have a more inviting and comfortable environment. There were also the St Lawrence Neighbourhood Health Services (1979), the services devoted to trauma (1981), and the centre for the care of adult haemophiliacs (1982), all of which will now be described in greater detail.

The Multiple Sclerosis Clinic

This centre developed out of the interest and initiative of Dr Trevor Gray, FRCP (Canada), chief of the division of neurology and chairman of the medical advisory board of the Ontario division of the Multiple Sclerosis Society. Prior to the establishment of the clinic in 1980, patients from Toronto (estimated to number about 1500) had to travel to Hamilton or London for regular supervision and care. Now Dr Gray 's team – neurologist, nurse coordinator, social worker, physical and/or occupational therapist – would be responsible for the primary care of these patients, reporting their findings and intervention to the patient's family physician. From the first, Gray set in place all the requirements for enquiry into the manifestations, diagnosis, prognosis, and cause of this chronic disease which affected so many young adults in the prime of life. Operating costs of the new clinic were borne by the Multiple Sclerosis Society, with the hospital providing the space, furnishings, and equipment, all located on 2-D south.

The Centre for Occupational and Environmental Health

With 10,000 industries in Metro Toronto subject to the regulations of Ontario's new Occupational Health and Safety Act, Dr James Nethercott, chief of dermatology, submitted a proposal in 1980 to the minister of labour which would provide consultation services, investigate conditions of work, conduct toxicologic studies, and serve as a resource base for these industries and their employees. The proposal was accepted, and in 1981 the first multidisciplinary clinic in Canada for occupationally related illnesses was opened at St Michael's under Dr Nethercott's direction.[47]

Dr Nethercott's team was among the most wide-ranging in the hospital: a joint venture of the University of Toronto's faculties of medicine and of engineering and of St Michael's Hospital, the team included medical and surgical specialists, members of the university's department of chemical engineering, a certified industrial hygienist, statisticians, research assistants, librarian, and others. A computer terminal was installed in the hospital's medical sciences library to allow a rapid search of literature. Operating costs were partially borne by the Ministry of Labour ($400,000 over three years) plus a grant from the J.P. Bickel Foundation.

The scope of the centre's work quickly became as wide-ranging as its staff – from hearing loss to contact dermatitis, and from back problems to fume intoxication. Dr Nethercott was appointed professor and director of the university's occupational and environmental unit in 1982, while remaining director of the hospital's department; in 1988 he resigned from both, to assume a similar appointment at Johns Hopkins University, Baltimore.

The St Lawrence Community Health Centre

In a turn of events reminiscent of 100 years earlier, Toronto's medical officer of health approached St Michael's in 1979 with a proposal that the hospital team up with his department to provide health services for the new planned community of 10,000 people taking shape in the heart of the old town of York, to be called the St Lawrence Neighbourhood.[48] After months of negotiations, during which time the Ministry of Health gave formal assurance of the necessary financial assistance, this first community health centre jointly directed and staffed by a hospital and the city health department was opened in 1981.[49]

In a further replay of the events of 100 years earlier, a member of city council raised the question of religion and religious symbols: she objected to the crucifix mounted on the wall of each room. It had been traditional at St Michael's that each patient room and each treatment room have displayed on its wall a small crucifix, the reminder of God's abiding covenant with His people. Now the councillor was demanding that the crucifixes go but Sister June Dwyer, the centre's director, stood firm; she met with city officials, where she outlined the centre's enterprising plans and programs, and the objections disappeared. In the meantime, one of St Michael's doctors had strongly challenged the councillor and her supporters through the press.[50] In 1992 the centre is thriving, the crucifixes still mounted on the walls.

Comprehensive Care Centre for Adult Haemophiliacs

Recognizing that the care available to the almost 200 adult haemophiliacs in and around Toronto was fragmented and crisis-oriented, hospitals were invited by the Canadian Haemophilia Society in 1982 to submit applications to establish a centre for their care. After a study of all the hospital proposals, an external review panel acting for the society recommended that St Michael's assume this responsibility.

Dr Bernadette Garvey, as director of the new centre, assembled a broad-based multidisciplinary team (physicians, rheumatologists, surgeon, physiotherapist, social worker, dentist, coagulation therapists, psychiatrist) which would provide a comprehensive health-care service to the patient and his/her entire family, designed to assist them in living as normal lives as possible; not only their biological needs, but also their social, educational, employment, and emotional problems were to be addressed. The first two years' funding for the centre, including the salary of nurse-coordinator Ann Harrington, had already been raised by the Canadian Haemophilia Society when the centre was officially opened by a representative of the minister of health on 24 November 1983.

Department of Ambulatory Care

The clinics and services just described arose out of the hospital's efforts to respond to the Ministry of Health's repeated injunction that all hospitals must find alternatives to expensive inpatient care, without sacrificing the quality of care. While the ministry was hinting at reducing inpatient beds to 3.5 per 1,000 of population in Metro Toronto (down from 4.0), St Michael's had, early in the 1975-85 decade, already reduced its beds to 701, down from 900. Its outpatient volumes had risen from 75,000 visits in 1969 to 161,808 visits in 1984-85, and its day-care surgical procedures in the operating room had risen to 5,366 – more than 24 percent of the total operating room volume.[51]

Directing the development of ambulatory care from 1971 was Dr Peter Kopplin (University of Toronto, 1963; FRCP [Canada], and post-doctoral fellow at the Yale School of Epidemiology and Public Health in Medical Care, 1969-70). The hospital had entered the decade with clinics on four levels of the old C-wing, all under Dr Kopplin's direction with the exception of the obstetrics and gynaecology clinic which was adjacent to its inpatient research areas, under its own chief. The departure from the old centralized pattern would be further extended with the move into the new C-wing when the clinics for ophthalmology, otolaryngology, and the neurosciences were each established next to their inpatient units, each under its chief.

In addition to the highly specialized clinics within the hospital, there were the new primary care, family practice clinics; these grew rapidly and were responsible for much of the increased volume of the 1980s. About this time the department of family practice became involved in the treatment of political refugees who had been victims of torture, beginning with a number of Chilean refugees who were referred to Dr Philip Berger for counselling and treatment. The extensive documentation of these and other refugees cared for in the department was the basis for Berger's paper on refugee medicine at the Amnesty International Conference in Greece in 1978, and for publications at home designed to create among Canadian physicians an awareness of the spread of torture.[52]

The *Bond Issue* (the hospital's news magazine) of June 1980 and December 1983 record the action of others in the hospital community on behalf of refugees and political detainees. One of the hospital's night-elevator operators picketed the Polish Consulate in Toronto every day for three solid months in a successful bid to have exit visas issued to his two daughters detained in Poland. In 1980 a nurse and a medical resident from St Michael's became part of a team of three nurses and three doctors in a four-week United Nations relief program in Hong Kong, helping Vietnamese refugees in a prison camp of 15,000 persons. By 1983 the hospital itself had employed fourteen refugees, under a special refugee assistance program funded by the federal government. Many of these men and women – from Poland, Hungary, Latvia, Roumania, Cambodia, South Vietnam, Iran, and El Salvador – had been well-trained professionals in their own countries (chemical, civil, flight, and electrical engineers; land surveyor; industrial psychologist; opera singer). All were grateful for their new "very nice, very good, free country," cherishing especially their freedom to work, to travel, and to have a legal place of residence.

The other two areas of rapid growth were outpatient psychiatry (including a mental health day-treatment program), and the venereal disease clinic, which in 1979 was the largest in Ontario. All of the clinics, both hospital and satellite (Broadview, St Lawrence), provided much needed clinical material for the doctors who faced the challenge of accommodating their teaching approach to the shrinking number of beds.

Over this sprawling "archipelago" (Dr Kopplin's term) was nursing coordinator Sister Barbara Grozelle, who knew and was known by name by the large majority of the regular visitors to the clinic. She was a tireless advocate on their behalf – literally feeding the hungry and clothing the naked, as outpatient sister-supervisors had done all through the years.

The emergency department had long been almost an orphan within the hospital family; while a study of the city's emergency departments in 1977 revealed that St Michael's was the second busiest of them all,[53] the hospital had no one physician whose sole responsibility was emergency. In 1979-80 Dr Kopplin headed a small committee charged with advising the medical advisory board on the necessary action to be taken; as a result, Dr Thomas Estall was appointed in 1980 clinical director of emergency, responsible to the director of ambulatory care. The following year, emergency was given departmental status.

Dr Estall's initiative and leadership became immediately evident – mainly in his provision within the year for twenty-four-hour physician coverage[54] and establishment of teaching rounds for interns, but also in his obtaining a firm commitment from the police for ready action and help with the increasing incidence of violence in emergency, as well as his respectful message, even to senior colleagues, that he would not stand for abuse of the emergency as a "back door" to admitting. The expanded and vastly improved emergency department was planned during his tenure, with significant input into the development by nursing coordinator Catherine (Kelly) Jirsch, who drew on her background in emergency nursing at New York City's Polyclinic and at St Michael's.

Medical Education: Undergraduate and Post-graduate

Those of the medical staff involved in undergraduate teaching entered this decade on a confident note: both in 1976 and 1977 students from St Michael's ranked first overall among the teaching hospitals in Toronto on their LMCC scores; among the students entering their final year, a majority named St Michael's as their first choice for clinical internship;[55] and in 1978 Drs Kovacs and Horvath participated, by invitation, in a course in pathology of the endocrine glands at Harvard Medical School – two out of the first three non-Harvard people to be invited.[56]

The results of the clinical teachers' work were clearly evident, and agreed upon; there was little university-hospital staff consensus, however, on what constituted "full time clinical teacher" status in terms of time and activities, remuneration, and accountability. This became one of the most hotly debated issues of 1979-80, both at the university, and with and within its teaching hospitals.[57] Amidst the confusion and conflict, the voice of reason and moderation in the person of Dr Horsey stands out – reflective, conciliatory, and loyal, but also aware of the competing interests at work.[58] At the height of the debate, much of it tied to money, Horsey outlined the real priority: each chief must make certain that there be no confusion as to who was responsible in the teaching system. There must be the palpable presence of a staff member who was ultimately running the show and who could be held accountable at all times.[59]

Among the issues at stake, but by no means the central one, was entitlement for medical secretarial staff and their classification for salary purposes. With the recurring problem of a budget overrun for clinical education each year (by more than $200,000 in 1979), the hospital refused in 1980 the increased costs attached to reclassification of their secretaries by a committee of the medical staff studying the matter.

More serious, in terms of the future of the post-graduate teaching programs, was the intervention of the Ministry of Health in its efforts to control costs and the over-supply of physicians identified by the Hall Royal Commission of 1980. In late 1980 the ministry asked hospital boards to consider freezing staff privileges at existing levels for both general practitioners and specialists. It was acting on data from its medical manpower advisory committee which showed that the number of physicians billing OHIP (the Ontario Health Insurance Plan) in the past year had increased by 558 (instead of the projected 250-300), resulting in a shortfall in its 1980-81 budget of $30-50 million. Further, only 36 percent of the current resident posts were being used to train specialists who would be practising in Ontario.[60]

In September 1981 the ministry announced its plan to control costs: ministry funding for residency posts would be reduced by 2 percent of trainees in 1981-82, then 15 percent over the next three years in all five Ontario health sciences centres – 200 post-graduate trainees in all. The university was involved in choosing where the reductions would be made; those services showing the fewest "academics" (educational value to the resident, papers produced, and meetings attended) would be the first to lose resident staff.[61] In January 1982 cuts of twenty-five residents from the Toronto teaching hospitals were announced, effective 1 July 1982, among them one cardiovascular surgery resident from St Michael's.[62] To discourage departments from recruiting residents and paying them from departmental funds, the ministry warned that it would "consider" penalties, for example, loss of a training post for each landed-immigrant specialist recruited to Ontario.[63]

In August 1982, with reductions of 5 percent (sixty-five posts) still scheduled for 1983, the Ministry of Health changed course: as part of a national program of manpower planning for health care, it would allow medical schools to maintain their present enrolments of residents on condition that they produce more specialists in family and community medicine, public health, radiation oncology, psychiatry, anaesthesia, rehabilitation medicine, geriatrics, emergency medicine, and neonatology. That is, the ministry's thrust seemed to be away from hospitals and more toward environmental health and prevention of disease.

Within the context of these foreshadowings of what the future might hold, the medical staff began a comprehensive review, chaired by Dr Michael Shea, of its post-graduate programs and what it must do to preserve them. Meanwhile the undergraduate program had continued to be very successful under Dr Norman Struthers, program director from 1975 to 1981: ten of the thirty students obtaining top honours in 1981 had been at St Michael's for their final year, including the gold medallist, both silver medallists, and four women.[64] The hospital continued to rank high among the hospitals-of-choice for general and rotating internships, and to receive very favourable appraisal by the Royal College.[65]

Trauma

The treatment of patients with multiple injuries was a part of life at St Michael's since its earliest days. Suddenly in the 1980s, however, the development of the facilities required to care for adult "trauma patients" (patients who have sustained injury to two or more body systems) became an issue among Toronto's teaching hospitals, sparked by the rumour that the Ministry of Health was considering approval of a second level I trauma unit – in addition to the one at Sunnybrook which was being used to capacity. In late 1981 Dr J. Waddell, chief of orthopaedics, presented to the board of directors a proposal for establishing the unit at St Michael's. The board approved submission of the proposal to the DHC on condition that such a unit entail no capital cost to the hospital.[66]

Informed in February 1983 that both Toronto General and St Michael's had serious proposals before the DHC, the board made it clear that if St Michael's were chosen the matter should be brought back to the board for assurance of funding before any plans for establishing a unit were implemented. This directive was reinforced in June 1983.[67] In the interval, a survey team from the American College of Surgeons, which had been asked to review the two proposals for the DHC, recommended that St Michael's be the site. The DHC asked for a further opinion, that of a faculty of medicine task force. This body, too, recommended that St Michael's be designated and urged St Michael's medical staff to make trauma the main focus in its strategic planning;[68] the task force also recommended that the Ministry of Health designate major trauma as a life support program, eligible for special ministry funding. Six months elapsed before the DHC finally recommended to the ministry that both St Michael's and the Toronto General be designated.[69]

Meanwhile the board was concerned that trauma cases were already being referred to St Michael's, and the chairman advised the Ministry of Health by letter that St Michael's would not accept the status of a trauma referral centre unless full funding was assured.[70] In a February 1985 meeting with ministry officials, while it was admitted that St Michael's had experienced an immediate and dramatic increase in referred trauma cases once the DHC recommendation was made known, the ministry declined to confirm that the $4-million increase to the funding base, announced that day, was specifically addressing the trauma-unit funding situation.[71] In its April 1985 press release announcing the increased funding, the ministry acknowledged St Michael's "substantial growth in multiple injury and other trauma cases," but it indicated that the increase was intended as well to assist the hospital to continue to provide an expanded cardiovascular service and a haemophiliac care centre (funded by the Canadian Haemophilia Society until 31 March 1985).

This uncertainty around operating costs for trauma continued for a further three years until the Ministry of Health confirmed by letter in January 1988 the designation of St Michael's as a level I adult trauma unit, one of only two such trauma centres in Toronto, and eligible for ministry funding for costs incurred in its trauma program.[72]

Non-medical Programs

The attention to medical ethics begun by Dr Beirne and Professor Abbyann Lynch in the department of obstetrics and gynaecology in 1977 was broadened and given tremendous impetus by the appointment in 1982 of George Webster as the ethics coordinator to the congregation's health-care institutions. Webster held a bachelor of sacred theology degree, an MA, and MDiv, and was completing his doctor of ministry studies. To deal with the ambiguities resulting from the advances in medical capabilities, Webster established a number of ethics subcommittees – beginning with the critical-care and palliative-care units – initiated rounds of the intensive care unit devoted to ethical issues, and made himself available to individuals and groups for consultation related to their concerns in patient-care issues.[73]

There were continuing efforts in staff development. Historically, the person chosen to be manager or supervisor in any of the hospital's professional or service departments was one who had demonstrated competence in the technical requirements of the department. Recognizing that this person did not necessarily make the best manager, the hospital in 1979 initiated a program, in connection with George Brown College, designed to provide a basic level of training in supervision across all of the hospital departments.

With the appointment of Bronwyn Morgan as personnel officer (later director) in 1980, the work of the personnel department reached a new level of professionalism; gone were the days when a position could be terminated with the simple appearance of a disgruntled orderly at the door of the secretary-treasurer's office with the announcement, "I'm handin' in my pants."[74] Morgan tailored the employment, progress, and termination process along with the personnel files into a highly effective system. Among the early initiatives undertaken by this capable woman was an in-house, two-year program designed to further management staff's understanding of such concepts as decision-making, management of time, and handling conflict. Later, with the help of a steering committee with wide hospital representation, she undertook a broad assessment of staff needs and developed a program ranging all the way from workshops in motivation to the very necessary foundations of hospital funding and hospital budgeting – the latter an area in which managers were increasingly being held accountable.

Together with its "learning" salaried staff, the hospital had waves of students from all the health disciplines (up to 225 in a 1981 survey) descending upon it each September – fresh and young, some a bit apprehensive, almost all idealistic and enthusiastic. None paid a tuition fee to the hospital, which provided lockers, laboratory facilities, and access to the employees' health unit to all students in all programs – the hospital's investment in their future and its own, as well as in the public's health care. A large proportion of these students eventually joined the staff.[75]

And there were two other programs narrower in scope: in 1979 the hospital began to offer, in conjunction with George Brown College, courses in English as a second language, attended mainly by staff from the dietary and housekeeping departments; and interested staff were given an opportunity to upgrade their French-language skills in a program specially funded by the Ontario government.

Quality-assurance and Risk-management Programs

These two programs, closely connected and using much of the same data, were established in 1983 in response to the most recent requirements of the Canadian Council on Hospital Accreditation.

Through the quality-assurance program, provision was made for internally administered audits of the quality of care and service provided in every hospital department; the aim was to ensure that the necessary procedures were in place to meet their department's and the hospital's goals, and to correct any deficiencies. Some of the components were already in place – particularly in nursing, which had established formal audits ten years earlier – but the latest initiative provided a framework for refinement and coordination. Dorothy Ann Finlay was seconded from nursing staff development to assist Dr Platt in coordinating the hospital-wide effort.

The parameters of the risk-management program were deceptively simple: to identify, evaluate, and reduce the risks of losses, including financial. Its implementation involved the collection and analysis of data on a wide range of policies, practices, and functions – all the way from patient safety to product evaluation.

The Move into Computerization

The first[76] automated installation for hospital (non-medical) use was the General Electric "maxifile" installed in the radiology department in 1977. Capable of storing up to 2.5 million patient records, with an information-retrieval time of less than three seconds, the maxifile provided a giant step forward in the effectiveness, variety, and accuracy of radiology information previously available in the manual filing system. Terminals were installed at the film-storage building up the street at 209 Victoria. The whole system was leased for $35,000 a year but promised to make redundant three to five staff, thus becoming one of the earliest instances of staff being replaced by technology at St Michael's.[77]

Communication capability was significantly improved with the introduction in 1979 of bell-boys capable of sending a signal sixty miles, and also of by-passing the switchboard completely and communicating bell-boy to bell-boy if the sender was in the hospital.

In late 1979 a computer review committee, chaired by Larry Thalheimer, was established to assess the requirements for a planned, total hospital system. In mid-1981 selection from the computer market began, and by 1983 payroll, management reporting, and accounts payable became the first hospital functions to be computerized. Raymond Briggs assumed direction of the department of information systems in 1983 and four years later the medical records department became the first department in the hospital to be fully computerized, with a data base on 400,000 patients who had visited St Michael's in the past ten years.[78]

Expansions, Consolidations, and Closings

The detoxification unit on Adelaide Street, which was opened in 1973 and funded specially by the Ministry of Health through the hospital budget, was by 1982 admitting 2,500 men annually. Aware of their need for rehabilitation services, Sister Anne Marie Carey formed in 1975 St Michael's Half-Way House, Inc.; the following year she opened the first half-way house, funded 80 percent by the Ministry of Community and Social Services. Two years later Sister Anne Marie saw the need for housing for single elderly men who were drinking through loneliness and lack of community support; to meet this need, the city agreed to rent to the board of the organization, which had been renamed St Michael's Half-Way Homes, two semi-detached houses on Carleton Street which were christened Matt Talbot House. Here Sister Anne Marie and her staff continue in 1992 their efforts to help the chronic alcoholic towards increasing periods of sobriety, and eventually to total abstinence and a happy stable life.

The social work department in 1982 extended its services to take over discharge planning, together with ambulance bookings, for the ninety or more St Michael's patients discharged each month to nursing homes or chronic hospitals after waiting periods of up to four months for the former and six for the latter. The contribution (teaching, field supervision) of Les White and his staff to the university's school of social work continued to earn the school's grateful recognition.[79]

When the department of rehabilitation medicine lost its medical director, Dr James Houston, in 1979 it was fortunate to have in place a well-qualified staff of physiotherapists and occupational therapists under the direction of Inna Wester. The hospital's move into tertiary care called for specialization within this staff, together with special assessment tools and assistive devices: for the brain-injured, computer software to promote cognitive and perceptual retraining and facilitate visual-motor pursuits; for the patient after upper-limb reconstruction, ultrasonic therapy and a variety of electrical apparatus to promote nerve stimulation. Adequate ventilation for the patient in the intensive care unit was another area of emphasis. In 1984 this department became the first department of rehabilitation medicine among the general hospitals in Toronto to be accredited by the Canadian Physiotherapy Association. Dr William Horsey had assumed medical direction of the department in 1980, a position he held until his resignation from the active staff in 1985 to become co-director of the neurology clinic unit of the Workers' Compensation Board.

In 1984 the hospital consolidated several purchasing offices (surgical supplies, general supplies, and so on) into one central purchasing department, a move which its auditors had repeatedly recommended but which the hospital could not implement for lack of space. This was a significant step in providing better receiving, billing, and inventory control.

And finally, a ninety-year-old service was discontinued: in early 1984 the on-site laundry was closed down and the hospital contracted the service of a commercial laundry – a move that had been considered and reconsidered over a period of almost twenty years. The laundry space was renovated and became the west annex, home of several research laboratories.

Two Departments Caught between Boom Times

In records relating to St Michael's, there is a recurring instance of a department head labouring for years under difficult conditions only to have the situation change dramatically after his/her departure – either improved structures are set in place to correct the cause of some of the difficulties, or new technology becomes available, or staffing freezes are lifted, or improved physical facilities are provided.

For fourteen years (1965-79) Sister Pauline O'Leary ably directed the medical records department and its school, years when the work of the department grew steadily in volume and complexity. Despite a personal work-week of fifty to sixty hours, Sister Pauline maintained a collaborative and harmonious relationship with all, even those of the medical staff whom she sometimes had to call on the carpet for being delinquent in their charts. As mentioned earlier, within a year of her departure the first automated equipment was made available to her staff, and a few years later the department was fully computerized. The medical staff's quality-assurance program, which has been described, addressed the ever-elusive goal of a complete and accurate medical record.

A second illustration is that of Martha Andrasko, director of pharmacy from 1973 to 1985 – years that brought phenomenal advances in drug therapy: new drugs for cancer treatment and for raising or lowering blood pressure, new antibiotics, new methods of administration (for example, total parenteral nutrition), and so on. All of these had a large price-tag attached; in addition, their ordering could not be regulated by the chief pharmacist except by suggestion, and the extent of their use could rarely be accurately forecast in each year's budget. Also, there were the totally unexpected drains on the pharmacy budget, as in 1983 when hospitals were alerted to the advisability of protecting staff against the hepatitis B virus (at $123 per person) but the cost of which must be borne by the existing global budget.[80] And there were such one-time incidents as when a drug had to be flown, at a cost to the hospital of $75,000, from London's Heathrow Airport to control the bleeding of a haemophiliac man in need of open reduction of a fracture.[81]

One of the recommendations of the influential Dubin report of 1983[82] was that hospitals adopt the unit-dose system of drug dispensing and distribution (the cost for which would be an additional $1 million at St Michael's) and a central IV additive program (which would transfer from the nursing staff to the pharmacy the responsibility for adding drugs to intravenous flasks). Andrasko had long advocated development of the latter service, but because of the severe space constraints during the hospital's redevelopment program, pharmacy was forced to wait its turn until the space vacated by the dietary department should become available.

Up-to-date on the developments within her field and always conscientious about patient safety, Andrasko waited for the day when the necessary technology for producing patient-drug profiles would be available to her. In the meantime, she carried on heroically, through staff freezes, budget ceilings, and mounting demands for service, guiding her eager pharmacy residents in their research, taking on the difficult task of questioning those prescriptions unsubstantiated by the literature[83] – in short, holding together a very busy department during a time of dynamic developments. Andrasko left St Michael's in 1985, just a few months before the new pharmacy facilities made possible the implementation of some of the more advanced pharmaceutical methods.

Capital Equipment

The cost, and the difficulty in meeting the cost, of the new technology that became available during these years was evident as far back as 1971 when the university's department of ophthalmology investigated the feasibility of sharing the use of expensive instruments within the teaching hospitals.[84]

The medical advisory board formed a medical budget committee in 1977, charged with reviewing requests and recommending approval for major expenditures. Its effectiveness was greatly increased when Dr Bruce Bird proposed a systematic approach to budgeting, whereby each department was required to submit a statement of its current inventory which would be used by the budget committee as a basis for assigning priority to new requests.[85] While the doctors found the inventory method useful for assigning departmental maintenance funds, they found themselves "quickly overtaken by major needs in the cardiovascular laboratory and monitoring equipment in the I.C.U. [intensive care unit]."[86] Long-range planning, with careful stewardship of Ministry of Health capital funds, was recognized as essential. (In the meantime, individual doctors were looking to sources other than the budget committee; one of these doctors was L. Casella, who was very successful in obtaining outside funds for replacement equipment in the coronary care unit.[87])

Despite the 1980 establishment (and the cost effectiveness) of a biomedical department for the regular servicing of equipment in the 9-F cardiovascular laboratories, the operating room, and the critical care areas, effective planning for major equipment needs and the funding for same on any kind of long-term basis remained a difficult exercise – with the doctors generally declaring their allocation totally inadequate, and the director of finance repeatedly faced with requests that totally outran his resources.[88] The budget and finance committee of the board of directors began in 1983 to review leasing arrangements, rather than buying, even as it realized that its commitments to the new cardiology facilities and other projects would thrust the hospital into major bank borrowing.[89] The high cost of keeping abreast in the mid-1980s was everywhere evident.

In the midst of all this, the medical advisory committee's computer subcommittee, chaired by Dr David Briant, asked for consideration of a computerized ADT/CPI (Admissions, Discharge, Transfer/Central Patient Index) system, but was forced to acknowledge that the current funding situation would not allow for the significant costs attached. As in an earlier situation, some individuals and departments took their own routes, with several purchasing microcomputers and software.[90] It would be several years before the system recommended by Dr Briant would become a reality; in the meantime, his committee took some comfort in the knowledge that a consulting firm was analyzing the computer needs for all the sisters' institutions.

Funding for Operating Costs

As indicated earlier, in January 1976 Ontario entered into an agreement with the federal government to apply the latter's Anti-Inflation Act and Regulations. Promptly the Ministry of Health informed St Michael's that it must cut more than $1.2 million from its budget base in fiscal year 1976-77 – the constraints to take the form of staff reductions and bed closures – but that the ministry's approval would be required for all significant changes.[91]

To meet this target, the hospital froze staff salaries at October 1975 levels and cut 120 staff positions. Of the $935,000 to be saved in this way, nursing was asked to accomplish permanent lay-offs totalling $542,000 and temporary ones of $80,000[92] – despite the fact that a 16 percent increase in surgical procedures had been carried out over the past three years amidst a 12 percent decrease in nursing complement.[93] As well, for the ten months from June 1978 to March 1979, beds and bassinets were reduced to 657 and 54 respectively. This began what would become an annual ritual of summer-bed closures: an announcement by administration of the beds to be closed, vigorous protest by the medical advisory committee, followed by closure and eventual fall reopening. Even when the medical advisory committee's own admission and discharge committee began in 1984 the annual forecast of the summer situation, the bed closures continued as before.

In 1977 the Ministry of Health began to recognize, for funding purposes, that there were major "uncontrollable growth" programs: hyperalimentation, haemodialysis, peritoneal dialysis, pacemakers, open-heart surgery, and heart catheterizations; in the 1977 budget these programs at St Michael's were forecast to cost $2.75 million, more than two-thirds of which were costs connected with the cardiology-cardiovascular programs. That same year the operating costs of the CAT scanning, previously rejected by the ministry, began to be partially picked up. These two high-cost programs were identified as major contributors to the projected deficit in 1977-78.[94]

Staff reductions and bed closures had their desired effect and at the annual meeting of the board in 1978 its audit committee was able to announce that the hospital was in a strong position. The hospital, meanwhile, had increased its per diem rate to $306 for out-of-Canada patients and it faced 1978-79 confidently, except for clinical-education costs. It was a jolt when the Ministry of Health announced further budget cuts in late summer.

To meet this latest requirement, the hospital engaged Arthur Andersen and Company to do an objective analysis of areas of potential savings, directing attention to major fiscal departments – nursing, radiology, and laboratory.[95] The director of finance (L. Thalheimer) proposed to the medical advisory board that the consultants carry out as well an analysis of existing medical staff operations, but the doctors showed little enthusiasm; they elected instead to go the way of voluntary constraint via their own medical and surgical utilization committees. By year's end, the ministry acknowledged that the 4.5

percent increase it had earlier allowed was considerably short of the wages that unions had negotiated, and it made additional allocations covering 80 percent of the hospital's projected deficit.[96]

The consultants and the board pointed out what appeared to be ineffective control mechanisms in nursing (particularly its practice of replacing staff who had booked off sick or were on vacation – for which little allowance was permitted in the budget). Nevertheless, it was becoming increasingly clear to the board that, where there was no limit other than capacity to the number of patients admitted (even the 701-bed capacity was repeatedly exceeded, with extra beds set up in the corridors – a practice that was finally abolished only in 1987), cost control would always be difficult. Thalheimer realized this and emphasized the need to predict more adequately for each budget year any changes in treatment and their impact on cost. He proposed more active medical-staff involvement in cost containment, for example in drug expenditures, and he was the first at St Michael's to make a serious proposal that documentation of the cost implications of medical-staff additions be an integral part of the appointment procedure. It would be almost five years before the idea took firm hold.[97]

The hospital moved into its 1981-82 fiscal year with an anticipated deficit of $1.9 million; while the line was being held on staffing, inflation at the hospital – as in the entire country – was rampant, ranging from 11.8 percent in salaries and wages, to 13.5 percent in food costs, 15 percent in laboratory supplies, and 18 percent in radiology supplies. Buried within the finance department's calculations was a $1-million annual loss to the hospital in room-differential (the amount which patients were charged for private and semi-private rooms beyond the rate established by OHIP), on account of a move made several years earlier to a geographic distribution of beds by service.[98] Nonetheless, towards the end of the fiscal year, the new director of finance, Lloyd Larocque (Thalheimer having resigned to accept a position elsewhere), was able to announce that the Ministry of Health, taking into account the life-support programs, had approved full funding.[99] Along with its announcement of full funding, the ministry introduced its BOND Plan (Business-Oriented New Development Plan) whereby hospitals would be allowed to retain certain income which did not form part of the operating budget financed by the ministry. Private and semi-private room rates might now be established by the individual hospital, and the hospital would be allowed to retain any surplus funds so generated. The ministry warned that it would no longer pick up operating deficits. The hospital immediately raised its room differentials by 25 to 30 percent, charged patients for the use of telephones, and introduced dual rates for the public and staff in the cafeteria.

With the country, and indeed the world, still in recession in mid-1982, the staff-hiring freeze was reinforced and a system analysis of major departments was begun with a view to making further cost reductions. Nursing was again targetted.[100] (The idea of a freeze was not accepted equally by all: when pathology lost a resident it asked for three new staff members to replace him, a request that was immediately questioned by the board.[101]) But the Ministry of Health, realizing perhaps better than the internal reviewers that the problem was not necessarily, or only, one of excess nursing hours, fully approved the 1982-83 budget. Far from being sanguine about the approval, the board set itself to maintain strict controls, with extensive medical-staff involvement; at the same time, however, it questioned how successfully it could do so in view of the public's unlimited demand for care.[102]

The opening of the new C-wing in 1983 added another dimension: with no experience in forecasting staffing needs for the new, more elaborate facilities, a shortfall of $1.7 million in the operating budget was soon apparent. When rehabilitation medicine found that it needed three more technicians and respiratory technology needed four, because of the new wing and rising volumes, it was proposed at the medical advisory committee that the freeze on hiring these extra people might be handled by transferring bronchodilator therapy to nursing![103] By the time the 1984-85 budget was prepared, Larocque was forecasting a shortfall of $3.4 million before giving consideration to the impact of tentative commitments made to the expected new chiefs of general surgery and of cardiology. Faced with this sobering news, the board agreed that draconian measures might be needed,[104] and in May 1984, at Larocque's suggestion, engaged the consulting firm of Touche, Ross to do an operations review. When the medical advisory committee put before the board of directors for its approval in June 1984 seven new active-staff appointments, a concerned board asked Dr Platt to establish a protocol, backed by a cost-impact analysis, which hopefully would provide the financial data for prospective medical-staff appointments prior to implementation.

In September 1984 the consultants delivered their report. Nursing – the largest department, and by now the most expensive (annual budget of more than $26 million) because of negotiated union settlements – was again targetted.[105] Although certain members of the

medical advisory committee questioned the methodology and conclusions of the report, and cautioned that the reduction of nursing
staff necessary to reduce costs by $2 million (the potential savings
within the nursing department identified by the consultants) would
negatively affect quality of care, the department of nursing immediately cut thirty full-time positions, followed shortly by another twenty-five.[106] Within six months it was evident that the cut had been too
deep, and the nursing department was in serious trouble, trouble that
would continue for several years.[107]

Meanwhile, however, medical-staff appointments continued (one
cardiologist, one psychiatrist, one PhD endocrinologist in December
1984), prompting a board ruling that no commitments might be made
to any doctor without consultation with the board, and that any
future request for approval of appointments must include a written
outline of the financial implications involved in provision of space,
personnel, and support services. At the February 1985 board meeting
where the director of nursing outlined her staff reductions, the board
received without comment the doctors' medical manpower survey
for 1985-87 which proposed medical additions of fifty-one, medical
deletions of seventeen, plus additions of thirteen secretaries, thirteen
support staff, and nineteen offices.[108] A worried director of finance
warned that, even with nursing achieving its target, the operating
deficit would reach $4 million before the proposed appointments of
the new chiefs and the commitments made to them. A contingency
planning committee of senior management prepared plans for more
service cuts and possible sources of revenue, but before these could
be implemented the Ministry of Health approved the hospital's budget as submitted.[109]

Part of the hospital's difficulty in financial matters was its lack, as
yet, of adequate methods and technology for costing programs. Government, too, seemed not to have a clear hold on what the new programs should cost, and continually had to resort to funding "uncontrollable growth" or risk the political consequences of imposing constraints. The medical staff, for its part, was forced to keep abreast of
developments in the other teaching hospitals or lose its hard-won
place. The nursing department had tried to assess and cost its real
needs. Responding to CCHA surveyors' recommendations, the
department had in 1982 established a patient-classification system
(the Medicus system) designed to match work-loads to levels of
staffing. Jeanne (Doll) Foxwell, associate director of nursing, took the
leadership in launching the Medicus project; the new director of

nursing replaced it by the Grasp system in mid-1984. Thus for two years staffing was done on the basis of a methodology with which not all were as yet thoroughly familiar. And finally, in the larger picture, there was the problem of the division of authority and responsibility. While the board was acutely aware of its accountability in the matter of public funds, it had to acknowledge that it was the medical staff that faced daily the public's spiralling expectations in a publicly funded health-care system.

Nursing

These were not the best of times for the department of nursing, nor were they yet the worst. The pool from which nursing drew its staff had changed with the closing of St Michael's school of nursing; the needs had changed, too, with the increasing transformation of St Michael's into a tertiary-care facility. With the opening of the intensive and acute care units, the fine special-duty nurses (many of them St Michael's graduates) almost disappeared, and even though nursing registries in Toronto proliferated, the hospital's relationship with their nurses was different – less personal, less sustained. Outstanding among the exceptions was Louise Ritchie, a Wellesley Hospital School graduate who came on call from a registry to St Michael's intensive care unit for several years and then joined the permanent hospital staff to serve as St Michael's highly respected, first secular night supervisor – a position that had been held only by sister-nurses for more than eighty years.

This decade opened with registered nurses streaming to the United States because Ontario was over-supplied;[110] it closed with acute shortages of nurses, particularly in the critical-care areas[111]– not just at St Michael's but throughout Metropolitan Toronto. In between, there were wide fluctuations, closely tied to the academic year: for example, 700 nursing vacancies in Toronto in June 1981, but 3000 new nurses graduating in September, of whom St Michael's employed 90.[112] Also in between, as has been commented on, were the periodic nursing cut-backs, after prodigious efforts made by nursing personnel officer Claudette Brunelle, RN, and her staff to recruit – even from overseas, with all that that involved in the way of red tape.[113]

While the critical-care areas quickly absorbed any experienced new staff, the wards receiving the new two-year graduates required extensive support through the active orientation and in-service programs and the exhaustive reference manuals provided by staff development director Elaine Anderson, MScN, and her staff. This group also developed slide tapes to teach special techniques to staff (such as enterostomal therapy and tracheostomy care) and to patients (such as those scheduled to undergo heart surgery, and the new diabetic); the tapes were made available to other institutions through the Ontario Hospital Association library.

With increasing specialization in nursing (psychiatry, cardiology, orthopaedics, and so on), continuing education became a way of life for St Michael's nurses, almost 500 of whom were enrolled in programs outside the hospital in 1980. In both 1983 and 1984 St Michael's critical-care nurses, coordinated by Jim Soonarane, RN, arranged two-day seminars in critical-caring nursing, using St Michael's personnel as presenters. These attracted each year 150 registrants and turned away 100 – an indication of the predominance of tertiary care in Toronto and the surrounding area hospitals, and the eagerness of nurses to obtain this kind of help.

In a break with a kind of isolationism that prevailed in the past, nursing collaborated extensively across departmental lines in its educational efforts: for example, with pharmacy, to explain total parenteral nutrition, and with dietary and rehabilitation medicine for other specific topics. Nursing continued to offer the course in cardiopulmonary resuscitation begun in 1970 for the nurses; this course was expanded in 1977 to include, first, the cardiology residents and then other medical services, and finally it was opened to x-ray and other technologists.[114] The fees of these instructors, all of whom were certified through the Ontario Heart Foundation, was borne by the nursing department. Rosemary (Everington) Watkins, RN, who was central to the CPR training, was also central to the development of an improved medication delivery system by a joint nursing-pharmacy committee in 1983.[115]

Nursing was commended in the 1981 CCHA survey for its move to improve its methods of planning and evaluating nursing care through the Nursing Process, introduced by Linda Lee O'Brien, MScN, in 1980, followed by the introduction of Primary Nursing – two concepts with which the new baccalaureate graduates were already familiar. About this time the department engaged its first three clinical-nurse specialists (in cardiology, maternal and child health, and neurological nursing), each of whom added significantly to the future orientation of these nursing specialties. Admittedly, not everyone was impressed, for old patterns die hard. When staff had to be cut it was often with regard to the need for "those highly paid" nurses that the department was questioned.

Three developments pioneered by nursing in this decade became effective services. In 1976 nursing established the hospital's first porter pool, complete with its own separate central-despatch and pocket-pager system; while it was intended to provide primarily for the portering needs of the nursing units, its services were soon being tapped by other individuals and departments. In 1978 nursing struck a steering committee that included radiology and laboratory representatives to establish a pre-anaesthetic clinic (PAC).[116] Supervised and staffed by nursing, and strongly endorsed by the anaesthesia department, the clinic was conceived as a way of checking before admission the heart and lungs of patients scheduled for anaesthesia and thus streamlining the flow of surgery patients through the operating room; paradoxically, even though the PAC was judged highly successful, some surgeons remained lukewarm to the idea for some time and had to be repeatedly nudged by the anaesthetists.[117] Nursing coordinators Maureen Hart and Jacqueline Mulcahy were deeply involved in both of these developments.

The third and last of the innovations in this period was that of palliative care. In April 1977 the nursing department engaged, within its staff development division, Joan Foy – a graduate of St Joseph's (Toronto) School of Nursing and St Michael's critical-care nursing program – to offer teaching, support, and counselling to nurses working with patients terminally ill from cancer. Generously gifted with vision and initiative in her own right, Foy was also deeply inspired by the work and philosophy of Dr Cicely Saunders, FRCP and member of the Order of the British Empire – a woman who was, at the time, the world's foremost authority on care of the terminally ill; her emphasis was on the control of symptoms, especially pain in all its aspects. In early 1978 Dr John Scott joined the medical staff and, with Foy, formed a palliative-care consultation team which addressed the needs of St Michael's cancer patients and their families both during and following their hospital stay.

In 1982 the hospital made the decision to set aside a ten-bed unit on 4-FS for the terminally ill patients who, until this time, had been scattered throughout the hospital. Specially funded by the Sisters of St Joseph as a two-year pilot project, the furnishings and decor chosen with particular attention to the needs of these patients (including a microwave oven to cook patients' favourite foods, and overnight accommodation for next of kin), the unit provided a gentle and restful alternative to the busy nursing unit. Dr Scott resigned before the new unit was opened, but the hospital was fortunate to have Dr Kenneth

Butler, FRCP (Canada), assume the position of director. Foy elected not to become head nurse; Shirley Herron, who had done some instruction with the team, assumed the position. After a few months, with the need for the consultation team lessened, Foy left St Michael's and in 1987 became co-founder of "Interlink," an organization that provides the link between the cancer patient, the hospital or cancer centre, and community services.[118] The palliative care unit has been a blessing to hundreds of St Michael's patients; in the words of a St Michael's nurse, long a patient in the unit, "This is my only home now, and it's like having two comforting arms around me."[119]

In January 1984 the administration of the department of nursing changed: Louis Wilson became director, with Jeanne Foxwell and Elaine Anderson as associate and assistant directors; the remainder of the nursing structure remained essentially as the author and Elizabeth Mange – with wide input from the senior nursing staff – had developed it almost ten years previously. Nursing Personnel, however, was subsumed within the personnel department proper. Wilson developed a nursing advisory committee for coordination within the hospital and liaison with outside agencies involved with the department, and launched a comprehensive quality-assurance program.[120] Reference was made earlier to the difficult challenge she accepted in responding to the recommendations of the 1984 consultants' report. Wilson left St Michael's in early 1989.

Long-range Planning

In response to the Mustard report of 1974, the congregation formed in 1974 a health-services planning committee chaired by Sister Janet Murray, executive director of St Joseph's Hospital. This committee worked steadily towards coordinating the activities of the congregation's six health-care facilities[121] into one interlocking system which would preserve relatively intact the operational autonomy of each institution while, at the same time, reducing to a minimum any duplication of resources. The larger goal was to maintain the congregation's institutions as an essential component of the church's mission and as a part of the total health-care system of the province, all under one ownership and governance.[122] Increasingly, the sisters emphasized that their goals could be attained only with the full participation of their institutions' lay staff. To help interpret each institution's philosophy, group facilitators were appointed. At St Michael's, Sister Marie Christine Mulvaney began this work in 1982, a work later taken over by Sister June Dwyer in 1985 in a portfolio named "mission education."

The university, meanwhile, was struggling in the midst of funding cuts to find ways of maintaining its existing programs. Concerned about the implications of certain suggestions being made from that quarter, St Michael's medical advisory committee in 1981 struck a subcommittee (the Quo Vadis committee), chaired by Dr M. Shea, to define St Michael's role in relationship to the university and to undertake long-term planning for the clinical services.[123] Although this committee obtained from each medical department its plans for the next five years, with a view to developing a set of positions for negotiating with the university, the resulting "Quo Vadis Report" stopped short of this. It represents, rather, a concise but comprehensive overview of each department in 1982 – its strengths in patient care, investigative work, and teaching – together with a strong statement of the philosophy guiding (and which must guide) these activities in a Roman Catholic teaching hospital.[124]

While Dr Shea's committee realized that it needed to do more work to assess programs in terms of their relative importance, and also to plan for the use of budget and space on the basis of the emphasis to be accorded each, a joint board-administration-medical staff committee finally concluded that no service could be cut without jeopardizing others. It resolved to inform the university that St Michael's intended to remain strong in all its existing areas.[125]

Although it soon became apparent that this position was unrealistic, two further developments occurred to help the hospital shape its future. The congregation, concerned that some rationalization of activities might be imposed by government or the university, and in an effort to strengthen what had been begun by Sister Janet, established in 1983 a senior group called the corporate health planning group, consisting of the board chairmen, executive directors, and chairmen of the medical advisory committees of its member institutions, and chaired by Sister Virginia Varley, a member of the General Council. At the direction of this group, St Michael's (and each member institution) developed a strategic planning committee; board member L. Hynes chaired St Michael's committee.[126] Building on the base established by the Quo Vadis committee, the new committee ranked in order of priority all the clinical departments and divisions for purposes of allocating financial, physical, and human resources. This, together with a newly articulated statement of mission, represented a very significant step in what had come to be called "St Michael's preferred future."

Another Building-fund Campaign

It was recognized from the beginning of the redevelopment program that the construction begun in 1978 was just that, a beginning. With cramped and out-dated operating-room and intensive-care facilities, and with the awkward traffic problems between the new wing and the existing hospital, it was important that there be no delay in proceeding to the next phase of the original building plans. The Ministry of Health, however, would not authorize the start of working drawings until the hospital showed that the funds were available – funds to the tune of $24 million in 1984 dollars for building and furnishings, in addition to the remaining OHRDP funds.

A professional fund-raiser (G. Goldie) and a campaign manager (R. Merifield) were engaged in 1982. To recruit a campaign chairman was more difficult and became a major preoccupation of the board for a full two years.[127] Potential chairmen questioned the possibility of raising even $12 million in the prevailing economic climate of which these business executives were all too aware.

Finally, in April 1984, the board was told that one of its members, Alan Dilworth, had agreed to chair the campaign, with Conrad Black, Ian Sinclair, and George Eaton as co-chairmen and Allen Lambert as honorary treasurer. The Ministry of Health was informed that the hospital had set a target of $25 million in a campaign which would extend over five years. The earlier campaign had gone only to the corporations; this one would go also to the public at large, and St Michael's public, a large majority of whom were by no means rich and powerful, was more than generous in its response.[128]

And Finally

On 2 October 1984, St Michael's proudly welcomed Her Majesty Queen Elizabeth II, who unveiled the plaque that commemorates the first phase of the redevelopment. As well, she received from Dr Kenneth Money, Canada's first astronaut, an autographed picture of Canada's six astronauts, all of whom had been tested in the hospital's vestibular laboratory in preparation for their space flights. With their feet planted (and sometimes mired), in the practical concerns of earth, St Michael's people could yet allow their imaginations to soar to the realms of royalty and far-off planets.

10

Countdown to the Centennial Year

The decade immediately preceding St Michael's one hundredth birthday in 1992 was one of almost cataclysmic economic and social change throughout Canada, but particularly in Ontario, in Toronto, and in St Michael's Hospital itself.

The short, sharp downturn in the economy during 1981-82 was followed by a period of intense growth, especially in Ontario, and of conspicuous consumption – much of it financed with borrowed money. The cost-of-living in Toronto became by 1991 the highest in North America. In the hospital field, these were years of big expansion, big expense, and potentially big liability claims.[1]

The excesses of these years came to an abrupt halt as the 1980s closed with more than 75,000 Canadian companies or individuals in bankruptcy, the once-mighty Standard Trust Company in failure, and the colourful Robert Campeau's empire in collapse. This most recent recession was felt most strongly in Ontario where more than 200,000 manufacturing jobs disappeared during 1990-91;[2] across Canada the jobless rate soared to 10.5 percent, with 1.5 million Canadians out of work. In the hospital field, many former executives and staff alike were living on their severance packages, unemployment insurance, or savings. In the midst of this sagging economy the federal government instituted its 7 percent Goods and Services Tax in January 1991.

In Metro Toronto the welfare rolls ballooned by 83 percent between 1990-91, with 117,000 men, women, and children on welfare – twice the rate of increase during the recession of ten years previously.[3] Metro Toronto's 220 food banks were supplying emergency meals and groceries to 120,000 citizens each month, 43 percent of whom held high-school diplomas and 10 percent university degrees; even with such assistance, many were seeing doctors for illnesses directly attributable to inadequate diets.[4] At St Michael's tuberculosis clinic (the only one in Toronto), the 102 new cases of that illness seen during 1990 were, in the judgment of clinic director Dr Victor Hoffstein, related to the economic situation – lower standards of nutrition and living accommodations, and associated stress.[5] Although crowded hostels were considered to be a factor in the rise of tuberculosis, many of Toronto's homeless chose such crowding in preference to the doorways and grates of the open street; in the winter of 1991-92 several downtown Toronto churches opened their doors to provide overnight accommodation. St Michael's Hospital supplied clean bedding and towels to St Patrick's Church, used for this purpose.

Throughout the decade, health care for an aging population was a continuing concern, becoming one of the Ontario Hospital Association's top priority issues in 1986 and prompting occasional murmurs about the need to ration health care. AIDS (acquired immune deficiency syndrome), almost unknown in 1980, had by 1983 leapt to prominence as the newest health threat. Meanwhile, the demand for the usual kinds of health care and their related technology continued unabated.

To fund the ever-accelerating demands, institutions, including hospitals, turned to mergers in an attempt to realize some of the economies of scale. The Toronto General and the Toronto Western hospitals became in 1986 the Toronto Hospital Corporation,[6] but failed four years later to complete a further merger with Women's College Hospital. An attempt to relocate the Wellesley and Princess Margaret hospitals onto Sunnybrook Hospital grounds was put on hold after months of discussion when the minister of health announced that Princess Margaret Hospital would relocate to University Avenue.[7] Concerned about the possibility of two powerful conglomerates – a north campus (Sunnybrook-Wellesley) and a south campus (Toronto General-Toronto Western) – within the university's teaching-hospitals complex, the Sisters of St Joseph pressed ahead with their plans to merge St Michael's Hospital and St Joseph's Health Centre,[8] until everything came to an abrupt halt in 1991.

Internally, hospitals began to take on more and more the characteristics of big business: their senior executives became "presidents" and "vice-presidents"; head nurses, now known as "unit managers," grew organizationally and psychologically distanced from patient care, their nurses' uniforms replaced by street clothes; patients became "consumers"; and references to "marketing the hospital's products" started appearing.[9] The sheer volume of paper and statistics accompanying the advent of the new corporate climate and the computer was both blessing and burden. As an illustration, in 1987 a twelve-page document was deemed necessary to set forth St

Michael's affiliation-agreement with the twelve-bed AIDS hospice, Casey House,[10] compared with the two-page memorandum that represented the first written affiliation with the University of Toronto in 1914. Simultaneously, established patterns of hospitals were being threatened by the search underway by the Ministry of Health for better ways of managing the health dollar. In 1987 a review panel commissioned by the ministry tabled its report (the Evans report).[11] It reminded the ministry that themes and recommendations repeated by similar commissions over the previous fifteen years had never been implemented: finding alternatives to institutional care; a shift in focus to the community, with increased emphasis on prevention, health promotion, and health maintenance; alternative primary-care funding arrangements; a shift to care in the home; and multidisciplinary approaches to care. The revival of these and other recommendations (including New Brunswick's "extra-mural" or "hospital-at-home" concept, estimated to have the potential for lowering hospital-bed use by 40 percent)[12] introduced a note of uncertainty throughout Ontario's hospital system, an uncertainty exacerbated when Ontario's first NDP government came to power in 1990 and hospitals had to deal with three different ministers of health in a period of six to seven months.[13]

The new government reaffirmed its earlier preference for non-institutional alternatives to health care, and for a channelling of funds away from institutions and into an attack on social problems.[14] In short, it quickly demonstrated an intention to address the "shortcomings in the system" and to initiate "changes which would involve a fundamental rethinking" of many of the practices supporting health-care delivery in Ontario, as called for in the Evans report.[15] Change did happen, and quickly. By November 1991 almost 20 percent of Metro Toronto's 15,000 acute-care beds had been taken out of service.[16]

The new government immediately moved on two other planks of NDP policy, both introduced during the preceding Liberal regime – employment equity (equal access to employment opportunities), which was a re-emphasis of principles already in the Ontario Human Rights Code; and pay equity (legislation that provides for equal pay, especially for women, for work of equal value). These two legislated requirements became for hospitals a major drain in terms of staff time and operating budget. A further piece of legislation, the Employer Health Tax Levy, represented for St Michael's in 1990 an incremental dollar impact of $801,000 over the previous year's OHIP premium.[17]

At the same time, teaching hospitals were faced with the increased need to fund research and research space, as well as the accelerating costs of new technology, much of which was seen as the price to be paid for membership in a "world-class" health complex – for St Michael's, the University of Toronto and its affiliated hospitals.

It is within this fluid environment that the story of St Michael's Hospital in the seven years preceding its one hundredth birthday will be sketched – years of daunting challenges, bold initiatives, and an undreamed-of turn of events.

A Change in Governance and Administration

Sister Christine Gaudet assumed the office of executive director on 4 February 1985. Although her experience in a university-teaching hospital had been limited to her year's residency at the Kingston General Hospital in partial fulfilment of the requirements for her master's degree in health administration (University of Ottawa, 1972), Sister Christine brought several years of senior executive experience to her new position. After obtaining her masters in household economics at the University of Toronto in 1960 and completing a one-year dietetic internship at St Michael's, Sister Christine served for eight years as director of dietetics, first at St Joseph's Hospital, Toronto, and then at Providence Villa and Hospital (1961-69). Following completion of her masters in health administration – and her winning of the class award – Sister Christine was from 1971 to 1983 executive director of St Joseph's Hospital, Comox, British Columbia, a 250-bed community hospital for acute and chronic patients. During these years she held senior positions on the executives of various British Columbia health organizations and in the Canadian College of Health Service Executives, and she obtained her fellowship in the American College of Hospital Administrators in 1980.

Sister Christine's initiative and organizational skills, as well as her untiring efforts on behalf of St Michael's within the university and its teaching hospitals, were evident throughout her time as executive director. Evident, too, in all the records relating to these years was her considerable literary talent and public-relations skills. At the January 1990 board meeting where her resignation was announced,[18] the chairman of the finance committee reported that the hospital had completed the first nine months of the fiscal year with a surplus, before building depreciation, of $1.3 million.[19]

Sharing the challenges, hopes, and relentless demands of the years from 1985 to 1990 was the new board chairman, Alan Dilworth, elected 30 July 1985 after serving four years on the board. A year into the position, Dilworth, by then chairman of Touche Ross, addressed a wide-ranging memo to the directors[20] regarding "this very large, complex organization for which we are responsible." Reflecting the tremendous amount of thought, time, and energy that he gave to his responsibility as chairman, the memo expressed as well his desire to see all the directors similarly involved. He invited directors to review their collective effectiveness as a board, and he underlined the need for the board to have adequate information in order to monitor quality of care and utilization of resources in the exercise of its stewardship. In this connection, he subsequently told the board that the hospital's auditors had been asked to conduct an overview with a focus on control over, among other things, campaign funds and approval of major expenses.[21] As it turned out, despite the chairman's early expressed resolve, and despite the presence of board members on a whole range of major committees, in the rush of events certain decisions appear either to have been made without total board involvement or to have received less than adequate attention there – decisions that ultimately erupted in the crisis of 1990.

During the years 1985-1990 the board's membership underwent successive changes; in fact, a massive shift occurred within every major decision-making body connected with the hospital during those years:[22] at the ministry, as indicated, four different ministers; at the university, two different deans; within the board, a new chairman and vice-chairman and fifteen new directors, in addition to the two new directors appointed from city council and the *ex-officio* members, while twelve long-serving directors retired; in administration, a new chief executive officer was appointed, and five assistant administrators were replaced, including the director of finance; in the medical staff, the wave of appointments of the 1950s and 1960s became an ebb of retirees as eight chiefs of departments or divisions reached retirement age, and new heads were appointed to nursing, pharmacy, and personnel – all big and busy departments. And finally, the close of the decade brought a complete changeover, with one exception, of the congregation's General Council.

After taking six months to assess the situation, and with a view to freeing herself for planning and for productive liaison with external bodies (the ministry, the university, various associations), Sister Christine reorganized the senior management in September 1985. In the new structure, Sister Catherine McDonough (BComm, Queen's University; MHSc, University of Toronto) became associate executive director-operations, in effect responsible for all day-to-day activity, with five assistant executive directors (finance, nursing, professional services, hospital services, and human resources) reporting to her. With some variations in her responsibilities,[23] Sister Catherine served in this capacity for four very full years; the chairman's announcement in May 1989 that she was stepping down was received with deep regret, especially by the hospital staff by whom she was held in admiration and affection.

The Strategic Plan

The blueprint developed earlier by the strategic planning committee was further refined during 1986-87 in an exhaustive and sensitive exercise. Consultants were engaged to assist in reviewing all medical programs and, by means of internal and external interviews, to determine St Michael's clinical strengths and to rank all programs within the clinical services against the hospital's mission statement. Based on the identified existing strengths, there emerged a logical grouping into nine areas of concentration: first, three areas that already had a high level of maturity and organization and, consequently, an established recognition among their peers – disorders of the blood and circulation, of the neuromusculoskeletal system, and of the renal, endocrine/metabolic systems; secondly, trauma, oncology, and biopsychosocial medicine; and finally, three with a future orientation – aging, women's health, and community health.

Parenthetically, in these last three areas the hospital was committing itself, in the midst of its high-technology activities, to remain faithful to its founding inspiration – its call to serve "the *minimis*." The "least," or most marginalized, people of the twentieth century were widely considered to be women, the elderly, the AIDS patients, and, of course, the poor.

The plan was received with enthusiasm and adopted in November 1987. Confident now in the direction it wished to take into the future, the hospital believed that it had a firm basis for channelling its funds, for allocating space in the proposed building program, and for recruiting staff.[24] In retrospect, one would have to question whether an effective ranking of priorities had been done; it appears that none of the existing programs were eliminated, even though it had been acknowledged at the beginning that service could not be provided across the whole spectrum.

Implementation of the Strategic Plan:
The Nine Areas of Concentration

Disorders of the Blood and Circulatory Systems

It is significant that in 1988 the name of the hospital's newsletter was changed to *Pulse*, its print overlaid by an EKG tracing. The emphasis in cardiology and cardiovascular surgery did indeed continue strongly throughout the 1980s. Dr Paul Armstrong was appointed chief of cardiology at St Michael's and professor of medicine at the University of Toronto in 1984. Prior to this, Armstrong had undergone extensive training: MD, Queen's University, 1966; residencies at Toronto and Kingston General hospitals, Massachusettes General, Boston, and St George's Hospital, London, England; FRCP and FACC (1974). He was a prolific writer and researcher, publishing forty-three articles between 1970 and 1984, and was also much in demand as a lecturer – he made fifty-nine presentations on three continents between 1974 and 1983. After his appointment to St Michael's, Armstrong continued his earlier research thrust. In 1986 he obtained permission to use the new drug t-PA (tissue-type plasminogen activator) which, through dissolving the thrombus, minimizes the muscle damage caused by heart attack; within a week, the first heart-attack victim in Canada to receive this drug had made a strong recovery. The following year Armstrong headed an eleven-hospital study where the drug was administered to twenty-six patients; a 69 percent success rate in re-establishing a myocardial blood flow was demonstrated.[25]

Research in other areas was active. In 1989 Dr Robert Chisholm, director of St Michael's new $2-million cardiac-catheterization laboratory, headed a team that was successfully and dramatically demonstrating the balloon-catheter technique (angioplasty) as an alternative to the more expensive and, in some cases, higher-risk open-heart surgery for blocked coronary arteries.[26] Drs Armstrong, R.J. Howard, and Gordon Moe – generously supported by the Heart and Stroke Foundation – were doing pioneering research in the mechanisms and process of heart failure; and the Italian community in Toronto, through its link with, and pride in, Dr Luigi Casella, continued to raise money for cardiac research at St Michael's. Remarkable in the records of these years is the recognition given to players, other than the doctors, on the team – the perfusionists, pharmacologists, nurses. Each was, and was seen to be, essential to the success of every endeavour.

In cardiovascular surgery, Dr Tomas A. Salerno (MD, McGill University, 1971; FRCS [Canada] and FACS) came in 1983, after six years of senior work at Queen's University, McGill University, and their associated hospitals, to be chief of cardiovascular and thoracic surgery at St Michael's and professor of medicine, University of Toronto. Salerno was an avid investigator (almost $350,000 in research grants between 1984 and 1987) and widely sought as a lecturer (forty-five presentations between 1981 and 1986, from Toronto and Montreal to Switzerland and Brazil).[27]

In 1987 Dr Salerno became chairman of cardiovascular surgery for the university's affiliated hospitals. That year the university asked its affiliated hospitals to reconsider offering cardiac-transplantation services, since the potential for success was reported to have increased dramatically; St Michael's was specifically recommended for involvement in mechanical-heart transplants. While the medical advisory committee approved in principle such a move,[28] the emphasis appears to have remained on the aorta-coronary by-pass, possibly because the facilities and staff were already taxed to the limit.

Throughout 1987 St Michael's repeatedly met with Ministry of Health officials and expressed its inability to deal with the demand for critical-care beds. In 1988 the ministry approved an expansion of facilities which would require an additional forty-one hard-to-find specially trained nurses. By January 1989 thirty-nine of these had been recruited and assigned to the new cardiovascular intensive-care unit, where the number of CV-ICU beds had been increased from seven to thirteen. Yet the new fourteen-bed medical/surgical ICU still required an additional thirty-two specialty nurses![29] These are but two examples of the tremendous growth during these years.

Because of the relentless demand for CV surgery, valiant attempts were made to continue the service. However, the considerable media attention given to the post-CV-surgery death of a patient in December 1988, followed by a second death two days later, prompted the Ministry of Health to initiate an investigation into the scheduling of heart surgery at St Michael's.[30] The investigators reported that the challenges faced by St Michael's "within the context of the Hospital's documented excellence in patient care in cardiology, cardiovascular surgery ... were faced also by each of the nine hospitals in Ontario to a greater or lesser extent." It directed eight recommendations specifically to St Michael's and, among a further twenty-two, eleven were aimed at the ministry.[31] The investigators concluded, also, that no one, neither the ministry nor the hospital, knew the cost of one cardiovascular case.[32]

In the face of challenges to the clinical care of surgical patients, the hospital adhered to its strategic plan and arranged for a massive outlay for diagnostic equipment to replace aging and older technology; in 1989-90 the new cardiac-catheterization laboratory was equipped with a Philips bi-plane digital angiographic unit, the first of its kind in North America.

In sum, the quality of professional staff and of equipment appears to have been in place to fulfill the directions set for cardiology and CV surgery by the strategic plan, albeit serviced by operating-room space as yet totally inadequate to meet the demands and a nursing staff subject to periodic depletion from burn-out and other causes, all functioning in what the above investigator's report characterized as a "complex and uncertain environment."

Prominent within this same area of concentration were the hospital's activities related to blood disorders, particularly those carried out at its centre for adult haemophiliacs. By 1989 the centre had registered 90 percent of Metro's adult haemophiliacs, and Dr J.M. Teitel had assumed direction of the clinic from its founder, Dr Bernadette Garvey.

A farm girl from Mono Mills (near Orangeville, Ontario), Bernadette Garvey had proceeded through a BSc with gold medal, earned at St Patrick's College, Ottawa, to an MD *cum laude*, at the University of Ottawa, and finally a post-doctoral fellowship in haematology at the Walter Reed Army Institute, Washington, DC. In 1987 Garvey was promoted to professor of medicine at the University of Toronto and in June 1989 she was elected chair of St Michael's medical advisory committee, the first woman to hold the position at St Michael's.[33]

Dr Garvey began an active interest in AIDS soon after it made its appearance in Canada, serving on both federal and provincial advisory committees and as chair of the Ontario Advisory Committee on AIDS from 1984.[34] In 1989 she assumed overall responsibility for medical supervision of St Michael's new HIV outpatient clinic for AIDS and AIDS-related illnesses, established with some funding assistance from the Ministry of Health. Garvey remained, throughout all this activity, deeply involved in decisions regarding the research work of the National Institutes of Health and the National Heart, Lung and Blood Institute, both based in Bethesda, Maryland. As well, she continued to direct the care and treatment of her patients with various other blood disorders on 6A-south, where for more than twenty years Joan Cleminson was a valued head nurse-colleague.

In 1985 St Michael's was chosen by Metro Toronto's District Health Council to be the teaching hospital that would serve as an affiliated hospital for Casey House, the new AIDS hospice to be established in Toronto – the first AIDS hospice in Canada to be funded by a provincial government. Under the affiliation-agreement St Michael's assumed responsibility for the quality of care at Casey House, assisted in selection of senior staff and in formulation of policies, and had representation on the Casey House board of directors.[35] The Ministry of Health channelled the capital and operating funds through St Michael's to Casey House, which was officially opened on 1 March 1988.

Disorders of the Neuromuscular Systems

Two of the major developments in the neurosciences during this period were the pioneering work of Dr Paul Muller in the treatment of malignant brain tumours by means of medical laser – an area in which members of St Michael's pharmacy, nursing,[36] and biomedical-engineering departments were recognized as essential collaborators – and the world's first successful sciatic-nerve transplantation by Dr Alan Hudson and his team, already mentioned. By 1988 patients were arriving from all over the world for peripheral-nerve repair or graft, and physicians came from far and wide to learn the technique and treatment. The multiple sclerosis clinic directed by Dr Trevor Gray received enlarged and enhanced facilities in 1988 to accommodate its patients, now numbering 1,000 registered, and its research activities, now linked with twelve other MS Clinics.

To assist the neurologists and neurosurgeons, a new Tomoscan CT scanner was installed in 1988. In 1990 the Ministry of Health announced the development of an MRI (magnetic resonance imaging) centre at St Michael's, in response to a proposal submitted by the St Joseph's Health System two years earlier, at which time it was stated that St Michael's had the largest clinical volume of neuro patients in the city.[37] The nine-ton magnet of the MRI was lowered into place in May 1990, at below-ground level, on the site where the stage B redevelopment was expected to commence in the near future. This new technology, complementary to the CAT scanner, provides three-dimensional images of the interior of the body and better definition of areas shaded by bone such as the skull, spinal column, and hips. As such, it was to be particularly useful in showing head and spinal-cord injuries, in scanning the brain for cancer, and in studying the processes of multiple sclerosis.

The division of orthopaedics, headed by Dr James Waddell, chief and professor of surgery, and, until 1989, head of orthopaedics, was active and productive in research and its application. Dr Ensor Transfeldt was studying the neurophysiology of the lumbo-sacral plexus as well as the biomechanics of the spine; Dr Robin Richards, who replaced Dr Waddell as head of the division in 1989, was recognized as a leader in upper-limb reconstruction; and by 1988 more than half of all surgery for sarcoma (bone and muscle cancer) in Toronto was being done at St Michael's, under the leadership of Dr Robert S. Bell.[38]

The prevalence of degenerative-joint disease among his patients, as well as the inadequacies of the available prostheses, spurred Dr Waddell to undertake some original research in this area. After four years of study and animal experimentation, Waddell, working with a French manufacturing company, designed a total hip prosthesis in 1986. The "St Michael's Hospital Prosthesis," as it was named, was subjected to clinical trials in ten hospitals across Canada and was by 1987 approved for use in Australia, New Zealand, and several European countries.[39] In an extension of this research, Drs Robert Byrick and Waddell demonstrated that fat emboli released during the cementing process could cause lung injury and even cardiac arrest, a finding which directed the surgeons to a non-cemented prosthesis; this research earned for Drs Byrick and Waddell the Canadian Anaesthetists' Society prize for research in 1988.[40] To accommodate these and other research activities, and to conform to externally set standards, the hospital completed in 1987-88 a $1.5-million expansion of its animal-research laboratories and a $725,000 replacement of its bio-medical-waste facilities.[41]

And finally, Dr Shawn O'Driscoll, trained in elbow surgery at the Mayo Clinic, Rochester, Minnesota, in a first-of-its-kind procedure in Toronto, implanted a hinged artificial elbow, restoring the use of a woman's arm for which earlier physicians had suggested amputation. As in so many accounts of the research of these years, the primary actor credited the whole team – which in this case included the orthopaedic nurses and the physiotherapists – for the satisfactory outcome.[42]

Disorders of the Renal and Endocrine/Metabolic Systems

The division of nephrology's clinical and research activities continued strongly, with the number of dialysis stations increased from ten to seventeen in 1989; that same year Dr Norman Struthers performed the program's five hundredth kidney transplant. Dr Mitchell

Halperin's research in the fluid and electrolyte handling by the kidney was recognized in his appointment to the metabolism grants committee of the Medical Research Council of Canada.

In the division of endocrinology and metabolism, Drs Alick Little and Phillip Connelly received substantial grant support for basic research into atherosclerosis,[43] and their core lipid laboratory was safeguarded by moving it from the university's health sciences complex to St Michael's premises in 1989.[44] (The doctors feared an attempted takeover of the laboratory by another hospital.) In the related department of pathology, Drs Kovacs, Horvath, and Sylvia Asa maintained their international profile in research into the nature, function, and classification of pituitary tumours; in 1987 Dr Kovacs conducted a course in pituitary research in Beijing, Republic of China.[45] Again in a related field, this time gastroenterology, the number of TPN (total parenteral nutrition) patients approved by the medical advisory committee for treatment in the hospital at one time was increased from seven to fourteen, with concomitant cost increases.[46]

Drs Timothy Murray and Robert Josse continued their research into osteoporosis, receiving two hundred new patients annually in their metabolic bone disease clinic, the largest clinic in Canada for the treatment of osteoporosis. In 1987 Dr Murray was appointed director of the bone and mineral group of the University of Toronto, which had its core facilities at St Michael's. In 1988 Dr Murray presented at a twenty-country workshop the promising results from his study on the potential for increasing bone mass by means of additional daily sodium fluoride intake.[47]

Trauma

The five-year struggle to overcome the roadblocks erected in the path of establishing a level I treatment centre for adult trauma patients at St Michael's was discussed earlier. References to the equivocation, by the DHC and the Ministry of Health alike, and the rival campaign actively mounted by the Toronto General Hospital to have that institution designated as the site of the new centre are strewn throughout the records of those years.

The hospital was serious in its intent to offer trauma services: a trauma room had been incorporated into the new emergency department completed in the stage A construction of 1982; a dedicated operating room and critical-care facilities were included in the stage B plans underway; and in the meantime, a section of 4-F was renovated in 1989 to provide a five-bed trauma critical-care unit, with neurosurgeon Dr W.S. Tucker in charge.[48]

The trauma service was bedevilled from the first by the shortage of critical care nurses to staff it and by the struggle for funds to support it.[49] Although it was an expensive service, – using Sunnybrook's 1986 estimate of $13,967 per trauma patient, St Michael's costs for its trauma patients that year would have topped $2.1 million – St Michael's continued to accept a volume of patients that grew from 150 in 1986 to 220 in 1988-89. One has to wonder whether the trauma service's access to both staffing and funds was not squeezed by the aggressive growth of the cardiovascular service, which "was there first."[50]

Dreams of a Research Institute

Competition had been keen among the medical staff for the scarce research space available to carry out the studies in their various fields.[51] In June 1987 the board was informed that a donor had expressed the intention of making a significant contribution to the hospital on an annual basis, preferably to be directed to research; further, that the executive committee had decided to form two not-for-profit corporations – a research institute and a research centre – and to establish an interim board of directors for the two. The hospital board approved both decisions.[52]

In March 1988 Scott Griffin, who had agreed to spearhead a study into the setting up of a research institute, presented his report to a special meeting of the board.[53] He had reviewed the research being done within the eleven teaching hospitals, the research emphasis at each one, and the research space and support staff available to their investigators. He concluded that, although St Michael's had researchers "who can stand with the best in the city," their ability to maintain a competitive position in research – and ultimately, the hospital's ability to survive as a tertiary-care facility – was hampered by limited funds, insufficient space, and inadequate support staff. He requested approval to declare basic and clinical research a top priority at St Michael's and, among other moves, to commission a feasibility study to triple the current research space and to hire a director of research. The board approved.[54]

Work proceeded throughout 1988 under a steering committee chaired by Scott Griffin, and on which Dr Martin Hollenberg, associate dean-research, University of Toronto, and Drs Kalman Kovacs and Clifford Ottoway from St Michael's served. It was decided that the fund-raising campaign then underway would be for hospital redevelopment *and* research. A prospectus detailing the direction, scale, and research requirements of the research institute was prepared, indicating the substantial financial expenditure to which the hospital and its board must be committed if the project were approved.[55]

In his presentation of the grand plan to a special meeting of the board in August 1989, Griffin expressed the view that research could secure St Michael's long-term survival and its future within a hospital community increasingly under pressure for survival. The board approved the prospectus and called for a funding proposal and a search plan for a director.[56] Two floors on top of the planned stage B construction were tentatively allocated to research.[57]

It is unclear whether the donor mentioned in June 1987 was the same as the one who surfaced in March 1990, when the board was informed that the steering committee had obtained a commitment of $12 million for the institute from an anonymous donor, the committee's objective being $30 million. In a wrap-up one month later the board was told of the progress made towards the establishment of a major world-class research institute, and the search committee was working to engage a world-class director.

As will be explained, the situation at St Michael's changed dramatically in the summer and fall of 1990. In November 1990 the board was told that major funding had been withdrawn from this project, the search committee for a director had been disbanded, and the whole project had been placed on hold.[58]

Oncology

Mention has been made of the work of Dr P. Muller in the treatment of brain tumours and the work of Dr Robert Bell in treating cancer of the bone. Despite these advances, the future of oncology within St Michael's strategic plan was thrown into question in July 1987. At that time, the Ministry of Health announced that Princess Margaret Hospital would be relocated to University Avenue next to Mount Sinai Hospital,[59] where expanded modern facilities would be constructed. This announcement was followed by site visits by a ministry-appointed team (the Backley commission) to each hospital offering oncology services, with a view to recommending which services would be allowed to continue and which ones relocated. Once a week over a period of eighteen months, the Backley commission met with presidents of the university teaching hospitals. After reviewing the commission's report, ministry officials called the presidents together and informed them that, while they supported the report's concepts, no new funds would be available for transfer, integration, or expansion of oncology programs within the university teaching hospitals.[60] With the new Princess Margaret Hospital still not under construction (summer, 1992) some cancer research continues at St Michael's: in May 1991 Dr Bhagu Bhavnani of the department of obstetrics and gynaecology was awarded a substantial three-year grant from the Medical Research Council of Canada into the role of estrogen in human cancer.[61]

Biopsychosocial Medicine

Grouped hereunder in St Michael's strategic plan were those activities which contribute to the psychological, emotional, and social welfare of its patients. Outpatient psychiatry continued to be strong in this period; new to the scene was the retirement clinic offered under the umbrella of the mental health clinic. Family therapy became a key component of the services offered by the social work department. As well, the teaching program within this department was recognized by the University of Toronto as a prototype for other teaching centres.[62] The occupational therapy department, deeply involved in the treatment regimen of the psychiatric teams, received in 1988 a five-year accreditation as a student-training centre.

In 1986 the hospital invited an external review of its pastoral care department with a view to re-establishing a program for the training of chaplains in institutional ministry. Two years later an Anglican priest, the Reverend Floyd Green, who had headed the clinical pastoral education program at the Queen Street Mental Health Centre for nine years, was appointed director of pastoral care at St Michael's. In 1989 the training program was re-established.[63]

In the fall of 1988 Cardinal Carter formally appointed George Webster – who had been hired by the hospital as its ethicist six years earlier – as medical-moral theologian to St Michael's Hospital.[64] Dr Webster developed, in his work with and within the various clinical areas, important policies and guidelines for a dynamic environment. These ranged all the way from the traditional ethical decisions around the use of restraints on patients and the provision of nutrition and hydration, through the newly emerging policies about access to dialysis/transplantation in the context of scarce resources, to *Do Not Resuscitate* guidelines and ways of dealing with the periodic requests from relatives and friends of palliative-care patients for an "easeful death" (euthanasia) for their loved ones.[65] Lastly, to meet a need for more and better post-surgery communication between family and surgeon, the hospital established in 1990 a surgical information lounge near the operating room, staffed by specially trained volunteers.

Aging

The challenge and the needs of an aging population were recognized at St Michael's when, in December 1984, a proposal for establishment of a geriatric assessment unit was submitted to the DHC.[66] The idea took focus and shape with the appointment of Dr Barry Wilson to the division of internal medicine in 1985, and its place was further secured by its designation as one of the nine areas of concentration for the future in the strategic plan adopted in 1987. Wilson began immediately the work of coordinating geriatric care at St Michael's with that of Providence Villa and Hospital.[67]

Over the next two years a joint geriatric-assessment program was established for the two institutions, with a consultation service, an elders' clinic, and an in-house geriatric team at St Michael's and a seventeen-bed geriatric unit at Providence. Dr Wilson, director of the program, and Gail Mitchell, clinical-nurse specialist in gerontology, worked with the multi-disciplinary teams of both places. With an emphasis on helping the elderly to help themselves, and with attention to patients' medication, diet, and exercise, the teams interrupted the downward spiral for many an elderly person – restoring independence for those whose real problem was discovered to be fear of institutionalization.[68] In 1989 St Michael's board was told that the geriatric-assessment proposal had finally received ministry approval and funding.[69]

Women's Health Care

In the early 1980s many women were expressing a preference for giving birth, not in the conventional hospital setting, but in a relaxed, family-oriented, home-like environment. They wanted, as well, easy access to the medical facilities that might be required to deal with any complications. The hospital provided for such a "birthing centre" in its strategic plan of 1984 and submitted a proposal for its establishment to the DHC.[70] The proposal went through more than one revision, as Ministry of Health guidelines changed.[71] The final version incorporated a non-interventionist, shared decision-making philosophy. It also made provision for the special training of coordinating nurses who would replace the current three categories of nurses (labour and delivery, post-partum, and nursery), and the eventual introduction of midwives when these would become legal in Ontario.

Although St Michael's proposal was ranked first of the two proposals submitted,[72] the Ministry of Health decided to establish two hospital-based birthing centres at the extremes of Metro Toronto – Scarborough General Hospital and Peel Memorial Hospital. In this, and in other proposals, it would be of interest to calculate the time and money spent by staff, architects, and consultants on bids that were eventually passed over. St Michael's moved, nevertheless, on some of the concepts, instituting "combined care"– one nurse to attend to both mother and baby, in the mother's room; presence during labour and delivery was extended to husbands/partners, grandparents, and even children as the mother wished; the clinical look of labour rooms was softened by redecorating with wallpaper and easy furnishings, and the labour room became as well the delivery room. The former delivery rooms were still used for Caesarean sections, and the former nursery remained for sick and "boarder" babies. All of this required a considerable adaptation of attitude and practice, especially by those nurses who had trained and had faithfully adhered to the conventional mode – among them, those trained by Sister Vincentia and Marcella Berger.

When the new facilities in 61 Queen Street East became available in 1988 it became possible to house all women's services (with the exception of inpatient) under one roof. These services, located on the fifth floor of the new building, included all gynaecology care (including colposcopy, cryosurgery, and laser surgery – procedures previously carried out in the operating room); pre-natal care, including pre-natal classes; infertility services; natural family planning; fetal-assessment unit (ultrasound); menopausal services; and various support groups (abuse, infertility, and so on). Screening for breast cancer – handled by the department of surgery – was directly below on the 4th floor. Directing the whole effort (17,000 patients seen in 1989-90) was the team headed by Dr Anthony Cecutti and Charlene (McCaffrey) Shevlen, chief and nursing coordinator respectively. The program was financially assisted by a substantial donation ($266,000) from the city's health care fund;[73] of significant cost to the hospital itself was the mammogram installed in 1988-89.

After these relocations, all that remained occupied of the extensive renovations made to accommodate the department of obstetrics in 1966 was the research laboratory. In addition to the medical research going on there, some significant nursing studies were being done: one concerned with the "monitrice" (labour coach) during labour; and currently (1992) St Michael's is involved in a twenty-hospital study correlating the rate of various medical interventions with the active presence (or the absence) of a nurse during labour.[74]

Community Health

By mid-1980 the area served by St Michael's was populated by a diverse mix of low to high socio-economic groups, with an equally diverse range of health-care needs. To the east were the neighbourhoods of Moss Park and Regent Park, Riverdale, and Cabbagetown, with their many, mostly poor, elderly residents and a younger group that was largely unemployed and plagued by crime and substance abuse. From these neighbourhoods the area extended to the business corridor, peopled by the upwardly-mobile high achievers. Towards the north boundary of this corridor were immigrants from various countries, and at the south were the middle- and upper-income residents of Crombie Park and Harbourfront. Recognizing the multiracial character the city had assumed, the office of the mayor provided to St Michael's doctors in 1987 a medical information gathering kit which contained a translation in twenty-five different languages of questions that doctors commonly ask patients.

In addition to the area served by the hospital proper, there were those areas served by its two satellite clinics: the Broadview Clinic and the St Lawrence Health Services. Almost twenty years old, Broadview Clinic was still seeing in 1990 some of its original patients from an area that stretched from Danforth Avenue to the Lakefront and from the Don River to Coxwell Avenue; Broadview maintained, in addition to its special focus on women's health, a brisk family-practice outreach that included medical care to a community-crisis centre for immigrants, abused women, and others. Patient advocacy was also an important part of this clinic's service. St Lawrence Health Services, serving the area from King Street to the Lakeshore, between Church and Parliament streets, provided health care to two elementary schools, a home for handicapped children, a sheltered workshop, and a shelter for homeless teens. The ideal pursued by staff in both centres was that of offering very personalized, family-centred care (help with parenting was a prominent feature), with an emphasis on health promotion as well as health maintenance.

At the hospital itself, by 1989 the department of ambulatory care had grown to encompass 129 different clinics in twenty-two separate locations, which received a quarter-million patient visits annually.[75] Operating there, a department-within-a-department, the department of family and community health under its chief, Dr Sudi Devanesen, maintained its in-hospital clinics as well as a wide range of outreach services. These extended all the way from home visits to the shut-in elderly to attendance at a Youthdale Crisis Centre, and from a shelter for displaced women (Street Haven, established and managed by St Michael's graduate Peggy Ann Walpole, and meriting a recognition far beyond what this book can offer)[76] to the hospice for AIDS patients – and with a variety of other centres in between.

When the building at 61 Queen Street East was renovated in 1988, family and community medicine took up residence on the whole of the third floor. With the breast screening centre on the fourth floor, the women's health centre on the fifth, and the department of occupational health and environmental health (whose staff was available to assess and monitor safety and environmental conditions in the workplace) on the eighth, health care thus took a significant step out into the community – a full and integrated service, backed by the full resources of the hospital.

Straddling the departments of dietary services and medicine, and allied with the health-maintenance/promotion efforts of several departments, was the clinical nutrition and risk factor modification centre established on the sixth floor of 61 Queen Street in 1989-90. There Dr David Jenkins and a team doing research in lipids and nutrition collaborated with the hospital's clinical nutritionists to provide individualized assessment of the risk factors contributing to certain chronic diseases and to assist people to reduce such risk through lifestyle modification. The city provided a grant of $120,000 to St Michael's towards the funding of this innovative project;[77] the investigators received, as well, a substantial grant from the National Institutes of Health. The continued excellence of the department of dietetic services, under Judith Pratt-Jeffries, was recognized in 1991 by the Canadian Dietetic Association's award of five-year accreditation of the department's internship program.

"The Flagship Building," 61 Queen Street East[78]

In July 1987 the owners of a nine-storey building at 61 Queen Street East, opposite St Michael's, approached the hospital to explore the latter's interest in partnership or purchase of the property.[79] The hospital commissioned a firm to evaluate the property and received a somewhat negative assessment of the building which had been constructed only one year previously: poor workmanship in general, with some major deficiencies in the various systems, and discrepancies between the supporting documents and the building as constructed.[80] Nevertheless, a special joint meeting of the budget and finance committee and the building and property committee approved a negotiating team to represent the hospital in negotiations with the owner.[81]

The time was right for considering such a move: earlier the hospital had held talks with the medical staff with a view to the latter moving out of the hospital to commercial-office space, on leases partially subsidized by the hospital.[82] Now the board was told, at a special meeting called to discuss the possible acquisition of the building at 61 Queen, that the hospital suffered severe space restraints which would not be satisfied even by the proposed stage B construction.[83] The board was presented with an executive summary concerning the proposed acquisition which included assumptions that revenues from leased office space (by physicians) and increased growth-funding grants[84] from the Ministry of Health (based on volumes of patients) would bring the hospital to a break-even position within a two-year period. The board was of the opinion that the move was in accordance with the ministry's BOND plan whereby hospitals were allowed to retain certain income which did not form part of the operating budget financed by the ministry. At the 29 September 1987 meeting of the board of directors, it was resolved that "the Sisters of St Joseph, Diocese of Upper Canada, who own and operate St Michael's Hospital, purchase 61 Queen Street East." The board authorized "the short-term borrowing of $12,711,000 plus the necessary funds for leasehold improvements by issuance of Bankers Acceptance Certificates through the Bank of Montreal," and resolved "that St Michael's Hospital guaranty [sic] the Notes, and that the appropriate Directors ... sign and execute such forms and deliver them to the Bank of Montreal."[85]

The proposal for physicians to relocate to the new building, leasing office space there with partial subsidy by the hospital, met with resistance from those doctors who were currently occupying fully-funded office space;[86] the very complex and thorny question of what constituted "geographic full time entitlement" was under discussion at both the university and the hospital and was at an impasse. In what appears to have been an alternate plan for use of the building, the hospital prepared to move selected programs into the space. To ensure that the quarters were appropriate to the type and volume of patients and to meet building-code requirements for ambulatory-care patients,[87] in a building supposedly designed for medical offices and laboratories,[88] floors that had been renovated before the purchase had to be totally replanned, redesigned, and reconstructed – at a cost that soared to $4.3 million.[89] The resulting facility – tastefully arranged, decorated, and furnished, merging doctors' private offices with clinics – was confidently believed to be capable of generating the growth funds necessary to support itself.[90] Joe Lavoie, vice president of finance and administration, was credited with being a key figure in developing the strategy and financing package for this new "St Michael's Hospital Health Centre."[91] The building was fully occupied by May 1990 but by October 1990, as will be seen presently, the sale of the premises was being given serious consideration.

Nursing

For the department of nursing during the years 1985-90, the challenges posed by the tremendous growth in so many clinical services (cardiovascular, neurosurgery, trauma, orthopedics, nephrology) were daunting.

The recognition in mid-1985 that there was a "critical" shortage of critical-care nurses in Metro Toronto[92] became, by late 1987, an acknowledgment of an "extremely critical" shortage,[93] and in mid-1989 St Michael's critical-care areas reported 127 registered nurse vacancies. In the midst of all this, three of Metro's community colleges extended the length of their nurse-training programs to three years, thereby severely reducing the number of new nurses coming into the system in 1988-89.[94] One wonders how the hospital had the courage or temerity to forge ahead, as it did, with its plans for cardiovascular expansion and its bid for a trauma program.

The hospital did respond vigorously to the challenge. It offered to support nurses enrolled in critical-care programs at Ryerson Polytechnical Institute,[95] enlisted consultants to help with recruitment,[96] and developed a recruitment strategy. Comprehensive and ambitious, the recruitment strategy included the following features: specialty-education programs in critical care, operating room, obstetrics, and mental health at the hospital's expense; extensive advertising; overseas recruiting; relocation assistance; and temporary accommodation. Much of this was virtually unknown for St Michael's nurses in earlier years.[97]

Both the shortages and the measures taken to relieve them had a large dollar sign attached; one small example – to offset the cutback in resident-training posts, the nurse-intravenous team extended its daily coverage to twenty-four hours at an additional cost of up to $135,000 annually. The larger costs included those of training just one trauma nurse for the trauma teams, estimated to be $5,500. In September 1987 forty additional nurses were approved in the budget because of the type of patients and the acute nature of their illnesses in the OR, intensive care, and acute care. A total of $800,000 was paid in advertising and relocation for nurses brought from other areas of the country in 1988-89.[98]

Where had all the nurses gone?[99] In 1987-88 many nurses left the hospital and joined the staffs of a growing number of nursing agencies, which were offering greater flexibility of working hours and were paying double or triple the rate paid by the hospitals under a negotiated contract. These registries had wide variations in rates – from $33.60 per hour to $36.50 per hour for critical-care areas, in contrast with the $28 per hour charged by HNS (Hospital Nursing Service), the registry which had been established ten years earlier with the backing of the hospitals, and which the hospitals still favoured. During 1987-88 St Michael's paid out more than $1 million in additional funds to nursing agencies to supplement its staff; the experience of the other Metro hospitals was similar.[100]

Despite the comparative success of the recruitment efforts – including thirty-nine nurses from England in 1989 and sixteen from Australia in 1990 – and with recruitment continuing in the United Kingdom, Australia, and New Zealand even as American hospitals were busily targetting Canadian nurses[101]– beds had to be cut because of the staff shortages.

The pattern of bed closures during the summers was not new; what was new, however, was the inability to reopen beds even late into the fall, a situation that worsened to the point where closures extended throughout the year.[102] In May 1989 St Michael's had 105 beds closed, with an additional 36 planned for the summer, constituting 20.5 percent of its bed complement; other Metro teaching hospitals anticipated similar closures, reaching even 25 percent and 27 percent[103] of their total bed capacities. By November 1989 – short by 220 nurses – St Michael's vice-president for nursing reported that 106 beds, including 32 critical-care beds, were closed, and another 145 were being recommended for closure over Christmas. Throughout all of this, bed-management committees and resource-utilization committees – with the leadership of Sister Catherine McDonough and the heavy involvement of the medical staff – worked tirelessly to try to match patient needs with the ever-dwindling resources.[104]

Throughout the years of the recruitment/retention struggles, Anita Fisher (VP, nursing) worked to enhance nurse satisfaction and patient care through the appointment of clinical-nurse specialists in several areas. A growth in the professionalism of nurses (and indeed of several professional groups – dietitians, physiotherapists, pharmacists, social workers) is evident in the references in the hospital's newsletter to their published papers and their presentations at association meetings. All of St Michael's health professionals appear to have reached a new stage of maturity.

St Michael's Place: A Housing Initiative

Running throughout the accounts of staffing problems at this time are references to the difficulty in finding housing for recruits from afar, as well as the high cost of housing and transportation and the unavailability of parking at the hospital.[105]

The departments of finance and of human resources were energetic in their efforts, attempting to locate an apartment building for staff, employing a real-estate agent to help find housing, and discussing subsidized parking and public-transit passes with the city. Finally, a proposal to build on the former laundry site came before the board in January 1990 and received its endorsement.[106] By this time the hospital had 400 vacancies in its ranks; that is, the problem was more than a nursing problem.

With housing-vacancy rates running at almost the zero mark for the past couple of years, the Archdiocese of Toronto had been active in attempting to make some of its church lands available for public-housing developments. The archdiocesan housing office, by now experienced, teamed up with St Michael's and with the Ontario Ministry of Housing on the hospital's plan to meet its staff's need for accommodation; a plan was conceived to create 240 units of affordable housing in a building to be erected on the northeast corner of Victoria and Shuter streets. While the one- and two-bedroom apartments were to be primarily for hospital staff and their families, a number were to be allocated to the handicapped and those requiring subsidized housing.[107]

Plans moved ahead quickly; the sisters agreed to donate the land on which St Michael's Place, as the development was to be called, would stand, an architectural firm (Kelton and Lakka) was selected, and a date for beginning construction was set.[108] But within nine months of its conception the project was put on hold, and within the year the board was told that "although, strategically, the hospital recognizes the need for [such a building] to assist in recruitment and retention ... proceeding would not be prudent at this time."[109]

The Giant Step into the World of Computers

While automated financial and administrative systems had been installed at St Michael's in 1977-78, a serious step into the large-scale use of computers was taken in 1985 when the Sisters of St Joseph's corporate health planning group, chaired by Sister Janet Murray, agreed that the establishment of a multi-institutional automated-information system constituted a project worthy of exploration. Under the chairmanship of W.V. Moore, a strategic plan was developed for a fully integrated patient information system, an ambitious project to be phased in over a period of eight years. Ray Briggs was engaged as the group's director of information systems.[110]

Advised that an approach made jointly to the ministries of health and of community and social services had met with little encouragement as far as funding was concerned (institutions, they were told, were expected "to find" funds for computerization within their own resources), St Michael's board approved in 1985 a management-information system for the hospital, to be phased in over a four-year period at an estimated cost of $4 million.[111]

After two years of preliminary work by Ray Briggs, in a move that represented a significant escalation of the plans developed in 1985, a contract was signed with Unisys in mid-1987 for a system which included a powerful Unisys A-12 mainframe computer and up to 1000 terminals and printers throughout the hospital.[112] Beginning in October 1987, in an effort to remove some of the apprehension and mystery surrounding computers and to stir up enthusiasm as he raised the level of staff computer-literacy, Joe Lavoie, VP of administration and finance, began to edit and circulate monthly an excellent little publication entitled, appropriately, *CHIPS TODAY*.

In March 1988 medical records became the first hospital department to be fully on-line – providing, among other features, replacement of the 400,000 card-index file by a computerized data bank, and new electrical-mobile shelving that doubled the filing space. Dietetic services followed a month later, with five terminals capable of handling the menus, tracking inventory, and preparing purchase orders, as well as nutritional analysis and maintenance of patient records. By means of an admission/discharge/transfer terminal in dietetic services, a new accuracy and timeliness was built into the information necessary for patients' food services.

In late 1989 the pharmacy was provided with two separate computer systems, both linked to the hospital's mainframe system. By means of the Rx Manager, physicians' orders could now be entered directly into the computer to maintain an updated patient's drug profile, and checks could be made for drug interactions; pharmacists were alerted to automatic stop-order dates, and "fill lists" and labels could be generated. The second system, CIVA (central intravenous admixture), was linked to the location within pharmacy where intravenous drug mixtures were prepared. At this time, too, the unit dose drug distribution was begun, a system whereby each dose of medication is individually labelled and packaged in pharmacy and delivered to the nursing units in ready-to-administer form. Introduction of this system, recommended several years earlier in the Dubin report, required (and was based upon) pharmacy's capacity to maintain complete patient-medication profiles. The multiple check-points contained within the new computerized systems enhanced accuracy, lowered the risk of contamination, and reduced drug wastage. It constituted, also, a major reallocation of medication-distribution activities from nursing to pharmacy staff. To house its expanded activities, pharmacy had been relocated in 1988 to the section of the B-wing vacated by dietetic services, newly renovated at a budgeted cost of $440,000.[113]

In addition to the above installations, throughout 1988-89 "modules" were implemented for admitting/discharge/transfer, central-patient index, five laboratories (biochemistry, haematology, blood bank, microbiology, and pathology), materials management, and general-ledger and accounts payable. The system became a model for a number of hospitals contemplating installation of a large integrated system computer network.

In mid-1990, with its management-information system 70 percent complete, St Michael's appointed Dr Michael Guerriere, physician and computer scientist, to the position of vice-president of clinical affairs, in charge of the computer system and hospital records. Guerriere, working with Granville Technologies, moved quickly to write some of the software required to initiate a process whereby a doctor would enter his patient's file number into the computer, a steno-pool staff-person would call up all the basic information necessary, and a report emerged that could be faxed to the referring doctor within minutes. A backlog of 14,000 letters was cleared up even as the system was being installed, and an estimated future saving of $100,000 annually was projected.[114]

St Michael's Hospital and St Joseph's Health Centre: The Bumpy Road towards Integration

For twelve years, at regular meetings chaired by Sister Janet Murray, the senior sister-administrative personnel at St Michael's and St Joseph's Health Centre shared their insights and expertise and offered mutual support. Along the way this loosely knit group was strengthened by the addition of the board chairmen from the member institutions, becoming in 1984 the Sisters of St Joseph Corporate Health Planning Group. Despite the best efforts of Sister Janet and the backing of the new structure, only limited progress was made in nudging the institutions towards closer collaboration. While they were guided by a common underlying philosophy, their individual characters and foci were quite dissimilar.

The congregation moved in May 1986 to a still more structured arrangement whereby the Sisters of St Joseph Health System was established – a federated model with five member institutions, each governed by its own board of directors but with a parent board over the whole.[115] Sister Janet was appointed president of the new SJHS. For two years Sister Janet applied her talents and her vast experience in the health-care field to the development of the system. She monitored the rapidly changing environment (which included the emerging power-blocks within the University of Toronto health sciences complex), and initiated joint ventures in those areas where the member institutions showed a need and a willingness to cooperate. While a few shared services were initiated,[116] the progress was painfully slow. To develop a structure whereby the health system's board had extensive authority to monitor and coordinate activities and to determine policy, but with minimum loss of autonomy for the member institutions, proved to be difficult indeed.[117]

In the face of reservations that surfaced from time to time, Sister Janet persevered in her task. In an important address to St Michael's board in January 1988, out of her own deep commitment to the church's mission in health care she sketched a probable future in which the congregation might no longer be there as a symbol of the driving force and presence of the church in this field. The board, then, would be the driving force. Responding to Sister Janet's address, some board members expressed their satisfaction with a "holding company"-type model, as already established in the SJHS's board; Sister Janet was told, however, that doctors viewed a move toward integration with some trepidation, fearing negative consequences for their programs and loss of independence in budgeting matters.

The congregation next turned to a consulting firm for a complete review of the situation. The consultants, finding that the loyalties of the member boards, chief executive officers, management, and medical staff lay each with their own institution rather than with a distant SJHS, suggested a continuation of the federation model within which the SJHS might be sustained and strengthened. The consultants predicted, however, that it would take years to bring about change and create a sense of pride and ownership of the SJHS within the member institutions.[118]

While this was not encouraging, the congregation moved, nevertheless, to put names and faces on the structure and process which the consultants had suggested for the SJHS: Sister Marie Paradis, a member of the General Council, was appointed president; a board of trustees was named, chaired by Sister Imelda Cahill, the general superior; and various advisory bodies and task forces were created. After one and one-half years of intensive work within the new structure, and following a retreat at which several participants had expressed the view that sharing in clinical programs would not occur without a re-examination of the SJHS's structure, the General Council made its decision; in a moving address to the board in November 1989, Sister Imelda reviewed the congregation's long history in the health-care ministry and its hopes for the future, and announced the congregation's resolve to integrate St Michael's Hospital and St Joseph's Health Centre.[119] The move, she said, was viewed as a way of maximizing the considerable strengths of the two institutions, and of passing on the sisters' legacy in health care (even as their numbers dwindled) while retaining their ownership and confirming their mission in health care in Toronto. While the federated model had allowed for considerable autonomy in each institution, the integration envisaged in the new arrangement was one in which a single chief executive officer, responsible to a single board, would direct and govern the two institutions.

An interim board of directors was appointed, chaired by Alan Dilworth, and was charged with conducting a search for a president of the integrated hospitals. Neither of the two incumbent presidents, Sister Christine Gaudet of St Michael's and Sister Margaret Myatt of St Joseph's, chose to stand for appointment to the position.[120] The search committee was fortunate in engaging Roger Hunt to be president of the integrated organization, which would be called the Fontbonne Health

System.[121] The legal process of registration of the name, achieving its incorporation, and approval of a new by-law would be the next step.

On 19 March 1990 Sister Christine, after five years of dedicated effort and of creative and courageous response to a complex and rapidly changing health-care scene, resigned her position and embarked on a sabbatical leave. Joseph Lavoie, who had become executive vice-president in the fall of 1989, now became the chief operating officer; for the first time in its ninety-eight year history, St Michael's Hospital was without a sister at its head.

Roger Hunt (BA, MBA in health administration), who came with a solid record in senior administration in multi-institutional health settings, assumed his new position in September 1990. Sister Marie Paradis, whose belief in and enthusiasm for the concept of integration had not flagged throughout the long haul, remained for a further six months to assist him during the transitional period.

Progress on Other Fronts

Throughout these years, St Michael's vigorous participation in education for all the health disciplines continued. The numbers (more than 600 annually) and range of students are truly impressive, a testament to the commitment of all the disciplines to the teaching function of St Michael's: in the 1988-89 academic year the undergraduate population numbered 163 medical students, 156 nursing students, 37 dental students, 32 physiotherapists, 26 dietetic interns, 20 students in the various medical technology fields, 6 social-work students, and one pharmacy student. In addition, post-graduate students numbered 40 medical interns, 133 medical residents, 3 residents in dentistry, and one in pharmacy.[122] While the hospital sustained its long tradition of popularity and success in medical education at both the undergraduate and post-graduate levels, there were fears for the future: the predominance of acutely ill patients in many of the services made them less suitable for teaching undergraduates, and the declining number of funded post-graduate positions was becoming by 1989 a cause for concern about that level.[123]

With regard to its building plans, in early 1988 the hospital received the good news that the Ministry of Health would share the funding for the construction of phase I, stage B (the other half of the C-wing, running along Victoria Street). A year later, Mayor Art Eggleton, Health Minister Elinor Caplan, and Board Chairman Alan Dilworth donned hard hats and lifted the first shovel of earth in a ground-breaking ceremony. The plans called for a handsome first floor, housing a new admitting department and various amenities; second and third floors that would extend the laboratory and radiology facilities from the C-wing; critical-care areas and a desperately needed surgical suite on the fourth and fifth levels; a cafeteria adjacent to the main kitchens on sixth; and cardiology, nephrology/dialysis, and musculoskeletal nursing units on the seventh, eight, and ninth floors. The well-conceived plans were nurtured and ably carried forward by Graham Constantine, who had earlier proved himself in similar projects. Hopes ran high that the new quarters would be ready for occupancy in the spring of 1991.[124]

The start of construction was dependent upon the hospital's assuring the Ministry of Health that it had the funds to proceed. The campaign for building funds, with a target of $25 million, begun in April 1984 under the chairmanship of Alan Dilworth had, by June 1985, raised almost $11 million in pledges and contributions. Larry Thalheimer assumed direction of the campaign office at that time, the contract of the professional fund-raiser (G. Goldie) having expired.[125] For five years Thalheimer made regular and precise accountings to the board; by 31 March 1990 he was able to report more then $26 million received in cash and pledges – with 82 percent of the latter paid in full. Proceeds from the efforts of individual board members and from special functions gave tremendous boosts along the way. The annual dinner hosted by Cardinal Carter in May 1985, receipts from showings of the musical "Cats" and of the opera "Aida-at-the-Dome," and other events ranging from a golf tournament to a champagne ball – from such disparate sources does a hospital draw its financial support in the dying days of the twentieth century.

At the November 1987 meeting of the board, Dilworth had proposed the establishment of a foundation "for creating greater public focus and awareness of St Michael's need for financial support." A vice-president of development was recruited and the process of legal incorporation and recruitment of members was begun. In July 1989 the board of St Michael's Hospital Foundation (a fourteen-member board, chaired by Hartland MacDougall) held its inaugural meeting. A structure with a permanent commitment to annual fund-raising was finally in place.[126]

The Hospital Auxiliary

The proposal for a foundation, which had now become a reality, was not new; the Hospital Auxiliary (formerly called the Women's Auxiliary) had had plans for such an undertaking forty years previously. In February 1947 Dr Harris McPhedran suggested to the auxiliary the establishment of a research fund as a laudable objective for that organization to pursue. The auxiliary's response was characteristically energetic and thorough. For a full year there was exploration with the university's board of governors, the sisters' General Council, the cardinal, the hospital's board and its lawyer, and, of course, those doctors most interested in the idea's fulfilment – Drs E. Brooks and William Magner. In November 1947 the auxiliary membership approved a motion that $50,000 be raised in a special-names campaign, the money to be held in trust and administered by a board of trustees; a campaign committee was established, and plans for a foundation appeared to be underway. Despite these brave beginnings, the executive committee of the auxiliary decided in March 1948 to table the idea "as it appeared not to be within the scope of the Auxiliary," and at a subsequent general meeting $300 was made available for medical research.[127] Thus began the auxiliary's longstanding support of research at St Michael's; in 1990, for example, a $60,000 donation was made to the Research Society for studies in osteoporosis.

The roots of the auxiliary are closely intertwined with those of St Michael's. The Women's Auxiliary was established in 1920 when hospital superintendent Sister de Pazzi Smith requested assistance with the making of bedding and bandages for patients. On 12 April of that year the auxiliary's inaugural meeting was held and an executive elected: Minnie McKeown, president; Katharine Frawley and Isabelle King, 1st and 2nd vice presidents; Helena O'Brien, treasurer; and Mrs Charles Sheard, Jr, recording secretary. The husbands of these women were all prominent physicians on the staff of St Michael's Hospital at that time.

At this same meeting, the women suggested "Captains," who would bring helpers to sew; hours of work were set at 1:00 to 5:00 p.m. four days a week, and the membership fee was set at $1. Although the treasurer's report showed a debt of $4.82 after six months' operation, by the end of the year $1000 had been raised and presented to "Mother Superior" for linen for the new nurses' residence. At the first anniversary of its founding, the auxiliary's activities had broadened to include the formation of an automobile committee which would arrange to take the sisters driving every Friday during the months May through August. Later that year the auxiliary established a scholarship which was to be given to the graduating nurse with the highest standing in general proficiency to enrol in public-health nursing at the University of Toronto, with the auxiliary's stated wish that she remain in Canada for one year after graduating – not naive women, these. This scholarship continued throughout the life of the school of nursing.

A reading of the auxiliary's records all through the years reveals a vision, initiative, creativity, resourcefulness, fine business sense – as well as a generosity of spirit and capacity for hard work – which suggest that the majority of these women could have been highly successful business executives had they chosen to be. Composed primarily of wives of doctors in the early years, their numbers were soon widened to include board members' wives and friends of both groups; the same names appear in the records over ten, fifteen, twenty years, opening their homes for meetings and teas throughout all that time (Mrs Florence McPhedran even hosted a tea on an Easter Sunday to help raise funds).

From its original purpose of assisting with sewing (100,000 articles were made in the first eight years), the auxiliary moved to fund-raising for a variety of special projects, for example, to assist in furnishings for the new A-B-C wings in 1929. It became a source to which doctors turned for special pieces of equipment, such as a fluoroscope ($800), an infant bronchoscope, a portable incubator ($612), and a circuloelectric bed for burn patients ($650). In its work, the auxiliary showed a special concern for needy mothers and babies on the obstetrical ward, for whom layettes were regularly provided; for needy adults on the public wards and in the outpatient department; and for needy nursing students. In the two latter cases an emergency fund was made available to the sister in charge to be used at her discretion.

While all the auxiliary's members were volunteers, there were other women (frequently secretaries from offices roundabout) who wished to give some time to the hospital. In 1961 Mrs Marjorie O'Sullivan reported that "volunteer services" now numbered sixty members; the auxiliary decided upon a crest to be worn on a smock which would be presented to the volunteer workers after a required period of service. That same year teenagers were accepted as volunteers for the first time. Ten years later a department of volunteer services was established and a salaried director was recruited, paid by the hospital. Volunteers were eligible to join the auxiliary after a probationary period and payment of the membership fee.

When the F-wing was opened in 1965 provision was made for a gift shop, managed by the auxiliary, on the street level. There Mrs Marion Palmer, who began as a volunteer "day Captain," became the salaried manager in an auxiliary initiative which raised (after expenses) $675,000 in the ensuing twenty-five years.[128] Beginning with Eleanor Healy in 1973, incumbent presidents of the auxiliary served as *ex officio* members of the hospital's board of directors. The long involvement of the auxiliary in the provision of reading material to patients reached a new level in 1979. Ever since 1922, volunteers from the Newman Club of the University of Toronto had staffed a mobile lending library, making rounds from ward to ward;[129] the auxiliary contributed money from time to time to restock their cart. In 1979 an auxiliary committee headed by Mrs Margaret Casella, with funds from the auxiliary matched by funds from the Ministry of Culture and Recreation, established a gracious and well-stocked permanent library in space given over by the hospital on 5-E, the sisters' former community room.

Apart from its special projects the auxiliary has supported financially such initiatives as redecorating the hospital's lounges, lobbies, and visitors' waiting-rooms. Its special direct-patient-contact activities were most apparent in the admitting department, the dental clinic, and the palliative-care and gastro-intestinal units. Further evidence of the same has been their longstanding involvement in the breast diagnostic centre, which Mrs Eileen Murray took a leading role in founding.

Between 1965 and 1990 this special group of women contributed – in addition to the gift of each one's very self in time and energy – a total of $2 million to the hospital,[130] including $200,000 in June 1991 to the redevelopment campaign. Clearly where there is character and spirit, and love of one's neighbour, a little red ink on the books in the early phase does not constitute reason enough for quitting.

The Evolving Financial Situation

The initiatives taken during these years to respond to a dynamic and demanding health scene have been noted; there remains to be examined the steps taken to fund the developments underway.

The era began with a good financial picture: the extra $4 million of the Ministry of Health's allocation, plus the restraint program of 1984-85, left the hospital with a tidy operating surplus which was transferred to the capital budget.[131] In September 1986 Lloyd LaRocque resigned as assistant executive director of finance. Joe Lavoie assumed this senior position in February 1987, and held it until he became executive vice-president in November 1989.

During these years both operating and capital costs were staggering. Prime examples include a cost overrun of $1 million for contrast media in diagnostic imaging for a single year (1986); a cost overrun of $400,000 in renovation costs (1986), not related to 61 Queen Street East; and, late in the period, major expenses that ranged all the way from a changeover from a single- to a dual-chamber pacemaker, at a cost of $5,000 per patient (which brought the cost of the 189 pacemakers inserted in 1988-89 to more than $900,000), to the undertakings that set in place a tremendously expensive, but effective, magnetic-resonance-imaging installation and an integrated computer system.

Tertiary-Care Programs

The escalating costs of the various tertiary-care programs were still more alarming. Requests from department heads and chiefs for expansion of these programs for the 1988-89 budget were 24 percent over the previous year's request, all subject to ministry approval. The situation appears to have been general throughout the Ontario health system. During that year twenty-three hospitals were undergoing operational review by the Ministry of Health, and St Michael's was not one of them.

In June 1988 the minister of health announced that St Michael's would increase its heart-surgery caseload by two hundred patients a year, and would add nine additional critical-care beds for cardio-vascular surgery, with ministry grants of $2.1 million and increased operating funds of $6.4 million. Because the additional funding still fell short of what was required to implement recommendations of the 1989 cardiovascular surgery investigation report, a line-by-line review by the ministry's area team was carried out.[132] At what was reported as a very productive meeting in mid-1989, St Michael's administrative and finance personnel presented to the Ministry of Health a costing methodology that was new to the Canadian hospital scene (Case Mix Groupings), which, St Michael's board was told, was received enthusiastically and accepted by the ministry.[133] St Michael's staff present at the meeting estimated that funding adjustments might now be made, even as high as from $8 to $14 million. In March 1990 Lavoie reported to the board on the appeals that had been successfully completed: $4.4 million would be awarded to cover additional cardiovascular and trauma costs; $3.6 million would be made available for further reimbursement of 300 open-heart procedures; and continued efforts were being made to secure funding for the years 1987 and 1988.[134] Also reported as successfully appealed were a $4-million figure for workers' compensation cases and $.3 million for a perfusionist-training program.

As with the cardiovascular program, the trauma program was under Ministry of Health review from August 1988. In May 1989, after the hospital protested that it was underfunded for a program costed at $2.7 million, trauma became subject to a line-by-line review.[135] The ministry's eventual response was contained in the additional funding reported immediately above. Big money, it can be seen, was involved in these two tertiary-care programs, but it was money for exceedingly complex care. In September 1990 Lavoie asserted that the volume of acutely ill patients at St Michael's had risen from sixth to third highest in the province; however, its costs were still $14 million below those of its peers.[136]

The Dispute over WCB Charges

One of the longest-running controversies of this period revolved around the amount to be paid for Workers' Compensation Board patients (while the services provided were paid for by the WCB, Ministry of Health approval had to be obtained by the hospital for the rates charged). In August 1987 the approved per diem rate was $434; Lavoie requested approval to raise this to $850 – invoking the ministry's own policy which encouraged hospitals to generate maximum revenues from third-party sources; non-approval of the request, it was stated, represented an annual potential loss to the hospital of $2 million. The debate see-sawed among the hospital's finance department, the ministry, and the WCB throughout 1987 and 1988.[137] St Michael's board was told in September 1988 that revenue increases that were being shown in the financial statements were the result of increased WCB rates, and in January 1989 the finance director was commended by the board for his persevering efforts in obtaining recognition of the new rate, $900 a day for WCB patients. The issue was complicated by reason of the fact that the ministry concurred with St Michael's data supporting the rates of $850 and $900 for fiscal 1988 and 1989. Although the WCB declined to increase its rates, even when faced with this information, the requested increase was incorporated into the hospital's financial statement. However, by September 1990 the hospital had still not had any success in collecting the WCB payments in dispute.[138] Meanwhile, as indicated above, they were being carried on the financial statements as revenue, in expectation of their eventual receipt.[139]

Possible Sources of New Revenue

The search for other new sources of revenue was active throughout these years. These included partially subsidized office space for the medical staff, the sale and lease-back of major equipment, and "growth funding."

From 1987 and into 1990 debate continued with regard to entitlements under the geographic full-time policy for university-teaching, medical-staff appointments. A variety of arrangements had grown like Topsy over the years, and now the hospital was trying to arrive at a consistent and equitable practice of allocation of space and amenities which would provide a firm basis for future negotiations with medical staff. The vast majority of medical staff paid no rent for office space; this was a situation that would prove difficult to change, but not for lack of effort.[140] In June 1989 the board approved a policy whereby department chiefs and laboratory directors would be allowed offices rent-free; no rent would be charged for offices used exclusively for research, teaching, or administration; and the hospital would provide up to 50 percent subsidy for office and secretarial space to each geographic full-time physician, beginning 1 October 1989. In March 1990 the issue was still unresolved and still under discussion between the finance department and the medical staff.

With regard to the sale and lease-back of capital equipment, the board was told in June 1987 that recent tax-reform measures held the potential for significant cost savings with regard to capital-equipment purchases. The board approved a motion from its budget and finance committee to proceed with sale and lease-back, subject to all necessary clearances being obtained from the General Council and legal counsel; the Ministry of Health approved the arrangement. In January 1988 documents were being prepared on the sale/lease-back of hospital assets to the value of $40 million, with net proceeds from the transaction amounting to $975,000.[141] This transaction went ahead. Lastly, with regard to "growth funding," it appears that an important consideration underlying the 61 Queen Street East development was the hospital's expectation of obtaining Ministry of Health "growth fund" grants based on the volume of inpatients, outpatients, and ambulatory-care patients.[142] Since the hospital's capacity for growth would peak by mid-1988 owing to space constraints, the need for such a facility was thought to be pressing. As it turned out, however, any increase in the number of clinic visits was offset by declines in inpatient volume and, as a result, the hospital did not obtain the anticipated growth revenues.

Stewardship

Throughout all of these developments there was some effort – by the Ministry of Health as well as by the hospital board and by its administration –

to impose controls. The ministry announced in 1987 that requests received in 1988-89 would be ranked in 1990, for implementation only in 1992-93, a policy which, if adhered to, should have substantially retarded the rate of growth. The board, for its part, announced its intent to approve no programs until ministry approval had been obtained. It also asked for an accounting of programs that had been eliminated, instructed its auditors to report on what controls were in existence within the hospital (with regard to redevelopment, computerization, campaign funds), and attempted to get answers as to where any savings had been realized.[143] The administration, finally, made provision for department heads to enhance their understanding of budget planning and control methods, and efforts were made to receive more complete estimates of the financial impact of new medical-staff appointments.[144] All that said, there appears to have been no sustained follow-through on these important initiatives. While extensive reports from all board committees throughout these months of intense activity are filed with board minutes, it is unclear to what extent, and to what depth, questioning and discussion of the contents of committee reports, including those on finances, actually occurred at board meetings.

Yet savings were realized in some areas. The hospital's safety record improved in 1987-88, earning a rebate of $228,149 in WCB premiums, and there were also savings of $5.5 million from 1975-88 as a result of energy-conservation programs initiated by Al O'Brien, director of environmental services, which won for the hospital an award from the federal government for "the most outstanding achievement in Ontario" in energy management. Administration had not been rewarding itself excessively: in 1989 a professional review of executive salaries revealed that, by comparison with salaries paid in industrial and financial organizations, St Michael's vice-presidents, executive vice-president, and president were being short-changed in both salary and non-cash compensation.[145]

On the other hand, there is little evidence of requests – for equipment, for staff (especially medical staff), or for facilities – ever being denied.[146] The words "it is anticipated" occur repeatedly, and assumptions and expectations of unlimited growth abound. The Ministry of Health, like a parent who cannot say No and stick to that position, may have encouraged hospitals in this attitude by its past record of making funding adjustments on appeal. And at the board level, a strong case could usually be made for going ahead with a new program, invoking the hospital's past experience with the ministry. In the dynamic, demanding years of 1987-90 it appears that sometimes decisions were made before the details were clear – for example, does "announcement" (by government) assume "approval"? Does "approval" assume "funding" and even "full funding"? Reviewing the events of those years, one is caught up and exhausted in the rush of events and cannot help wishing that someone, somewhere, had set limits. Yet it appears that there were few limits, outside those imposed by the lack of nursing staff, and the limits that did exist were often circumvented.

Warning Signals

The hospital's auditors drew attention in March 1989 to accounts receivable from the Ministry of Health ($6.4 million for *anticipated* funding for new programs and services), and $2.4 million in other *receivables* which in fact represented amounts in dispute and which, if not eventually funded, would reduce accounts receivable by $8.8 million and the unappropriated balance of equity would be reduced from $72.7 million to $63.9 million. The auditors recorded that management was of the opinion that the costs and rates were justifiable, and would be recovered – a perception that later proved to be erroneous.[147]

A year later, in February 1990, the board was told by the hospital's finance department that budgeted costs were overrun for many reasons, including the expense of consulting fees and the high cost of advertising and medical/surgical supplies (cardiovascular-pump cases and angioplasties, both heavy users of medical/surgical supplies, had increased from 665 to 990, and 240 to 300 respectively). Interest rates, too, were above the budgeted levels, reflecting the interest allocated on the amount borrowed from the campaign fund, as well as interest charges on equipment leases. (The board was told that a $1.7-million reduction was made that month in the amount owing to the campaign fund, and further repayment would be made as funds became available.[148])

The board was confidently informed that, despite these aberrations, the hospital was ending the year 1989-90 with a surplus, before building depreciation, of $220,000 on gross revenues of $155 million, but that appeals for the years 1987-89 remained under negotiation.

This was in February 1990. A month later the hospital's auditors drew the board's attention to accounts receivable from the Ministry of Health of $11.9 million (one-half of this for 1989), which represented anticipated funding for costs of new programs and services, and $3.99 million from the WCB and other amounts in dispute. If not funded at all, the operating deficit for the year would be $8.3 million, and the accounts receivable and unappropriated equity would be reduced by $15.9 million.[149] Again the auditors noted that management was of the opinion that all these costs and rates were recoverable; and again, management's opinion turned out to be erroneous.

The Shocking Revelation of St Michael's Accumulated Debt

In mid-1990 the sisters serving as audit committee for the congregation's finances raised concerns with the General Council about parts of St Michael's 1990 financial statement. At about the same time the general superior was alerted that a problem existed when the hospital's auditors requested written confirmation from her of the $5.3 million receivable (presumably from the congregation) on the hospital's books. The ministry's area team responsible for reviewing St Michael's budget became concerned when it received, in the fall of 1990, the hospital's budget for fiscal 1990-91, which, in the ministry's view, incorporated assumptions regarding operations, revenues, and expenses in excess of the hospital's true anticipated activity. Meanwhile, in discussions between the General Council and the hospital board, the latter recognized the real extent of the problem – the hospital had accumulated a debt of $50 million. In late 1990, with the assistance of a chartered accounting firm, the hospital's board and management developed a ten-year recovery plan which called for substantial financial assistance from the Ministry of Health and for disposal of some congregation assets, primarily the 61 Queen Street East property. Upon receipt and discussion of the recovery plan, the minister of health announced that the government would, under the provisions of the Public Hospitals Act, appoint a team of investigators to "investigate and report on the quality of the financial management and governance of St Michael's including an explanation of the change in the hospital's financial condition, why it was not detected at an earlier stage, and to offer remedial recommendations."[150]

The investigators engaged forensic-accounting and financial-advisory services (the firm of Ernst and Young), as well as legal advisers (Fraser and Beatty). Interviews were conducted with thirty-eight individuals – from the Ministry of Health, the General Council, the board, hospital administration, the banks, the WCB, auditing, consulting, and legal firms – who had been involved with St Michael's during the years under review (1 April 1986 to 31 December 1990).

Report of the Investigating Team

The lengthy report, released to the government and the hospital on 30 August 1991, is here highlighted only, and the points made are the views and conclusions of the investigators – not of the author, and not of the congregation.

The report revealed a startling fact: St Michael's was in debt to the amount of $65 million, and its operating deficit for the year ending 31 March 1991 alone was $16.6 million. The investigators attempted to give an explanation of how this situation had developed.

For more than a century, the sisters had owned the property where their various works were conducted (in the case of St Michael's, both the hospital at 30 Bond Street and its satellite clinic on Broadview Avenue), and this had never caused confusion. In terms of St Michael's problems in 1990, however, the investigators concluded that the issue of ownership was fundamental to an understanding of why St Michael's debt was not discovered earlier.[151] They took the position that confusion about who really owned 61 Queen Street East and its debt was a major factor in causing the hospital's financial difficulties. In their judgment, because St Michael's – owned and operated by the Sisters of St Joseph – was not separately incorporated, and therefore had no separate legal existence apart from the sisters, the hospital could not own the shares of the numbered company which "owned" 61 Queen Street East, the building that constituted more than one-third of the total debt.

The investigators concluded that further uncertainty about the ownership of 61 Queen Street East stemmed from the fact that the hospital's by-laws do not authorize the board to borrow on behalf of the hospital; St Michael's was able to finance the 61 Queen Street transaction only because it could do so based on the credit of the sisters. Notwithstanding the sisters' supposed control over banking and borrowing, dealings with the banks were primarily handled by hospital management. Still further cause, or indication, of confusion was that, while St Michael's financial statements for the years 1987-90 did not reflect the assets and liabilities of the numbered company which owned 61 Queen Street East, the accounts (revenues and expenses) of that company were maintained by St Michael's finance department, although the board was never presented with them. The amount of money concerned was substantial: purchase price of the building was $12.7 million; financing of the debt to 31 March 1991, $5.9 million; cumulative cost for renovations and furnishings to 31 March 1990, $5 million.

In the area of governance, while the appointment of the hospital's president and executive vice-president is contained among the powers of the sisters set forth in the by-laws, in practice the sisters nominate only and the board appoints. Nonetheless, it appeared to the investigators that the hospital's governing structure created uncertainty regarding whether the chief executive officer was primarily responsible to the board or to the sisters. The sisters, for their part, expected the board to exercise a supervisory function with respect to the operation of the hospital.

While noting the possible ambiguity of the board's role, the investigators criticized the board's functioning with regard to its committees. The committee structure, they said, did not ensure that all significant decisions were ultimately considered by one knowledgeable group of board members; the flow of information between its committees, and from them to the board, resulted in a level of information at the board level that was quite inadequate in some important instances. Too, there was a suggestion that the executive committee, rather than the full board, was used too freely in arriving at decisions. The investigators noted some board members' remarks, during their interviews, about being disinclined to challenge management on complex health-care funding issues. Yet they were critical of the board in that there appeared to have been no meaningful consideration at the board level of the qualified auditors' opinions that accompanied the 1989 and 1990 financial statements – opinions which indicated that amounts totalling $24.7 million might not be recoverable.[152]

In their critique of the quality of financial management[153] the investigators recorded that, at the time of her appointment as president, Sister Christine had made it clear that she did not consider one of her strengths to be in the financial area. Lavoie was engaged as vice-president, administration and finance, in February 1987, reporting to the president through the executive vice-president, Sister Catherine McDonough. Sister Catherine left St Michael's in June 1989 and in November 1989 Lavoie became executive vice-president.

The investigators noted that over the period 1986-1990 the president assumed less direct responsibility for decision-making, which became more diffused than it had been before. A style of financial management developed that emphasized revenue generation at the expense of managing costs. When costs began to overrun, rather than cutting costs to avoid deficits, management chose to pursue aggressively additional funding, sometimes at considerable extra expense.

Criticism was sharp with regard to management's handling of major capital acquisitions, especially of the building at 61 Queen Street East where the lack of financial reporting to the board (resulting, at least in the investigators' view, from confusion over ownership) allowed the growth of a $23.6-million debt to go largely undetected. The original rationale for acquiring the building assumed a break-even cash flow within two years and the potential for growth funding of up to $2 million annually. Plans for the use of the building changed, with the original commercial-rental space (doctors' offices, laboratories) evolving into a health-care facility providing new and expanded facilities, publicly funded – that is, the original objective of alleviating space shortages gave way to revenue-producing endeavours. In addition to the severe flaws that the investigators found in the business plan for the building, they cited failure on the part of management to do appropriate planning and timely reporting to monitor and control renovation costs, failure to obtain ministry approval for the building's use as a health facility, and an inadequate approach with respect to financial reporting – in short, a failure of management to exercise prudent financial management.

A second major acquisition during the reference period was the magnetic-resonance-imager, purchased without ministry approval. When the ministry eventually did announce operational funding to a maximum of $200,000 annually, the hospital was left with the responsibility for the capital costs, thereby assuming a commitment of $1.1 million in fiscal 1987 and $1.2 million for each fiscal year from 1988 through 1991. In the investigators' view, while management was imprudent to proceed with the purchase when ministry funding was doubtful, its action was consistent with a pattern that the hospital had developed of incurring expenditures and then attempting to secure funding.

Then there was the computer-information system. The original plan by a selection committee for a phased, conservative approach was changed following the new management put in place in 1987; a more comprehensive computer-information system was installed within a compressed time-frame and without, in the investigators' judgment, sufficient consideration of the operational impact.

Finally, in at least one instance proper channels were bypassed: an $800,000 piece of cardiology equipment was approved, not through the capital equipment committee, but rather through the office of the chief operating officer, with the result that senior management and the board were not aware of the commitment.

In the view of the investigators, one of the primary reasons why the growth of St Michael's debt was not detected earlier[154] was the manner in which certain disputed revenues and accounts receivable were recorded in the financial statements. These totalled $15.9 million in fiscal years 1988, 1989, and 1990 – amounts under appeal or in dispute, which were recorded as revenues, and which gave the appearance that expenses during those years were funded, when in fact the hospital was operating with significant deficits.

The debt associated with 61 Queen Street East – its acquisition, financing, and operational losses – was not reflected in the financial statements, nor was the corresponding asset. The full amount of St Michael's capital-lease obligations was not included in the annual financial statement for fiscal years 1988 to 1990 inclusive, nor was the actual position with regard to the use of certain designated funds until fiscal year 1990.

In sum, in the investigators' view, by the way facts were presented or omitted, the usefulness of the financial statements was reduced. As a result, the problem of the hospital's poor financial performance went undetected.

The Ministry of Health did not escape the investigators' criticism: they charged that, by its prolonged discussion over a period of years concerning the funding under dispute, the ministry contributed to the size of the problem and the failure to deal with it.[155]

In thirteen pages of recommendations,[156] made with a view to helping to prevent a recurrence – either at St Michael's or any other public hospital – of the problems they had uncovered, the investigators proposed a financial recovery plan for St Michael's. This plan addressed the hospital's governance structure and management policies, and recommended changes to the regulatory environment in which St Michael's and other hospitals operate.

Briefly, the investigators recommended a recovery plan for implementation over five years, with allocation of the debt divided almost evenly among the sisters, the hospital, and the Ministry of Health. They recommended incorporation of the hospital, a refining of the board's role and responsibilities (including committee structure, reporting relationships to the sisters, appointment of the chief executive officer and signing officers, authority over banking and borrowing), and establishment of an internal audit department to enhance the credibility and integrity of the budgeting, financial reporting, and control systems.

They recommended, as well, immediate amendment of the Public Hospitals Act which, in their view, is "virtually mute on the subject of the role of the board of directors of public hospitals"; mandatory filing of accounts of designated funds with the ministry; equitable funding for peer-group hospitals; and finally, regulations to prevent the launching of new programs without ministry approval.[157]

The Public Reaction

The investigators had declared that "St Michael's needs a fresh start."[158] It appears that the public agreed. For several days after the report of the investigation was made public on 7 November 1991, the Toronto papers covered the details and offered their suggestions of what should have been done, or what should now be done. The media were, in general, sympathetic and gentle, speaking of "a sick hospital," "a pioneer in medicine," "a hospital with a reputation for shrewd and careful management," and declaring that "a strong community bond fuels St Michael's." A year later, with the accounts of St Michael's necessary but painful recovery plan well publicized, a group of civic leaders and celebrities spearheaded plans to raise $5 million over three years to help the hospital. The group's name bespeaks the sentiment that St Michael's elicits in the hearts of Torontonians, "The Friends of St Michael's."[159]

Developments to May 1992

The hospital had taken major steps toward recovery before the investigators' report was made public. Roger Hunt, who had been engaged to head the planned merger of the St Michael's/St Joseph's Health Centre operations, assumed the position of president and chief executive officer of St Michael's on 1 December 1990.

Under Hunt's leadership a recovery plan was developed by January 1991 (that is, before the investigation was mandated by government) to reduce the operating deficit, restructure the debt, and re-establish sound management practices and processes. The plan is too intricate to review in detail, and it is too early to assess how effective it has been. The recovery plan was given a new impetus with the arrival in September 1991 of Jeffrey Lozon as chief operating officer.[160] Among the developments has been an arrangement with the Ministry of Health whereby the latter will maintain St Michael's base level of funding while the hospital repays its debt from within its own budget.[161] The sale of 61 Queen Street East is under consideration. Fund-raising efforts by the hospital and its supporters have been vigorous and quite effective – $100,000 from a direct-mail campaign by St Michael's Foundation in 1991; $150,000 from a ball at the Ontario Jockey Club and a Classic Golf Tournament; significant proceeds from art auctions sponsored by the Italian community.

Although revenues were thus being supplemented from a number of sources, it has been necessary to reduce expenses by closing beds, amalgamating units, and laying off staff. These tough measures, taken to ensure the hospital's survival, began with a reduction of thirty management positions in February 1991, followed by fifty staff positions and a closure of fifty-eight beds in December 1991, and a further 110 positions and a reduction to 450 beds in March 1992.

One cannot walk through or around the hospital today without feeling deeply and personally the losses that have followed the tragic errors in judgment – whole units are closed; the best of the large private rooms are padlocked; the sorely needed stage B redevelopment remains little more than a hole in the ground. But by far the deepest losses have been those of the more than 200 staff members, some with more then twenty-five years' experience, including several whose contributions to St Michael's are recorded in this book. That said, the signs of recovery are clear. A new strategy is in place to define and balance St Michael's patient care, teaching, and research objectives with the requirements of its eight-year financial-recovery plan; no treatment programs have been eliminated, though some have been pared down; St Michael's traditional commitment to medical education has been reconfirmed, and St Michael's will become one of the senior "medical schools" within the University of Toronto's radically new curriculum to be put in place later in the year; the debt has been reduced by more than one-quarter over the past year, without reducing the number of patients treated; the Ministry of Health has reconfirmed its intent to support phase B of the hospital's redevelopment plans, construction to begin in early 1994; and best of all, there is a growing feeling among staff that St Michael's will be preserved and will prosper.[162]

In the months leading up to this centennial year the cross has been keenly felt at St Michael's. Now is the time for all who have loved this great institution to recall in faith another cross which was followed by a glorious Resurrection.

Preparations for the opening of St. Michael's Hos...

In 1890 A fire broke out in Notre dame Insurance C...
expenses. At the time the hospital was unthought of...
needless expenses. — The following year perceiving th...
need of a Catholic hospital Pervines to Work. I M. d...
called the attention of three sisters asking their advice...
the probability of changing Not dame to a Hospital...
The sisters immediately Agreed — One having more...
perience of business than the other two sisters spo...
up and said, what a loss to have spent so much...
on repairs. however M. de C. was not to be discou...
She quietly said to sister there is no use in talking...
mistakes of the past it will not help us in our...
what do you intend to do for the hospital sister...
answered I will make shirts the second sister an...
to the same question I will make bread bags...
third sister a little more timid said I will Col...
it. — All right said M. de C in the name of God...
speak of it tomorrow to Rev. Mother. Finally perm...
was granted and the work Commenced In a...
after sisters went out to Collect after making th...
of a C. Hospital X the people were delighted and ga...
according to their Means the smallest donation...
5.00 10.00 20.00 25.00 50.00 1 00.00 500.00 God eve dev all...
the work and put it firmly on its feet — The year...
the Devil was enraged and did his powerful best...

...work of God...but His Sat—Majesty was... to over... what God built up.—... Col William...
...the first donation for the hospital a Chair...
...—The proceeds of the 1st days begging was furniture
...Blankets 35.⁰⁰ Cash 100.⁰⁰...three or four...
...enabled us to begin M. de C. was answer...
...the least sum but as it was for the poor it was...
...it was decided to go to the well off only...
...day a sister accompanied M. de...Call on a...
...liberal but not understanding the need...
...hospital gave a Cheque for 100.⁰⁰ also a prepos...
...horse and buggy to enable sisters to... her...
...soliciting donations as she was tired already...
...walking Mother objected to the kind offer saying...
...not the where with to board it:—
...Gentleman the late Hugh...gave the 26...
...after the Surg—Building was proposed a Sister...
...again went among the Citizens to furnish...
...Building and succeeded in Collecting 300.⁰⁰
...worth of Sheeting & Covering and toweling
...also 150.⁰⁰ Cash for fitting Yard
...Thus ending the Collection for Hospital...

Source: ASMH, Ad, H-1-1. no. 106.

Appendix B
Financial Statement, 1892-93

Appendix C

Report of the Inspector of Prisons and Public Charities, 1895

Copy.

OFFICE OF THE

Inspector of Prisons and Public Charities, Ontario,

PARLIAMENT BUILDINGS.

re Inspection of **Toronto** 27 Feby. 1895.
St. Michaels Hospital,
Toronto.

[stamp: ST. MICHAEL'S HOSPITAL A-1-1 ARCHIVES 075 TORONTO]

Sir,

I made an inspection of the St. Michaels Hospital, Toronto on the 15th January 1895. There were then 49 patients under treatment.

At the beginning of the official year there were 80 patients in residence, and since that date 218 have been discharged and 15 have died.

The operating room, dispensary, dining room, reception room, kitchen, laundry and furnace rooms were all in good order. The bath rooms, wash rooms and water closets were also in good order. All departments were clean and well kept, and the building was in good order generally. There is good drainage and ventilation.

The new wing is nearing completion, and will afford additional accommodation that is much required. The hospital is well supplied

338

supplied with competent nurses, and there is a resident medical practitioner and good staff of doctors in attendance.

The sick from the city or elsewhere are received, and non-paying or poor patients are cared for as if they were paying patients.

Last year out of a total of 765 patients, 246 paid nothing for their care and treatment, besides which relief was given to 469 outdoor patients.

All classes, nationalities and creeds are admitted to this hospital, and it is well worthy of the support and assistance of all who take an interest in the welfare of the sick and the afflicted.

I have the honor,
To be, Sir,
Your obed't servant,
(Sgd) T. F. Chamberlain.
Inspector.

The Hon,
The Provincial Secretary,

Source: ASMH, A-1-1, no. 075.

Appendix D

Medical Staff Appointments, 1895

Visiting Physicians

    A. McPhedran, M.D.; J.E. Graham, M.D.; F.F. McMahon, M.D.;
    C. McKenna, M.D.; M. Wallace, M.D.; A. Garratt, M.D.

Visiting Surgeons

    R.B. Nevitt, M.D.; I.H. Cameron, M.D.; W. Oldright, M.D.;
    E.B. King M.D.; L.M. Sweetman, M.D.

Assistant Surgeons

    W. McKeown, M.D.; J. Amyot, M.D.; C. Temple, M.D.

Specialists

    Gynaecology.......J.F.W. Ross, M.D.
    Neurology.......D.C. Meyers, M.D.
    Laryngology......M. McFarlane, M.D.
    Ophthalmology and Otology..A.M. Roseburgh, M.D.
    Dermatology......N. Allen, M.D.

Pathologist

    R.J. Dwyer, M.D.

*Electrician**

    C.R. Dickson, M.D.

*C.R. Dickson, M.D. was appointed to Toronto General Hospital in 1889 as a specialist in electro-therapeutics. Electrotherapy at this time had a broad use in the treatment of many conditions – neuralgia, angina pectoris, locomotor ataxia, bladder paralysis, and migraine. See W.G. Cosbie, *The Toronto General Hospital 1819-1965: A Chronicle* (Toronto: Macmillan, 1975), 115.

It appears that he held appointments at both hospitals, as did several of the doctors listed here.

Source: ASMH, AC no. 396.

Appendix E

Memorandum of Negotiations for Affiliation
with the University of Toronto, 1914

Toronto, January 30, 1914

The Committee appointed by the Board of Governors of St. Michael's Hospital to place before the Committee appointed by the President of the University of Toronto the consideration of the present and future relations of St. Michael's Hospital to the Medical Faculty of the University begs to set forth the following facts:

While the Representatives from St. Michael's fully realize that the University Representatives appreciate the importance of their Hospital as a field for Clinical teaching, yet, in as much as the deliberations of the Committee will be subject to review by the Governing Bodies of both Institutions, feel it well to embody in this memorandum some of the subjects already taken up at a previous meeting.

The acquisition of sufficient clinical material for the training of the students in Medicine, as represented by the present General Hospital, which to all intents may be regarded as a University Hospital - represents to the University a very large outlay. The amount of money apportioned or spent by the University of Toronto since the founding of its Medical Faculty may be set down in round numbers as $800,000.

The relative amount of clinical material available at St. Michael's as compared with that at the General Hospital, taking the Report of the Medical Health Department for the year ending December 31, 1913, as a basis of comparison, is as follows:

Toronto General Hospital
Orders issued.......................2,527
St. Michael's Hospital
Orders issued.......................1,736

In other words, over forty per cent of the total is contained in the beds of St. Michael's Hospital.

For this material, which has been freely offered and of which avail has been made, the University has, in contrast to the cost of the material in the General Hospital, paid nothing.

The representatives of St. Michael's Hospital viewing the above facts, feel that the consideration, kindness and value of their Hospital has not been sufficiently recognized and that further through perhaps rather indifference than intent, their Hospital has been placed in a decidedly inferior position in the minds of the Profession generally and the student body in particular.

The only possible reason the Representatives from St. Michael's can advance to their Board for the continuance of the present relations between the Hospital and the University is that the Association of their Hospital with the University lends a certain prestige to their Hospital.

We beg specially to draw attention to the fact that the University authorities assume the right to appoint whomsoever they will at St. Michael's Hospital for the purpose of utilizing the clinical material there available for the instruction of students.

Bearing these facts in mind, we wish to make the following suggestions as a basis for our future relations:

1. Competition or rivalry on a proper foundation is good for both Institutions.
2. Absolute autonomy of St. Michael's Hospital. It is inconceivable that the head of a Department in a competing Hospital should have the power to appoint the Staff of another Hospital engaged in the same line of work.
3. We, on the other hand, freely admit the impossibility of the Board of the Hospital having any power to appoint anyone to the Teaching Faculty of Medicine in the University of Toronto.
4. Following this, we suggest that the Hospital be free to accept or reject such nomination.
5. It cannot be reasonably disputed that students sent by the University to St. Michael's for clinical training should have the same advantages as students sent by the University to the General Hospital, and that laboratories and such other facilities necessary for this purpose should
be established and manned at the Expense of the University.
6. It is suggested that the University which now complains of the inadequacy of the facilities offered by St. Michael's should, in addition to stating such fact, make a vigorous and honest effort to materially aid in the improvement of such facilities.
7. We believe that St. Michael's Hospital may be fully equipped as a Clinical Hospital by the following comparatively inexpensive additions to its facilities:
    (a) A Hospital Museum
    (b) A resident Pathologist
    (c) Clinical laboratories, readily accessible from the wards
    (d) One or more large rooms suitable for clinics (e) A properly fitted post-mortem room

Finally we wish to note the remarkable analogy on general conditions between St. Michael's Hospital in its relation to the University of Toronto and the relation of the Montreal General Hospital to McGill University. A full consideration of these relations will, in our judgement, prove of great value to guiding those who have to take up the final solution of the present problem.

Source: ASMH, H-1-1, no. 080.

138

1919 - 1920

Salaries & Wages

		$	
	Superin	3000	00
	Assistant Superin	2000	
	Supt. of Nurses	1500	
	Supervisor of Out-door Dept.	1200	
	Night Supervisor	1200	
	Secretary	2000	
	Assistant Secretary	1000	
	Instructor of Nurses	1500	
	Sister in Receiving Office	1200	
	Asst. in Receiving Office	800	
	Registrar	1000	
	Pharmacist	1800	
	Asst. Pharmacist	800	
	Sister in charge of X-ray Dept.	1200	
	Laboratory Technician	1000	
	Head nurse in Operating room	1800	
	Procuratrix	1800	
	Asst. Procuratrix	1500	
	Matron of Nurses' Residence	900	
	Hospital matron	900	
	Asst. Hospital matron	800	
	Sister in charge of Kitchen	1000	
	Sister in charge of Laundry	1000	
30	7 Ward Supervisors @ $ 1000.	7100	
	Chaplain	300	
	Pathologist	1125	
6	30 third year Nurses	2252	06
5	30 Second year Nurses	1800	
4	45 First year Nurses	2160	
50	6 Ward Tenders	3600	
35	Janitor	420	
35	Night Watchman	420	
90	Engineer	1080	
80	Night Engineer	960	
70	Fireman	800	
22 dis	Launderer	1140	

30 – 45	7 Assistants	2604 50
85	Cheff	1020
45	a 2nd Cook	540
40	Assistant	480
35	Pastry Cook	420
113	3 Elevator Operators	1356
	Window Glass Cleaners	835 99
30	2 Telephone Operators	720
	Seamstress	480
	"	298 50
	8 Cleaners	4227 28
30	6 House maids	2060
30	10 Pantry maids	3600
		72594 03

Source: ASMH, A-1-7.

344

Appendix G
Memorandum Regarding Hospital –
University Relationship, 1920

November 15, 1920

At a recent meeting, held in the office of the President of the University of Toronto, to discuss the University-Hospital relationship between the University of Toronto and St. Michael's Hospital, Father Bench requested that a summary of the views expressed by the Heads of the Departments of Medicine, Surgery, Obstetrics and Gynaecology in the University, be forwarded to him for presentation to the Board of Governors of St. Michael's Hospital.

The University desires to continue its present teaching privileges in St. Michael's Hospital, but it is essential that the students, attending this Hospital be provided with adequate facilities for their work, and that the clinical instruction given by the staff be in accord with the educational policy as determined by the heads of the various clinical departments of the Faculty of Medicine of the University.

To meet the requirements with reference to clinical instruction, it is advisable that heads appointed by the hospital to administer the various services, viz., Medicine, Surgery, Obstetrics and Gynaecology, and any other medical service of the hospital in which medical teaching is carried on, be willing to co-operate with the heads of these various departments in the University, in the development of work both in the University and in the Hospital. The head of a service must fulfil all the requirements demanded of him by the hospital, but at the same time, he should be a teacher and a man capable of developing younger men to be competent clinicians, clinical teachers, and if possible, investigators.

In order to maintain a staff of a University standard, on the hospital, due regard must be given to the development of younger men as clinicians and teachers. To meet the present day requirements in practice and teaching of modern medicine, the Faculty of Medicine have outlined a definite course for men wishing to join the staff as teachers. A preliminary training of two years, as an Interne in a recognized hospital plus one year in a University laboratory, is demanded. After the completion of this training, application may be made for a position on the staff, probably as a resident Physician or Surgeon, in one of the teaching hospitals. Applicants receiving this appointment, will engage in hospital work, teaching and research, and receive from the University, a salary of $1000.00 per year. If the applicant does satisfactory work as Resident Physician or Surgeon, he would be considered eligible for any new or additional appointment to the attending staff. During his first few years on the attending staff, he would be required to devote the major portion of his time to the service of the hospital and University, only being allowed a limited time each day for private practice. He would receive a salary from the University of from $1500.00 to $3000.00 per year.

The above plan is already in operation in the Department of Medicine, as it applies to the staff of the Toronto General Hospital and the Hospital for Sick Children, and it is hoped to extend this plan to other departments, when sufficient financial assistance is obtained, and to hospitals other than the Toronto General Hospital and the Hospital for Sick Children, when adequate clinical and laboratory facilities are provided.

In the appointment of new members to the staff, who may wish to become clinical teachers, it is important that their preliminary training conform to that required by members in a similar medical service in the Toronto General Hospital.

345

With reference to the standard of hospital equipment, etc., which might be considered satisfactory for a teaching hospital, the standard laid down by the Committee on Hospital Standardization of the American College of Surgeons, and known as "the minimum standard" constitutes a very satisfactory beginning if fulfilled in all details. The following is "the minimum standard":–

(1) That physicians and surgeons privileged to practice in the hospital be organized as a definite group or staff. Such organization has nothing to do with the question as to whether the hospital is "open" or "closed", nor need it affect the various existing types of staff organizations. The word "staff" is here defined as the group of doctors who practice in the hospital inclusive of all groups such as the "regular staff", the "visiting staff", and the "associate staff".

(2) The membership upon the staff be restricted to physicians and surgeons who are (a) competent in their respective fields and (b) worthy in character and in matters of professional ethics; and in this latter connection the practice of the division of fees under any guise whatever, be prohibited.

(3) That the staff initiate and, with the approval of the governing board of the hospital, adopt rules, regulations, and policies governing the professional work of the hospital; and these rules, regulations and policies specifically provide:

(a) That staff meetings be held at least once each month. (In large hospitals the departments may choose to meet separately).

(b) That the staff review and analyze at regular intervals the clinical experience of the staff in the various departments of the hospitals, such as medicine, surgery, and obstetrics the clinical records of patients, free and pay, to be the basis for such review and analysis.

(4) That accurate and complete case records be written for all patients and filed in the hospital, a complete case record being one, except in an emergency, which includes the personal history; the physical examination, with clinical, pathological, and X-ray findings when indicated; the working diagnosis, the treatment, medical and surgical; the medical progress, the condition on discharge with final diagnosis; and, in case of death, the autopsy findings when available.

(5) That clinical laboratory facilities be available for the study, diagnosis, and treatment of patients, these facilities to include at least chemical, bacteriological, serological, histological, radiographic, and fluoroscopic service in charge of trained technicians.

It is important that the teaching staff of the hospital have complete charge over all cases used as clinical material for teaching purposes, and that all cases in any ward used for teaching, be subject to clinics if their physical condition permits.

There are many other details in connection with organization in a teaching hospital that might be mentioned, but the above constitutes in our mind, the essentials for a satisfactory working arrangement in which both hospital and University will benefit.

Amendment–

The clause beginning with the words "It is important" was amended to read as follows:

"It is important that the teaching staff of the hospital in conjunction with the attending physician have charge over all cases used as clinical material for teaching purposes, and that all cases in any ward used for teaching, be subject to clinics if they so consent, and their physical condition permits".

Source: UTA, Office of the President,
A67-0007/063a/224.

Appendix H

Chairs of the Board of Directors,
Chief Executive Officers of the Hospital,
Chairs of Medical Advisory Board/Committee

Chairs of the Board of Directors
Most Rev. John Walsh 1892-99
Most Rev. Denis O'Connor 1899-1908
Most Rev. Fergus P. McEvay 1908-11
Most Rev. Neil McNeil 1912-34
Most Rev. James C. McGuigan 1934-40
Mr John J. Fitzgibbons 1940-63
Hon. T. D'Arcy Leonard 1963-69
Mr Robert Adair Davies 1969-75
Mr Anthony G. S. Griffin 1975-85
Mr Alan J. Dilworth 1985-90
Mr Patrick Keenan 1990-

Chief Executive Officers of the Hospital
Sister de Chantal McKay 1892-93
Sister Assumption Keenan 1893-1902
Sister Demetria McGregor 1902-05
Sister Irene Conroy 1905-08
Sister Victoria Devine 1908-15
Sister de Pazzi Smith 1915-22
Sister Teresa Aquinas Stritch 1922-26
Sister Juliana Mitchell 1926-28
Sister Othilia Maguire 1928-30
Sister Margaret Phelan 1930-32
Sister Norinne Pollard 1932-38
Sister Zephyrinus Lyons 1938-44
Sister Louise Carey 1944-48
Sister Margaret Phelan 1948-50
Sister Maura McGuire 1950-56
Sister Janet Murray 1956-63
Sister Mary Zimmerman 1963-85
Sister Christine Gaudet 1985-90
Mr Joseph Lavoie (executive vice-president) 1990-91
Mr Roger Hunt 1991-92
Mr Jeffrey Lozon 1992-

Chairs of the Medical Advisory Board/Committee
Dr Edmund E. King 1913-30
Dr Joachim Guinane 1930-36
Dr D'Arcy Frawley 1936-39 and 1945-47 (Meetings suspended 1939-45)
Dr William Magner 1947-51
Dr Edward F. Brooks 1951-69
Dr William J. Horsey 1969-84
Dr James Waddell 1984-89
Dr Bernadette Garvey 1989-91
Dr David Briant 1991-

Notes

Chapter 1

1 The sketch of early Toronto presented here is drawn principally from J.M.S. Careless, *Toronto to 1918, An Illustrated History* (Toronto: James Lorimer & Company and National Museum of Man, National Museums of Canada, 1984).

2 Careless, *Toronto to 1918*, 41.

3 Many, with the active encouragement of city officials, pressed on beyond Toronto to the country roundabout.

4 Careless, *Toronto to 1918*, 73.

5 Sister Mary Agnes, *The Congregation of the Sisters of St. Joseph* (Toronto: University of Toronto Press, 1951).

6 J.M.S. Careless, *Brown of the Globe* (Toronto: Macmillan, 1959), vol. I, *The Voice of Upper Canada, 1818-1859*, 155-79.

7 Ibid.

8 M.W. Nicolson, "The Other Toronto: Irish Catholics in a Victorian City, 1850-1900," in *Meeting Places: Peoples and Neighbourhoods of Toronto*, R.F. Harney, ed. (Toronto: Multicultural History Society of Ontario, 1985), 65.

9 By 1851, the year the Sisters of St Joseph came to Toronto, the Roman Catholics formed 25.8 percent of the population of Toronto; 90 percent of these were Irish (Nicolson, "The Other Toronto," 53, 66). See also Elizabeth M. Smyth, "The Lessons of Religion and Science: The Congregation of the Sisters of St. Joseph and St. Joseph's Academy, 1854-1911," PhD thesis, University of Toronto, 1989.

10 Careless, *Brown of the Globe*, vol. 1:33, 179.

11 Sister Mary Bernita Young, *Silent Growth, The Life and Times of Sister Bernard Dinan* (Toronto: Utlas, 1986).

12 It is not known how the house got its name, for the French influence within the congregation in Toronto would have ended with the death fifteen years earlier of its foundress, Mother Delphine Fontbonne. The name may have been suggested by Bishop Lynch who had earlier (1856) founded a seminary in Niagara, N.Y., which he called Our Lady of the Angels.

13 With the exception of the material cited in notes 15 and 16, the information presented here regarding Notre Dame des Anges is taken from ARCAT, Sisters of St Joseph Papers: General Correspondence, St Michael's Hospital; Notre Dame Home, Series L AE04 and L AE05.

14 The archbishop bought the church in 1875 for $9,354; he sold it to the sisters in 1884 (ARCAT L AB04). The sisters borrowed $10,000 in February 1885, probably to purchase the property (ASMH, HX-468, Ledger of Receipts and Expenditures). The mortgage was redeemed 28 April 1890.

15 Careless, *Toronto to 1918*, 76.

16 In September 1890 the motherhouse property was mortgaged again for $12,000 — once more for "the Bond Street property" — and the mortgage was redeemed in September 1902 (ASSJ, B 90 A). See also *Jubilee Volume, the Archdiocese of Toronto and Archbishop Walsh 1842 - 1892* (Toronto: Geo. T. Dixon, 1892).

17 CTA, City Council Minutes, 1891, Appendix A.

18 ASSJ, Council Minutes, 26 November 1891.

19 These went almost immediately, and in their response to their call for help, were joined a week later by a fourth sister. The four were relieved from time to time by other sisters.

20 *Women at Work, Ontario 1850-1930*, Janice Alton, Penny Goldsmith, and Bonnie Shepard, eds. (Toronto: Canadian Women's Educational Press, 1974), 38.

21 CTA, City Council Minutes, 11 April 1892 and 14 February 1894. The first house officer at the new Isolation Hospital was Dr Frederick Fenton, who would become in 1909 the first chief of the combined obstetrics and gynaecology department at St Michael's Hospital (*The Municipality of Toronto, 1923*, 3 vols., Toronto: Dominion Publishing, Chapter 12, "The Hospitals of Toronto," by John N.E. Brown).

22 CTA, City Council Minutes, 14 February 1894, 163, 256.

23 CTA, City Council Minutes, 14 February 1894.

24 CTA, Annual Report of Medical Officer of Health to Local Board of Health, 15 November 1893.

25 ASSJ, Council Minutes, five entries from 8 May 1890 through 30 May 1892.

26 ASSJ, *Annals of the Sisters of St Joseph*, 176.

27 ASSJ, Council Minutes, 1 May 1892.

28 ARCAT, Sisters of St Joseph Papers: General Correspondence, 1855-99; *Canadian Freeman*, August 1868. See also W.G. Cosbie, *The Toronto General Hospital 1819-1965: A Chronicle* (Toronto: Macmillan, 1975), 70.

29 See, for example, CTA, City Council Minutes for 1868 and 1890, which show grants to the "Sisters of Charity, House of Providence" – an institution operated by the Sisters of St Joseph; see also ASMH, reports of early inspections by provincial government inspector, which use the words "Under the management of Sisters of Charity."

30 ARCAT, Sisters of St Joseph Papers: General Correspondence, St Michael's Hospital, L AE04: 24 October 1865; 26 February 1873; and 5 March 1873.

31 ASSJ, Council Minutes, 3 October 1890; 26 November 1891; 1 February, 29 February, 20 April, and 1 May 1892. On the last date Notre Dame was finally decided upon as the preferred site.

32 ASMH, Admissions Register.

33 ASMH. Financial support was beginning to flow, for a sister was making the rounds, begging (ASHM, H-1, 106). Notre Dame des Anges ledger entries for May and June 1892 show "Donations for Hospital" to be $103 and $392.75, and a July entry of "Donations" – probably for the hospital – gives the figure of $1,049.30.

34 ASSJ, Council Minutes, 1 July 1892 and 16 August 1892.

35 UTA, P.78-0071 (05), calendar of University of Toronto's faculty of medicine for 1893-94.

36 ASSJ, Council Minutes, 1 July 1892.

37 ASSJ, Council Minutes, 3 October 1892.

38 CTA, City Council Minutes, 1891, Appendix A. The recommended annual salary for Dr Allen was $2,400. Dr Allen was dismissed in March 1893 (City Council Minutes, 1893, Appendix A).

39 For a thorough examination of the struggles of public-health practitioners in Toronto at this time, see Heather Anne MacDougall, "Health is Wealth: The Development of Public Health Activity in Toronto, 1834-1890," PhD thesis, University of Toronto, 1981.

40 ASMH, Board Minutes, 4 October 1916; 11 October and 23 November 1917.

41 Obituary, *Globe*, 5 October 1922; for the account of the inquest, see *Globe*, 21 October 1922.

Chapter 2

1 Careless, *Toronto to 1918*, 201; the total of 144,000 was later revised to 181,216 (source for both figures is *Census of Canada*, 1851-1921).

2 Academy of Medicine, Minutes of the Toronto Medical Society, 1892-96.

3 UTA, the university's medical faculty calendars, as well as *100 years of Medicine at University of Toronto*, a special magazine issue of the faculty of medicine, Fall 1987.

4 Dr Nevitt was dean at the Ontario Medical College for Women (OMCW) from 1887 until it was absorbed into the University of Toronto in 1906, at which time he held the rank, also, of professor of clinical surgery at the OMCW. Also among the first faculty appointments at the OMCW were Drs I. Cameron and A. McPhedran. Later Drs Dwyer, McKeown, and McMahon had faculty appointments there.

5 CTA, Council Minutes, 1895, Appendix C. The financial statement for year ending 31 December 1894 shows that payments to St John's Hospital ended the previous 31 July, as did payments to St Michael's.

6 *Globe*, 14 June 1893, "Charity Reform."

7 Nicolson, "The Other Toronto."

8 Rt. Rev. Msgr. Treacy, "Reminiscences of Early Days in St. Michael's," ASMH, NS-6, *Alumnae News*, January 1940.

9 ARCAT, W AA05.07. The following spring the archbishop ordered a special collection to be taken up on Sexagesima Sunday in aid of the hospital. St Michael's ledgers show entries of $1,155 received from church collections in February 1895 and $242.26 in March 1895.

10 The *Catholic Register*, 22 June 1893.

11 Letters to the *Globe*, 3 June 1893, and to the *Evening News*, reprinted in the *Catholic Register*, 29 June 1893.

12 Cosbie, The *Toronto General Hospital 1819-1965*, 135.

13 Note that this was a private view, and one not in tune with the official position of the General Hospital.

14 Council may also have been persuaded that restoring the grant was a matter of simple justice. In a letter to the city council, dated 25 February 1895 from the Sisters of St Joseph in charge of St Michael's Hospital, council was reminded that "the Catholic minority ... are [sic] forced to pay a double burden; as no portion of the taxes collected from Catholic ratepayers for the support of City Charities is appropriated

to St. Michael's, Catholics are in consequence obliged to maintain the Hospital by contributions" (ASSJ, Box 90).

15 CTA, Council Minutes, Appendix C, 1895, and Appendix C, 1896.

16 ASMH, Box AD, H-1, N0.106, memoirs of one of the founding sisters, wherein she recounts that "perceiving the need of a Catholic hospital ... Mother de Chantal called the attention of three Sisters asking their advice as to the probability [sic] of changing Notre dame to a Hospital." Their response seems to have been cautious; "however M. de C. was not to be discouraged," and she said, "I will speak of it tomorrow to Rev. Mother." She pressed them further with the question, "Sister, what do *you* intend to do for the hospital?"

17 Mother de Chantal was at the motherhouse for her annual retreat in August 1903 when she suffered a heart attack in the chapel at three o'clock on 10 August. She died two hours later.

18 Some accounts give Brampton as Dr Dwyer's birthplace. However, the author has secured Dr Dwyer's baptismal certificate from St Patrick's Church, Napanee, Ontario. It states that he was born at Napanee on 25 October 1867 and baptized there 20 June 1868. The author has also obtained a document from the Ursuline Archives, Chatham, Ontario, concerning Dr Dwyer's sister Josephine, who entered the Ursuline Order. The document gives her place of birth as Napanee, Ontario. The parents' names are the same on the two documents. Their mother's name (Rennie) is well known in the Napanee area. The office of the registrar general for Ontario has told the author that births were not registered at the office of the registrar general until 1869, and that baptismal certificates are the usual documents for confirming place and date of birth before 1869.

19 Academy of Medicine, Minute Book of Toronto Medical Society, vol. 4, 1890-92, and vol. 5, 1892-95.

20 ASMH, H-3-1, no. 112.

21 The autopsies were carried out in a little brick building in the yard behind the hospital, furnished with a stove in one room and an autopsy table in the other (ASMH, Dr Malcolm Cameron's notes).

22 Although the eulogies expressed at the time of Dr Dwyer's death unfailingly speak of his medical skills and his contribution to St Michael's Hospital, they speak, too, of his other accomplishments and traits – his grasp of history, philosophy, and Egyptology, and his brilliant wit and humour.

23 ASMH, Mr Ryan's remarks at the opening of the new wing.

24 Mrs Ryan's contribution was acknowledged by naming the first nurses' residence, opened in 1898, the "Margaret Ryan Home for Nurses." In 1923 the board arranged for a light to be placed on a portrait of Mr Ryan, with a tablet outlining his work on behalf of the hospital (ASMH, Board Minutes, 29 November 1923). The tablet was later mounted on the outside wall of the A-wing on Bond Street. In addition to the new wing, Ryan bequeathed in his will an annuity of $500 a year for twenty years to St Michael's.

25 The details are taken from a *Globe* article covering the opening day ceremonies, 21 November 1895.

26 A good description of "Hollydene," Ryan'shome, is contained in Lucy Booth Martyn, *Aristocratic Toronto: 19th Century Grandeur* (Toronto: Personal Library Publishers, 1980).

Chapter 3

1 ASMH, *News*, 30 December 1896. Only the General, the Victoria Hospital for Sick Children, and St Michael's are mentioned in the calendar of the University of Toronto's faculty of medicine.

2 See Careless, *Toronto to 1918*, 122, 136-7, 147.

3 Carlotta Hacker, *The Indomitable Lady Doctors* (Toronto: Clarke, Irwin, 1974). See also *Canadian Who's Who*, 1990, and ASMH, letter of 18 May 1992 from Dr Pearl Smith Chute's daughter to Dr Peter Kopplin, uncatalogued, June 1992.

4 ASMH, Box A-1-7 and AX, *Junior and Senior Internes*, 1892-1953. In fact, in the roster of interns for 1904-05 two women are listed, along with four men: the women are Dr Mary Callaghan (Mrs McCarthy) and Dr Pearl Smith (Mrs J.E. Chute). It would appear that Dr Chute had returned to Canada after almost ten years for, perhaps, a furlough and refresher course; see also letter from her daughter, above.

5 ASSJ, Council Minutes, 20 February and 19 September 1911; 19 September and 11 October 1912; and 14 August 1913. See also Mary Ryan Smith, "Reminiscences," *St. Joseph Lilies*, centennial issue, 1851-1951, 202.

6 ASSJ, Annals, September 1904. The sisters who had gone to staff new foundations in Hamilton, London, and Peterborough became permanent members of those dioceses and are not included in this figure.

7 Smyth, "The Lessons of Religion and Science," 91.

8 ASSJ, Annals, 324, 435. Reading the enthusiastic accounts of the congregation's schools and their achievements during these years, one is struck by the "bare bones" entries regarding the hospital. It is as if the latter was regarded as foreign territory, the domain of doctors and nurses only. One is left with

the impression that the source of energy and support for the hospital sisters was the hospital community, rather than the congregation as a whole.

9 ASSJ, Council Minutes, 11 August 1899, and ASMH, H-3, no. 166.

10 ASSJ, Annals, 325; opening ceremonies of new wing, *Globe*, 21 November 1895. Also: Peter G. Goheen, *Victorian Toronto 1850 to 1900, Pattern and Process of Growth* (Chicago: University of Chicago Press, 1970), 213.

11 ASSJ, *Annals*, 212.

12 Cosbie, *The Toronto General Hospital 1819-1965*, 129, 130.

13 ASMH. Beginning in January 1893 the expense account shows wages for "washerwoman," and by 1894-95 there were thirteen auxiliary helpers. From the wages listed – for example $72 annually for laundress – it appears that these people received room and board on the premises.

14 It is difficult for the author to present an account that is entirely free of bias. Some of the conclusions drawn here are based on the author's familiarity with the lives and legends of the early congregation, not all of which can be documented with hard data. However, with regard to the dispensing of charity, evidence is available: during the first several years, the ledger of accounts regularly lists outlays for clothing for patients greatly in excess of outlays for sisters' wardrobes.

15 ASSJ, Council Minutes, 2 November 1905 and 11 September 1907.

16 ASSJ, Obituaries.

17 ASMH, Scrapbook no. 5:34. Sister de Sales's biographer records that she was "known to, and revered by thousands" and was "one of the best-known religious in the Province of Ontario." Sister de Sales was one of the three sisters appointed to the first executive board of St Michael's (replacing the advisory board) in 1913.

18 It was a later Sister de Sales (Fitzpatrick) who recounted this incident of her training years.

19 ASMH, Book of Admissions, Q-shelf, no. 550.

20 At this time in Toronto's history the highest incidence of prostitution among women was found among domestics and factory workers (Acton, Goldsmith, and Shephard, *Women at Work, Ontario 1850-1930*).

21 AO, *Statutes of Canada*, 1854-55, 18 Vict., Chapter 225, "An Act to Incorporate the Sisters of St. Joseph for the Diocese of Toronto in Upper Canada," assented to 19 May 1855.

22 AO, *Statutes of Ontario*, 1898, 18 Vict., Chapter 76, "An Act Respecting the Sisters of St. Joseph for the Diocese of Toronto in Upper Canada," assented to 17 January 1898.

23 AO, The Charity Aid Act, 1874.

24 AO, Prison and Asylum Inspection Act, 1868.

25 Richard P. Splane, *Social Welfare in Ontario, 1791-1893: A Study of Public Welfare Administration* (Toronto: University of Toronto Press, 1965), 210.

26 ASMH, AC no. 396. Account of meeting of representatives from the Ontario Hospital Association, including J.J. Foy, MPP (St Michael's solicitor), with representatives of the provincial government.

27 ASSJ, Box 90.

28 Splane, *Social Welfare in Ontario, 1791-1893*, 209.

29 ASMH, AC no.396. Accounts of opening ceremony, Hugh Ryan wing.

30 ARCAT, Sisters of St Joseph Papers: St Michael's Hospital, 1893-1914. The agenda for an advisory board meeting on 28 June 1901 included "Request of Registrar of Women's Medical College that a deputation from that College meet with this Board"; the 30 June 1904 agenda includes "Report of meeting with representatives of Toronto University, October 22, 1903"; also, "Report of application by the hospitals to City Council for increased maintenance."

31 The composition of the board was the same from 1895 through 1897. In the fall of 1898 Archbishop Walsh died, followed by Hugh Ryan in 1899. In June 1899 Archbishop O'Connor assumed the presidency, and John Ryan replaced his brother Hugh. In 1901 Sir Frank Smith died, and was replaced by T. Flynn. In 1902 John Ryan died. The roster of 1906 showed Archbishop O'Connor, Flynn, O'Connor, and Hugh T. Kelly providing a thread of continuity despite the considerable losses suffered through death of members.

32 ASMH, AC no. 396, newspaper article, 5 June 1902: "The trustees of St. Michael's Hospital are said to contemplate the erection of a wing to the north of the present building, running from Bond to Victoria Sts."

33 Splane, *Social Welfare in Ontario, 1791-1893*, 210.

34 John Murray Gibbon and Mary S. Mathewson, *Three Centuries of Canadian Nursing* (Toronto: Macmillan, 1947), 158. Five years later the Grey Nuns opened St Boniface in Winnipeg, then in 1899 the Sisters of St Joseph of Hamilton opened their school at Guelph, and finally in 1900 three other orders founded schools in Montreal and Victoria.

35 Mary Agnes Sniveley was the respected and influential "Lady Superintendent" of the Toronto General

Hospital School of Nursing at this time. A native of St Catharines, Ontario, and a graduate of Bellevue Hospital, New York, she may have been instrumental in recruiting Harrison from her alma mater.

36 Isabel Maitland Stewart, *The Education of Nurses* (New York: Macmillan, 1943), 87-90.

37 Annie K. Spitz (class of 1895) wrote at the time of the celebrations honouring fifty years of graduations in 1944, "I was Rev. Mother Assumption's first probationer, and the last pupil nurse to get in on the two years training ...." (ASMH, NS-6, *News*, vol. 8, no. 3 [August 1944], 10. (Mother Assumption became superior in 1893.) Students listed in the 1894-95 records –Boyne, Lavery, and Kelly – became the graduating class of 1897, three years later (ASMH, A-1-7-1, no. 114).

38 The reference is probably to Dr Dwyer, medical superintendent, and Dr John Roche, who was the first house doctor with Dr Dwyer.

39 From an interview printed in St Michael's *News*, August 1942, and reprinted in Gibbon and Mathewson, *Three Centuries of Canadian Nursing*. The probationary period was later increased to four months. Once a week the students had an afternoon off, beginning at 2 p.m., and euphemistically termed "a half-day."

40 The chief nurse is referred to in the early records (for example, the payroll) as head nurse or, more often, operating-room nurse. Doyle is pictured in the graduation photos of 1897 and 1898, evidently in charge of the school.

41 ASMH, AC no.396.

42 ASMH, graduation pictures. The sisters, meanwhile, wore their traditional black habit, with white apron, depending on their work. All-white habits were first worn in the early to mid-1930s; however, for some time it remained the practice to wear the black habit to Mass, and then to change into white. See ASMH, H-1, no.077, notes on operating room by Sister Amata Charlebois, O.R. supervisor from 1931 to 1941; also, ASSJ, Council Minutes, 10 November 1935, and Ordinances of the General Chapter, Section IX, 1938. Interns were wearing white-duck uniforms as early as 1914 (ASMH, A-12-1,010: Rules and Regulations of St Michael's Hospital, 1914).

43 The graduation pin of Elizabeth O'Leary (1894) is among the treasures of the ASMH.

44 However, some schools voluntarily underwent inspection by the New York State Board of Nurse Examiners as a means of securing for their graduates registration and entrée to positions in the state of New York. St Michael's invited such an inspection in 1924.

45 ASMH. This fiscal period is chosen for comment because it includes entries (for example, government grants), which will begin to appear regularly but are not in the first financial report (Appendix B). Expenditures are not examined in detail here. "Butcher's meat," eggs, butter, and groceries constitute the big items. A smaller, but consistently appearing, item is "Surgical Instruments," indicating the emphasis placed on building up this service.

46 Sisters apparently bought material from which they made and sold shrouds for the dead, making a small profit on the transaction. The item appears monthly in the ledger from April 1894 for several years.

47 ASMH, AC no, 396, account of the meeting. This was the beginning of united efforts by the hospitals of Toronto, and later of Ontario, to improve the funding basis for their operations. In 1902 the Ontario Hospital Association was formed for the purpose of mounting united action for guarding the interests of the hospitals and obtaining increased government aid for indigent patients, as well as increased county and city aid.

48 ASMH, AC no. 396, account of the meeting.

49 Every overview of the Toronto hospitals of this time refers to the superior facilities for surgery in the Hugh Ryan wing. Yet by 1911, and again in 1913, the provincial inspector was calling for a new surgical suite, citing the disadvantages under which surgeons were working.

50 ASMH, A-1-7-1, no. 114.

51 As early as 1881, nursing students at the Toronto General were going out in this way to private homes, and as late as 1915 Wellesley Hospital students had this experience. See Cosbie, *The Toronto General Hospital*, 107, and Joan Holloban, *The Lion's Tale: A History of the Wellesley Hospital, 1912-1987* (Toronto: Irwin, 1987), 94.

52 It is unclear how long St Michael's continued the practice of "Outdoor Nursing." By 1914 students were no longer going out to the homes, but apparently still provided special-duty nursing in the hospital (ASMH, A-12-1, Rules and Regulations of St Michael's Hospital). That same year Mother Victoria mentions that there were ordinarily ten nurses providing such nursing to patients in serious cases "for which we receive no remuneration" (ARCAT, Sisters of St Joseph Papers, St Michael's Hospital: General Correspondence). In November 1917 the superior general met with the Nurses' Alumnae Association to hear its complaint that the privilege of attending very ill patients was being given to pupil nurses instead of to them (ASSJ, Annals). The allowances for student nurses are recorded in ASMH ledgers, A-1-7.

53 At the same time three small houses were acquired for the help (ASMH).

54 ASMH, H, no. 1170.

55 Communication received by the author from the faculty of pharmacy, University of Toronto, 21 May 1990.

56 ASSJ, Annals, 524. Sister Columba was in charge of the pharmacy when St Michael's first pharmacopoeia was prepared in 1916. It is preserved at the Academy of Medicine, Toronto.

57 The inspector in 1903 observed, "We cannot but especially mention the splendid ventilatory system in the new part of St. Michael's, as we consider this very important in such institutions (ASMH, newspaper clipping, February 1904).

58 Dr Dwyer delivered the first baby born in St Michael's Hospital on 6 December 1893 to Helen Dowdy. She remained in the hospital until 27 December (ASMH, Admissions Register).

59 ASMH, A-7-6, Account of the official opening.

60 G. Harvey Agnew, *Canadian Hospitals, 1920 to 1970: A Dramatic Half-Century* (Toronto: University of Toronto Press, 1974), 70.

61 The names of these doctors appear regularly in the admissions register during the hospital's early years.

62 ARCAT, W AA05.07. It appears that a staff of four physicians was being considered: "one from Toronto, one from Trinity, one from Women's, and one Independent." Four surgeons, one from each school, were also listed. In addition, the names given for other services were listed: "Eye and Ear, Dr. G.H. Burnham, oculist and aural at Toronto General Hospital [who later became chief of the eye service at St. Michael's], and Dr. Trout; throat and nose, Dr. James Thorburn, consulting physician at the General; diseases of women, Dr. Ross; chloroform and ventilation, Dr. Oldright; consulting, Drs. Cameron and Teskey; external or dispensary, assistant doctors attend to this [and] afterward go on staff."

63 Registrars were young physicians, not on the active staff, appointed annually, and responsible for the compilation of medical and scientific data. Registrar appointments became much sought after.

64 Dr Leslie Sweetnam, a surgeon on the staff of the Toronto General and an associate professor of clinical surgery at the University of Toronto, had been one of the most active surgeons at St Michael's from at least 1895 onwards. In November 1901 Sweetnam amputated the gangrenous arm of a public-ward patient who had been shot. He was scrubbing his hands afterwards when a bristle from the scrub brush penetrated under his nail. Blood poisoning quickly developed, and he was taken to John Hopkins Hospital, Baltimore, where the eminent Dr Halstead, under whom he had studied, attempted unsuccessfully to save his life. Dr Sweetnam died in December 1901 at forty-two years of age.

65 See also UTA, A 67-0007, Box 56, nos. 187, 174.

66 ASMH, A-7-5, no. 106, a newspaper of 29 June 1901 carried the announcement of Dr MacMurchy's appointment to the General, and of Dr Margaret Macollum's to the Hospital for Sick Children, and added that possibly a third woman might be appointed – to St Michael's – but that the matter had been left in abeyance at the board meeting earlier. It appears to have been dropped, for no woman was appointed to St Michael's that year.

67 Very senior university officials composed the committee: President Loudon, Vice-Chancellor Moss, Dean Reeve, and Drs Cameron, Primrose, Ross, G. Bingham, and A. McPhedran. The committee held a similar meeting with the trustees of the Toronto General Hospital.

Chapter 4

1 The outdoor patients are to "receive the very best treatment ... whether they pay a cent or not" (ARCAT, Sisters of St Joseph Papers: St Michael's Hospital, General Correspondence, Archbishop McEvay to Mother Victoria, 30 January 1911.)

2 ASMH, Box A-1-7.

3 ASSJ, Council Minutes 20 February and 19 September 1911; 19 September and 11 October 1912; 14 August 1913; and 9 March 1914.

4 Abraham Flexner, *Medical Education in the United States and Canada: A Report to the Carnegie Foundation for the Advancement of Teaching* (Boston: D.B. Updike, Merrymount Press, 1910).

5 UTA, A 67-0007, Office of the President (Falconer), Box 56, nos. 185 and 191.

6 C.K. Clarke, *A History of the Toronto General Hospital* (Toronto: William Briggs, 1913), 126. Dr Clarke, who was dean of the medical faculty from 1908 to 29, writes, "The final agreement was made on December 1, 1910. The University, which had contributed $300,000 originally, undertook to make a further contribution of $300,000, and in addition to that agreed to put up a Pathological Building on a site deeded to them by the Hospital Trustees ...." Also UTA, A67-0007, Box 67.

7 ASSJ, Obituaries. Although Sister Irene Conroy was superior at St Michael's Hospital for only three years, her involvement there encompassed a much longer period. As late as 1926 she was chairperson

of three major committees established by the General Council, on all of which St Michael's had representation: building, cooperative purchasing, and hospital management.

8 ARCAT, Sisters of St Joseph Papers: St Michael's Hospital, General Correspondence, Hugh Kelly to Mother Victoria, 8 June 1909, regarding a call he had received from Professor I.H. Cameron and Dr Clarke, dean of the medical faculty.

9 ARCAT, Sisters of St Joseph Papers: St Michael's Hospital, General Correspondence, January 1910.

10 Professor Irving Howard Cameron had a long association with St Michael's. He occupied the chair of surgery and clinical surgery at the university from 1897 until his retirement in 1920, and received several degrees, both earned and honorary. He played an important part in building up the faculty of medicine. He operated regularly at the General and the Hospital for Sick Children, as well as at St Michael's, where he headed one of the two clinical services in surgery at the time of these negotiations. He was the only recorded member of St Michael's staff who preferred to be called "Mister" rather than "Doctor," following the British precedent for surgeons. See also *Canadian Medical Association Journal*, February 1934, 224.

11 ASSJ, Council Minutes, 19 November 1910.

12 Presumably, this was the proposal regarding the university paying the interest.

13 ASSJ, Council Minutes, 15 December 1910.

14 See calendar of faculty of medicine, University of Toronto, 1911-12. See also ASSJ, Box 90. The university was paying $15 per student annually to Toronto General, but only $5 to St Michael's and the Hospital for Sick Children.

15 At this meeting the president expressed his uncertainty as to whom he should address his correspondence. The mysterious territory of religious orders evidently complicated matters for him, since the archbishop, the superior general, the hospital superior, and the hospital lawyer were all involved in the negotiations.

16 ARCAT, Sisters of St Joseph Papers: St Michael's Hospital, General Correspondence, 13 March 1911.

17 ASSJ, Council Minutes, 31 March 1911; see also C.K. Clarke, *A History of the Toronto General Hospital*.

18 At this meeting it was suggested that "costs be separated for those parts of the new building which would be used exclusively by the hospital or by the University."

19 UTA, A 67-0007, Box 56, no. 173.

20 ASMH, H-1-1, no. 080. See also A-2-2, no. 081.

21 ASMH, A-2-2, no. 081. However, later that year the university's lawyer forwarded to F.B. Hayes, a member of St Michael's board, extracts from the agreement between the university and the Toronto General "which might be used as a model for a similar one for St Michael's Hospital and the University" – with the added clause, "further discussion to be carried out regarding the new addition at St. Michael's Hospital and accommodation therein to be afforded to the University ... and the consideration to be paid by the University for such accommodation ...." (UTA, Box 203).

22 UTA, Box 33, nos. 478, 479, 480; Box 38a, no. 84.

23 UTA, A 67-0007/063a/224; Agnew, *Canadian Hospitals, 1920 to 1970*.

24 UTA, Box 33, no. 115. A further half-dozen of St Michael's staff were at the front in 1915, "having left large and remunerative practices" (ASSJ, Box 90A, St Michael's Hospital Annual Report, 1914-15).

25 UTA, Box 33, no. 484, and follow-up correspondence in Box 33, no. 208 and 209 ; Dr Clarke had apparently passed over those applications which had not included references.

26 UTA, Box 33, no. 109, and ASMH, A-2-2, no. 081.

27 ASMH, photograph of first contingent of St Michael's nurses to go overseas, and wall-hanging with names of all who served with the armed forces.

28 This argument would be used again in the early 1970s when pressure was being put on St Michael's to relocate to Scarborough.

29 In 1904 a devastating fire had completely swept away the heart of the wholesale district (on both sides of Bay Street above and below Wellington), leaving 5,000 people out of work and $10 million in losses. Flying embers from an earlier fire at 135-137 Victoria Street had ignited the north wing of the hospital. From 1905 onwards organized fire drills were conducted at the hospital, and the provisions for fire protection were part of every report of the provincial inspector from 1905 to 1913.

30 ASMH, A-1-1; also A-1-2, no. 057.

31 ASSJ, Council Minutes, 19 September and 31 October 1911; also, ASMH, MAB Minutes, November 1922.

32 ASSJ, Council Minutes, 25 March 1919.

33 ASMH, Dr Cameron's notes; also, MAB Minutes. Dr Harrison (by then Dr Esther Loudon) was appointed assistant gynaecologist to the outpatient department, August 1922.

34 Seventy University of Toronto medical students were either killed in action or died of wounds (medical faculty calendars, 1916-17 and 1919-20).

35 ASMH, Dr Cameron's notes.
36 ASMH, Board Minutes, March and July 1917, and January, September, and October 1918. For the year ending 30 September 1920 the financial report showed an operating deficit of $8,589.33, prompting board members "to wait upon the Board of Control" to secure a grant. Assistance of $15,000 was received after an audit of the hospital's books by the city auditor – the usual procedure in hospital-city relations at that time (Board Minutes, November 1920, as well as February and December 1921).
37 ASMH, MAB Minutes, November 1915 and February 1916.
38 ARCAT, Sisters of St Joseph Papers: St Michael's Hospital, General Correspondence, 6 March 1914, and ASSJ, Council Minutes, 18 March 1914.
39 The reason for the delay can only be surmised. Probably the unsettled conditions and the shortage of supplies during the First World War contributed to the inaction.
40 ASMH, Board Minutes, 12 October 1919; 2 January 1920; 14 January, 10 June, and 22 June 1921. A board member raised at this time the question of the board's responsibility in the matter of finances for the hospital, and recommended that the board's position be clearly defined. The matter was dropped, but was destined to reappear, and with unsettling consequences, a few years later.
41 ASSJ, Council Minutes, 5 February 1910.
42 In the 1908 report of the inspector of hospitals, the name of "Mother Superior Victoria" is entered as superintendent.
43 Such approval rendered the congregation secure from any interference in its internal government, except from Rome (ASSJ, Circular letter from Sister Margaret Phelan, superior general, to the local houses, 13 January 1935). For an example of Mother Victoria's working relationship with Archbishop McEvay, see ARCAT, Sisters of St Joseph Papers: St Michael's Hospital, General Correspondence, 30 January 1911.
44 Archives of St Michael's College, letter to the author from the Reverend F. Black, 24 October 1990.
45 The title would become a subject of controversy fifteen years later, when it became necessary to clarify the nature of the board.
46 ASSJ, Council Minutes, 13 September 1913.
47 The archbishop, however, did not regularly attend; board members took turns conducting the meetings, a practice that continued until 1940 when J.J. Fitzgibbons became the first lay chairman.
48 ASMH, Board Minutes, 11 February 1915. A booklet entitled Rules and Regulations of St. Michael's Hospital, 1914 is preserved in ASMH, A-12-1.
49 ASSJ, Council Minutes, 17 April and 5 December 1914. See also Joan Holloban, *The Lion's Tale, A History of the Wellesley Hospital 1912-1987* (Toronto: Irwin, 1987), 34.
50 Kates, Peat, Marwick and Company, *Health Services Teaching and Research in Toronto Teaching Hospitals* (Toronto 1972).
51 ASMH, Board Minutes, 4 October 1916.
52 This was Dr T.A. Robinson, who subsequently served for many years in St Michael's department of surgery (see ASMH, board minutes, 13 October 1918).
53 Ibid., 21 February 1919.
54 Ibid., 3 October 11 January 1919, and 2 January 1920.
55 Ibid., 23 November 1920.
56 UTA, A67-0007/063a/224, and ASMH, Board Minutes 25 February 1921. The article originally read: "It is important that the teaching staff of the Hospital have complete charge over all cases used as clinical material for teaching purposes, and all cases in any ward used for teaching be subject to clinics if their physical condition permits." The article was amended by the hospital to read: "It is important that the teaching staff of the Hospital in conjunction with the attending physician have charge over all cases used as clinical material for teaching purposes, and that cases in any ward used for teaching be subject to clinics if they so consent and their condition permits."
57 ASMH, Board Minutes, 23 November 1922.
58 ARCAT, Sisters of St Joseph Papers: St Michael's Hospital, General Correspondence, 16 June 1927. See his letters to Archbishop McNeil, 24 January 1924 as well as 10 June and 1 November 1927.
59 ARCAT, Sisters of St Joseph papers: St Michael's Hospital, General Correspondence, letters to Archbishop McNeil, 10 and 16 June 1927 and 1 November 1927.
60 ARCAT, Sisters of St Joseph Papers: St Michael's Hospital, General Correspondence, Sir Bertram's letter to Archbishop McNeil, 4 April 1928. The question of finances was not all; Sir Bertram had had the impression for some time that the board's recommendations were not taken seriously by the hospital authorities.
61 ASMH, Board Minutes, 5 April 1928.
62 ASSJ, Council Minutes, 12 October and 24 October 1928, as well as an unofficial record of the latter

meeting, filed with the Council Minutes.

63 For the board's involving the medical advisory board before major decisions, see, for example, MAB Minutes for 8 December 1914 and August 1915 at ASMH.

64 Ibid., February 1918; 23 September and 28 November 1920; 6 and 7 December 1920; 10 January and 3 March 1921. The superior at the time was Sister de Pazzi Smith, who served from 1914 to 1922.

65 The university's medical faculty calendar for 1898-99 (UTA) shows Professor J.F.W. Ross as a gynaecologist at both adult hospitals. Professor J.M. MacCallum is listed as ophthalmologist-otolaryngologist in the 1901-02 calendar.

66 ASMH, AX.

67 See *100 years of Medicine at the University of Toronto*; also, *Canadian Hospitals, 1920 to 1970*.

68 ASMH, MAB Minutes, 13 May 1915. Evidently the idea was implemented, and with satisfaction, for four years later the doctors were ready to go to the archbishop in protest against a sister being transferred from the laboratory. Ibid., 26 February 1919).

69 ASMH, HX, Sisters' Council Minutes. In May 1924 the sisters' council made the decision to give one week's paid vacation to staff. In 1929 reference is made to a contract for ambulance service to be provided by one Trull, who would return to the hospital fifty cents for each call handled.

70 ASMH, interview with the superintendent, Sister Teresa Aquinas, published in the *Toronto Star*, 7 April 1924.

71 Copies of *St. Michael's Hospital Medical Bulletin*, 1922-1935, are, with a few exceptions, among the holdings of the library of the Academy of Medicine, Toronto. Publication apparently lapsed after 1935; in 1938 the possibility of reviving the *Bulletin* was discussed but no action was taken because of the expense involved (ASMH, MAB Minutes, 19 January 1938).

72 W. Magner, "The experimental production of cholecystitis in the rabbit," *St. Michael's Hospital Medical Bulletin*, vol. 9, no. 2 (December 1930). The C-wing, completed in 1928-29, had a small laboratory on the roof.

73 ASMH, Scrapbook no. 5:27, announcement of September 1929. Later newspaper accounts quoted a registration of 250, "the largest medical convention ever held in the Dominion."

74 ASMH, E-19, and MAB Minutes – for example, 23 January 1938 and 2 March 1939.

75 Eighteen months before his death, Dr Silverthorn published an article entitled "Acute Appendicitis" in the April 1925 issue of *St. Michael's Hospital Medical Bulletin*, in which he observed, with regard to doctors awaiting developments in cases of suspected appendicitis, "Some lessons are dearly learned."

76 The advent of the new machines introduced a new question: who was entitled to the fee charged the patient? The hospital records show that, in the early days, the physician was to get 50 percent of the cash receipts for the ECGs performed, and $9 out of every $15 charged for the BMRs (Basal Metabolism Rate). (ASMH, Sisters' Council Minutes, 3 March 1928.) The radiologist received, in addition to his salary of $300 a month, 20 percent of the net profits of the department (ASMH, Board Minutes, 28 May 1926).

77 ASMH, H-3-13, no. 226.

78 ASMH, H-3-4, no. 351, notes by Dr William Magner. The second surgical service was headed by I. Cameron, who also operated at the Toronto General.

79 Miss Graves married Dr P.W. O'Brien, who became the hospital's first paediatrician. Miss O'Connor remained a prominent member of the alumnae, as president for two terms, and as well was active in local and national nursing organizations (ASMH, NS-6, History of the Alumnae Association).

80 ASMH, Board Minutes, Sister de Pazzi Smith (superior), reporting to the board, 7 September 1918. See also MAB Minutes, 24 September 1918 and 15 June 1925. Also *Canadian Nurse*, vol. 21, no. 9 (September 1925), 474.

81 ARCAT, Sisters of St Joseph Papers: St Michael's Hospital, General Correspondence, Report of Inspection of 10 September 1924.

82 Ibid., letter from McGill University, 22 September 1924, and telegram from Father Moulinier, 29 September 1924. Sister St Philip, who was a graduate of 1895 and an instructor from 1921 to 1928, would have been sixty years of age at the time and probably declined to go to university.

83 ARCAT, Sisters of St Joseph Papers: St Michael's Hospital, General Correspondence, Report of Survey of School of Nursing, 21 May 1928.

84 ASSJ, Council Minutes, 14 August 1928. Reading reports of these and other inspections by various outside agencies, one is continually reminded of how seriously the sisters considered recommendations and tried to correct deficiencies. See also ASSJ, Box 90-A, *Souvenir Booklet of Silver Jubilee, 1892-1917*.

85 ASMH, NS-6, *Alumnae News*, December 1959.

86 Miss Foy authored a complete history of the Nurses' Alumnae Association for its twenty-fifth anniversary in 1929 (ASMH, NS-6).

87 ASMH, GS-2, no. 335, Annual Report of St Michael's Hospital, 1928.

88 ASMH, GS-2, no. 334, Janet Neilson, "History of Public Health Nursing in Toronto," Zada Keefer, ed. Submitted in 1945 to Mary Mathewson for use in compiling a history of nursing in Canada. The author of the present work is at a loss to explain the discrepancy between this date and that shown in the MAB Minutes of 1915. It may be that a small beginning was made in the various clinics, as reported by Neilson (*who was there*), and then a more formal and comprehensive establishment of each clinic was made on the dates reported in the MAB Minutes. The 1907 date for the opening of the chest clinic at St Michael's is corroborated in a biography of the first nurse to staff it: Marion Royce, *Eunice Dyke; Health Care Pioneer*, (Toronto and Charlottetown: Dundurn Press, 1983).

89 A copy of the booklet published to explain the endowments is preserved at the Academy of Medicine, Toronto.

90 J.P. Hynes, architect, submitted plans for the board's review on 25 March 1925 and 23 August 1926, (ASMH, Board Minutes).

91 ASSJ, Annals, 14 April 1923.

92 ASSJ, Council Minutes, 28 January 1926.

93 ASMH, Board Minutes, 26 April 1926, and ARCAT, Sir Bertram Windle to Archbishop McNeil, 1 November 1927. The hospital applied to the Province in 1926 for a grant of $150,000 and renewed its request two years later, increasing the original amount by $50,000; it is unclear whether the grant was made, even though the hospital had threatened that, without a grant, it would have "to put in the windows and allow the new wing to stand as it is until funds are available" (ASMH, A-2-1, no. 075).

94 ASMH, Scrapbook no. 5:8. *Toronto Star*, 28 March and 5 May 1924.

95 ASSJ, Annals, 656, 657, 694. Dr John Amyot was instrumental, along with Sir Bertram Windle, in bringing Dr Magner to St Michael's.

96 ASMH, A-2-2, no. 081. President Falconer to Father Cline, secretary of St Michael's board, 15 June 1921.

97 ASMH, taped interview, Dr Adrian Anglin with Sister Camilla, hospital archivist, August 1981; see also taped interview with Dr W. Keith Welsh, February 1978, wherein he states, "Dr. Magner was very influential in the organizational structure of the hospital."

98 ASMH, Account ledgers, December 1901. These ledgers show an entry of $259 for x-rays.

99 Cosbie, *The Toronto General Hospital*, 184-5, and ASSJ, Council Minutes, 31 October 1911.

100 Cosbie, *The Toronto General Hospital*, 190.

101 ASMH, campaign literature, Scrapbook no. 5.

102 ASMH, Scrapbook no. 1:29, and Scrapbook no. 5:24.

103 ASMH, Scrapbook no. 5.

Chapter 5

1 Michael Horn, *The Great Depression of the 1930s in Canada* (Ottawa: The Canadian Historical Association, Historical Booklet no. 39, 1984). See also Pierre Berton, *The Great Depression, 1929-39* (Toronto: McLelland & Stewart, 1990).

2 See *Five Great Encyclicals* (New York: The Paulist Press, 1939). In his "Quadregesimo Anno" of 1931 Pope Pius XI built upon and further developed some of the principles of the social and economic doctrine of Pope Leo XIII.

3 See, for example, *Catholic Register*, 16 April 1931 and 21 May 1931.

4 *Catholic Register*, 17 September 1931 and 31 December 1931. The archbishop's appeal grossed $111,615.

5 ASSJ, Council Minutes, 25 April 1931, regarding extension to nurses' residence; ASSJ, Council Minutes, 2 May 1931, regarding change from DC electric power to AC "as more economic"; ASMH, Local Council Minutes, 27 August 1931; ASMH, A-1-7, Financial Reports to Province of Ontario, 1931-1948.

6 ASMH, Local Council Minutes, 27 August 1931 and December 1924; ASMH, A-1-7, Financial Report to Province of Ontario, 1935.

7 ASMH, MAB Minutes, 29 March 1933.

8 ARCAT, Sisters of St Joseph Papers: St Michael's Hospital, General Correspondence, Invitations to a meeting to discuss forming a union, 1 November 1934.

9 ASMH, Board Minutes, 14 May 1940.

10 Author's interview in the fall of 1989 with Sister Louise, who helped draft the initial agreement.

11 ASSJ, Council Minutes, 9 October 1930 and 16 November 1935. As well, the archbishop urged the congregation in 1936 to become involved, in a social-service capacity, in the poor sections of the city (ARCAT, Sisters of St Joseph Papers, General Correspondence, exchange of letters between the superior general and the archbishop, 20 November and 16 December 1936).

12 ASSJ, *St Joseph Lilies*, centennial issue, 1851-1951, 277.

13 ASSJ, Council Minutes, 6 April 1934; 2 May 1934; and 11 October 1934.

Notes

14 Sister Othelia McGuire, who had been appointed superior in 1928, resigned two years later because of serious ill health; this may have accounted in part for the board's revival having been delayed. Doubtless there was discomfort, too, among the remaining board members, and possibly the Depression was a factor with those members totally engaged in keeping their own businesses afloat. One is also tempted to surmise that the old approach-avoidance behaviour which had been manifested earlier towards the university was surfacing again – this time towards sharing power with the board.

15 ASSJ, Council Minutes, 2 May 1931.

16 Dr Peter Moloney, OBE, served on St Michael's board for twenty-six years until 1962. Holder of a number of degrees, both earned and honorary (MA, PhD, LLD, FRSC), Moloney was, during this time, a member of the team that solved the problem of the crystallization of penicillin; as well, Moloney did landmark research on diphtheria vaccines and on insulin. The Moloney Building of Connaught Laboratories was named in his honour.

17 Author's interview with Sister Louise, fall 1989.

18 Agnew, *Canadian Hospitals*, 1920 to 1970, 125.

19 ASMH, MAB Minutes, 3 May 1938, and 6 October 1938. Copies of the Clinical Society's Proceedings for 1938 are preserved in ASMH.

20 MAB Minutes (ASMH) contain a handwritten note that states, "no minutes from 1939-45."

21 Dr Geraldine Moloney served as a senior intern in gynaecology. She later went on to a distinguished career at Women's College Hospital.

22 UTA, Medical Faculty Calendars, 1909-10, 1923-24, 1929-30, 1935-36; also, ARCAT, Sisters of St Joseph Papers: St Michael's Hospital, Archbishop McNeil, chairman of the board, to members of the staff, St Michael's Hospital, 21 May 1927.

23 The reorganized department was described in *St. Michael's Hospital Medical Bulletin*, June 1931.

24 ASMH, H-3-3, no. 1104.

25 Moved by the need for such equipment during an outbreak of poliomyelitis in England, Lord Nuffield decreed that every hospital within the empire which might have a reasonable expectation of the use of a respirator should be supplied with one (*British Medical Journal*, vol. 1, 14 January 1939, 84); also, ASMH, MAB Minutes, 2 February 1939, and NS-6, *Alumnae News*, June 1940.

26 ASMH, Board Minutes, 14 May 1940.

27 ASMH, B-1, History of the Biochemistry Department.

28 In 1927, for the first time, a resident surgical officer and a resident medical officer were appointed, the salary of the former paid by the university, that of the latter by the hospital (ARCAT, Sisters of St Joseph Papers: St Michael's Hospital, Sir Bertram Windle to Archbishop McNeil, 1 November 1927). Among their duties was that of "helping, encouraging, and instructing the young internes."

29 UTA, Medical Faculty Calendars, 1929-30 and 1935-36.

30 The author is indebted to the Reverend William O'Brien and James O'Brien for many of the details of Dr O'Leary's life. In 1991 the Frank O'Leary Community Health Centre (not a project of St Michael's Hospital) was established by former patients of Dr O'Leary and their children.

31 In 1945 the maternal death rate in Canada was 2.3 per 1000 live births; in the city of Toronto the rate was 2.1; at St Michael's Hospital the rate was .53 per 1000. In 1945 the death rate of infants under one month in Canada was 28.0 per 1000 live births; the city of Toronto's rate is not known, but St Michael's was 8.7. ASMH, *Alumnae News*, vol. 12, July 1948.

32 ASMH, *Pulse*, vol. 3 no. 4, 15 March 1991. This was the Dr S. Gordon Ross Memorial Fund which, in addition to commemorating Sister Vincentia, "from whom he had learned so much" (ASMH Foundation/Development Office files), will provide scholarships for the staff of St Michael's or their children pursuing studies in a health-care-related field.

33 ARCAT, Sisters of St Joseph Papers: St Michael's Hospital, Archbishop McNeil to staff of St Michael's Hospital, 21 May 1927, and MAB Minutes of 27 May 1927.

34 UTA, Medical Faculty Calendar, 1929-30. The scholarship was awarded to the student who, at the end of the fifth year of the six-year course, had taken first-class honours in at least three-quarters of the subjects of that year and had obtained the highest marks in the examinations.

35 ASMH, H-3, no. 178, and Academy of Medicine, Biography Files, Dr E.F. Brooks. See also article by Drs Pratt and Brooks in *Canadian Medical Association Journal*, September 1938, vol. 39:240-3.

36 ASMH, U-4, no.176.

37 George Ewart Wilson, *Fractures and Their Complications* (Toronto: Macmillan, 1930; also, ASMH, Board Minutes, 22 April 1941, and E-7/077, description of course in *Bulletin of American College of Surgeons*, 1941, 717-19. The author has many memories of Dr Wilson in his later years, including his habit of continually flexing his fingers as he walked about; they had become badly scarred from his frequent use of the fluoroscope.

38 It was said that among Dr Wilson's rules for his staff was one that prohibited their going to the floors in scrub-suit and laboratory coat.
39 *Sixty Years of Service: A History of the Ontario Hospital Association*, 1924-84, 6.
40 *Canadian Hospital*, May 1928, vol. 5, no. 5:9.
41 *Sixty Years of Service*, 6.
42 Interview with Sister Louise, fall 1989: "Representatives from the Boards, administration, and staff got an appointment with the Mayor; we were in and out in ten minutes, with our request granted – numbers count!"
43 ARCAT, Sisters of St Joseph Papers: General Correspondence, 5 September 1939.
44 Agnew, *Canadian Hospitals*, 160.
45 ARCAT, Sisters of St Joseph Papers: General Correspondence, Sister Margaret Phelan to Archbishop McGuigan, 20 October 1941, in which she noted that Dr Magner, sitting on a committee of the Ontario Medical Association, expressed his opposition to any plan that might mean government control.
46 ASMH, Sisters' Council Minutes, 22 July 1945.
47 ARCAT, Sister Margaret Phelan to Archbishop McGuigan, 20 October 1941.
48 *Canadian Hospital*, March 1928, vol. 5, no. 3:33.
49 ASMH, H-1, no. 169: Operating Room 1918-41, by Sister Amata Charlesbois, also, author's interviews with Jean Watson, December 1991, and with Marion Finegan and Sister Helen Bradley, June 1992.
50 ASMH, D-7, no. 173, "Ethics, 19 hours, Sister St Philip." The same file contains notes for a course in microbiology, and a detailed set of notes for a three-month course in anatomy.
51 ASMH, NS-6, *Student News*, May 1947.
52 Statistics from the Department of Health, Ottawa, published in *Canadian Nurse*, April 1928, vol. 24, no. 4:180.
53 Sister Vincentia's reminiscences to the author several months before her death.
54 ASMH, Reprints of November Examination Papers for Registration of Nurses in Ontario, 1926-1941. In 1926 nurses wrote examinations in anatomy and physiology, children's nursing, medical nursing, general-orthopedic and gynaecological nursing, obstetrical nursing, preventive medicine and hygiene, and principles of nursing technique.
55 However, the head dietitian, a sister student-pharmacist, a priest-psychologist, and a masseur taught in their respective fields (ASMH, Reports of Inspections by Nurse from Department of Health).
56 In 1937 the student had a sixty-hour week if on days, sixty-nine and a half hours if on nights. She had a half-day off weekly if on days; if on nights, one night off every two weeks. In 1947 graduate staff were on a divided eight-hour day, but students still had a fifty-one-hour week on days and a fifty-seven-hour week on nights, with a day off each week. In 1950 the school moved to an eight-hour day for students.
57 With the movement out of the residences and the introduction of the eight-hour shift, there was concern for the safety of nurses. In 1947 the hospital purchased a ten-passenger station wagon to take nurses home at midnight (ASSJ, Annals, 8 January 1947).
58 ASMH, framed wall hanging with names inscribed of those nurses who served in the armed forces.
59 This was the first of the committees that would become a way of life in the school of nursing and the hospital; its members were Sisters St Philip, Colette, Vincentia, Hieronyme, and Jeanne.
60 In 1952 the two component parts of nursing – complementary, but each with its own focus – were separated for administrative purposes into nursing education and nursing services, each with its own director and support staff.
61 This was the Sodality of the Blessed Virgin Mary, prominent for many years in guiding the religious, social, and recreational side of school life.
62 *The Dietetic Profession in Canada*, Margaret Lang and Elizabeth Upton, eds. (Toronto: The Canadian Dietetic Association, 1973), 16.
63 Ibid, 17; also, author's interview with Sister Mary Francis Peck, February 1991.
64 Marilyne Telford, "Dietetic Internship Programmes in Canada: A Comparison between 1935 and 1985," *Journal of the Canadian Dietetic Association*, vol. 46, no. 4 (Fall 1985), 259. (The staff and student dietitians lived in a small house provided by the hospital.)
65 ASMH, Q-1, no. 469.
66 MAB Minutes, 26 January and 13 May 1915.
67 Ibid., 27 December 1926.
68 A few months later a second school was opened at Hôtel-Dieu Hospital, Kingston; for many years these were the only schools in Canada for preparing medical-record librarians (Agnew, *Canadian Hospitals, 1920 to 1970*, 146).
69 ASSJ, Box 9, a record by Sister Carmella Fischer, who lived at the hospital at the time. Attempting to

locate the window, the author discovered that the Park Road Baptist Church had been destroyed by fire in 1961, but that its stained-glass windows were rescued and removed to Yorkminster Park Baptist Church, where, in 1991, some of them were still in crates.

70 Sister Edana Ryan supervised the setting up of the new operating rooms (ASSJ, Obituaries). Sister Mary Kathleen recalls that Sister Edana, who had had extensive experience in both the operating room and emergency, "would guide a new interne's hand when he inserted his first tracheotomy tube; she was a great person." During the construction of the new E-wing, patients travelling to the operating rooms in the D-wing had to be transported across a "bridge" suspended five floors up linking the C and D wings.

71 "People came from all over to see it" – interview with Sister Alice Marie, September 1989; also, ASMH, newspaper clippings of the opening-day ceremonies.

72 The Nurses' Alumnae Association made a substantial contribution to the cost of the chapel; its financial statement of 20 March 1939 makes reference to "a balance of $500" towards the cost of installing two windows in the chapel (ASMH, NS-6). The provincial government and the city gave grants of $50,000 and $60,000 respectively to the cost of constructing the new wing (ASMH, A-1-7).

73 ASMH, H-885, letter to Sister Camilla Young, archivist, regarding the Toronto Historical Board's walking tour of Queen Street downtown, landmark no. 21, St Michael's Hospital.

74 ASSJ, Council Minutes, 5 February 1938.

75 ASMH, H-V.2:2.

76 Sister Norine became secretary of the Catholic Hospital Association of the United States and Canada in 1933, and in 1937 was elected a member of the Canadian Hospital Council, precursor to the Canadian Hospital Association.

77 ASSJ, Annals, August 1938.

78 ASMH, taped reminiscences by Dr Arthur L. Hudson, who began his association with St Michael's in 1937, working there in his spare time as a medical student and continuing through his internship. Hudson returned in 1947 to head the division of dermatology. The Dr Stuart MacDonald mentioned by Hudson was a son of famous Canadian author, L.M. Montgomery; he was for thirty years a staff obstetrician at St Michael's and assistant professor on the faculty of medicine.

79 ASMH, minutes of meetings of the board of governors during the war years.

80 Barry Broadfoot, *Six War Years, 1939-45* (Toronto: Doubleday Canada, 1974).

81 Interviews with Sister Frieda Watson and Sister Louise, both of whom were in the business offices during those years. Also, ASSJ, Annals, 1265.

82 ASMH, A-1-7, no. 123, Statistical Reports to Province of Ontario, 1941, 1942, 1943, and Board Minutes, 20 April 1943.

83 *Official History of the Canadian Medical Services, 1935-45, Volume One: Organization and Campaign*, W.R. Feasby, ed. (Ottawa: Queen's Printer, 1956). The details regarding the 15th General Hospital are from 163, 210, 312-13 of this source. In March 1945 the 15th General returned to the United Kingdom and was disbanded.

84 ASMH, NS-6, *Alumnae News*, August 1944, Letters from Margaret Hunt, Margaret Conlin, and Marion Pallett, graduates of 1932, 1941, and 1938 respectively.

Chapter 6

1 *Canada One Hundred, 1867-1967* (Ottawa: Dominion Bureau of Statistics, 1967).

2 ARCAT, Sisters of St Joseph Papers: General Correspondence, Sister Juliana to Cardinal McGuigan, 17 April 1952.

3 At the Museum of the Academy of Medicine, Toronto, a sales record of tthe Cambridge Scientific Instrument Company, Cambridge, England, for 1 July 1913 to 31 December 1913 shows an einthoven string galvanometer dispatched on 11 July to "Univy. Toronto (Dwyer)" – Dr Dwyer was physician-in-chief at St Michael's. On 15 September one was dispatched to "Univy. Toronto", and on 24 December one to Montreal General Hospital. The Montreal General's galvanometer, for which $1,100 had been paid, was installed some time in 1914 (*Canadian Journal of Cardiology*, vol. 3, no. 8 (Nov./Dec. 1987), 358-61.)

4 *Medical Post*, 7 October 1969, vol. 5, no. 20. Dr Loudon's article, "Clinical Electrocardiography," was published in *Canadian Practitioner and Review*, vol. 39, no. 7 (July 1914), 407-17.

5 Academy of Medicine, Local Biographies. Also, ASMH, notes by Michael O'Sullivan, director of biochemistry.

6 ASMH, correspondence surrounding Dr McPhedran's appointment, also Board Minutes and correspondence relative to Dr Welsh's appointment.

7 Cosbie, *The Toronto General Hospital*, 206, 248, 260; according to Cosbie, Shenstone was a "comprehen-

sive general surgeon" and a pioneer in thoracic surgery.

8 ASMH, tape prepared for the archives by Dr W.K. Welsh, 23 February 1978.

9 Author's interview with Alice McNamara, who was a theatre supervisor at the hospital during the years 1946 to 1964.

10 In a survey conducted in 1949, the American College of Surgeons had recommended greater specialization within the department of medicine, a recommendation that Dr Brooks was at first inclined to dismiss (ASMH, MAB Minutes, 1 June 1949).

11 Academy of Medicine, Local Biographies. Also, ASMH, taped interview with Dr A. Anglin.

12 ASMH, MAB Minutes, a marathon meeting of the medical advisory board, 15-17 September 1947.

13 ASMH, see, for example, MAB Minutes, 13 April 1950.

14 ASMH, MAB Minutes, 13 December 1948: the opinion of interns was to be sought before deciding on housing some of them at Elliott House as a way of easing the space shortage at the hospital.

15 Ibid., 7 October 1946.

16 Ibid., 4 April and 3 May 1948. Junior interns' salaries were raised to $300 annually in 1953 at all the Toronto teaching hospitals. At a 12 December 1955 meeting it was reported that two post-graduate applicants had been lost to the United States, where the salary was triple that offered at St Michael's. St Michael's MAB acknowledged that all intern salaries were inadequate.

17 ASMH, Board Minutes, 13 December 1946.

18 ASMH, MAB Minutes, 2 February 1948 and 6 December 1954.

19 ASMH, Board Minutes, 17 June 1948.

20 ASMH, D-7, Report by Dorothy Riddell of a five-day visit, 1950.

21 ASMH, D-7, Joint Report by Dorothy Riddell and Dorothy Dix of a three-day visit, 1956.

22 Among the leadership positions Sister Mary Kathleen held were: board of directors of the Canadian Nurses' Association (1946-48); Provincial Council of Nursing, Ontario Department of Health (1952-58); executive of Ontario Conference of Catholic Hospital Association of United States and Canada (1944-59); president of same (1947-49) and (1956-57); examiner for the Evaluation of Catholic Schools of Nursing in Ontario and Quebec (1944-48); and official visitor to Manitoba schools of nursing in the 1958 pilot project evaluating Canadian hospital schools of nursing.

23 See visit of General Alexander of Tunis to St Michael's Hospital, *Catholic Register*, November 1949. By then governor-general of Canada, the former Allied Forces leader in North Africa was shown a letter he had written to a little girl, who by 1949 had grown up to be a student at St Michael's, in response to one she had written to him at the front.

24 One of the leadership positions held by Sister Mary Kathleen's students was the presidency of the 141,000-member College of Nurses of Ontario. First Dorothy Wylie, and then Ann Ford, graduates of 1950 and 1955 respectively, occupied this post.

25 Author's interview with Sister Mary Kathleen, Fall 1989.

26 ASMH, MAB Minutes, 1 April 1946 to 2 April 1956, especially 29 October 1948 and 6 December 1954.

27 Ibid., 18 December and 29 December 1950.

28 ASMH, Z-1.

29 ASMH, Board Minutes, 11 May 1950. Previously only a few students from each class had been able to take advantage of affiliation at the much-in-demand Toronto Psychiatric Hospital.

30 ASMH, MAB Minutes, 30 April and 18 December 1950, and 7 May and 11 September 1951.

31 Ibid., 14 December 1953; 5 July 1954; 7 March 1955.

32 Ibid., 5 and 12 December 1955; 16 January 1955.

33 Ibid., 10 January 1949. It appears that pathologists at the other Toronto hospitals had similar reservations at this time. So did those contacted in Vancouver and Victoria, despite the fact that the Canadian Medical Association approved the plan in principle (ibid., February and March 1949).

34 ASMH, Board Minutes, 11 June 1957. The Toronto General entered into a contract with the Red Cross at about the same time (Cosbie, *The Toronto General Hospital*, 302).

35 ASMH, MAB Minutes, December 1949 through March 1950; also, 7 March 1955 and 3 October 1955.

36 Ibid., 2 April 1956.

37 Ibid., 28 April 1947.

38 ASMH, Board Minutes, 20 April 1949. Certain third parties – for example, the Workman's Compensation Board – paid the hospital $1 for x-rays of patients covered by their plan; the hospital was allowed to collect $1 from patients not covered by any plan.

39 Ibid., 30 August 1946.

40 Ibid., 17 June 1948.

41 ASMH, MAB Minutes, 7 May 1951 and Board Minutes, 31 January 1952. In its 7 March 1955 meeting the Medical Advisory Committee agreed to send Dr C.B. Baker for a refresher course in cardiovascular

surgery and Dr J.K. Wilson for one in cardiology.

42 ASMH, MAB Minutes, February 1955; 16 April 1956; and Board Minutes, 18 and 25 April 1956.

43 ASMH, Board Minutes, 17 February 1956.

44 ASMH, MAB Minutes, 16 April 1956.

45 Ibid., 26 June 1956. The medical advisory board and the board of directors saw the danger of the public wards being used for private gain under the proposed constitution, and even the end of the hospital as a teaching hospital affiliated with the university (ASMH, Board Minutes, 18 April 1956). In addition to the conflict in roles (between the medical advisory board and the medical staff organization) posited by the proposed constitution, the whole question of the medical staff fund was a sore point.

46 ASMH, Board Minutes, 17 November 1955 and 17 February 1956.

47 For example, in 1954 space was provided on the wards for interns to do their charts, and dictaphones were provided in the chart room.

48 ASSJ, Papers of Sister Margaret Phelan, her Christmas letter to the congregation, 1943.

49 See "Catholic Hospitals of Ontario form Conference of Catholic Hospital Association," *Canadian Hospital*, October 1931, 16; see also ASMH, H-3, no. 178.

50 ASMH, taped account by Sister Maura of construction of the cafeteria.

51 ASMH, Board Minutes, 5 April 1945.

52 Ibid., 11 May 1950.

53 ASMH, Sister Maura's tape. The final cost was $139,486 (ASMH, A-1-7, no. 079).

54 ASMH, Board Minutes, 20 April 1949. Sister Margaret appears to have kept the board informed, but did not seek its formal approval, as her successor would do. She had arranged for the purchase of this property in 1945, at a cost of $70,000 (ASMH, "Extra Expense 1945-61" notebook).

55 UTA, Faculty of Medicine Calendar, 1941-42. When relocated to 1-AS in 1950, seven qualified physiotherapists were added to the staff; the number would double within the next two decades (ASMH, GM-13, no. 067).

56 ASMH, Dr Bardawill's research.

57 ASSJ, Box 93, report prepared by Sister Maura, 1956 for presentation to the congregation. Also, UTA, Faculty of Medical Calendar, 1949-50. This calendar showed that, among the teaching hospitals, St Michael's had the largest volume of outpatients; and among the three adult teaching hospitals, the largest number of emergencies (28,346).

58 ASMH, H-19, no. 227; Q-1, no. 556; H-19; and NS-6 *Alumnae News*, vol. 13, no. 4, October 1949.

59 ASMH Board Minutes, 28 January 1953.

60 ASMH, Sister Maura's tape regarding construction of cafeteria.

61 A statement published in the *Toronto Daily Star*, 14 February 1955, as part of the hospital's fund-raising campaign showed government grants received as $2.6 million. This is the figure shown in Sister Maura's report of the years 1950-56 (ASMH).

62 ASMH, A-1-7, no. 079, "St. Michael's Hospital Capital Expenditures, 1945-1954."

63 *The Canadian Who's Who*, 1936-37, and ASMH, account of opening of E-wing, 1937.

64 ASMH, *Toronto Daily Star*, 14 February 1955.

65 ASMH, *Globe and Mail*, 16 and 21 February 1955. Dr W.J. Horsey, neurosurgeon, performed a "first" by severing certain nerves to save the life of a man who was dying from exhaustion by thrashing his arm and leg, a condition caused by a blood clot at the base of the brain. Dr C.J. Bardawill's research into the use of growth hormone in the treatment of leukaemia appeared to hold great promise for the future control of this disease, as did Dr C.B. Baker's present and future surgery for artery and heart-valve replacement.

66 ASMH, Board Minutes, 18 May 1955. To express its appreciation the board commissioned an oil painting of McDougald, and invited him to sit on the board. As well, a committee composed of McDougald, Sister Maura, and Fitzgibbons, Roesler, Stewart, and Jolly was formed to administer the distribution of campaign funds.

67 ASSJ, Box 94, letter to Sister Maura from Stan Martin, executive-secretary of the Ontario Hospital Association.

Chapter 7

1 *Canadian Hospital Directory*, vol. 26 (1978), August 1978.

2 St Michael's lost even a parking-lot attendant, who followed his favourite doctor to one of the new hospitals.

3 ASMH, Board Minutes, 11 June, 57. The item appeared on board or medical advisory board minutes twenty-three times between 1956 and 1962.

4 ASMH, MAB Minutes, 18 July 1960 and 9 January 1961. In 1961 the beginning rate was raised to $1,800

with $500 steps through the ranks to the resident, and similar adjustments were made for the new 1962 intern staff.

5 The three commissioners were A.J. Swanson, former administrator of Toronto Western Hospital; Msgr John G. Fullerton, long associated with the St Michael's board and with the Catholic Hospital Association; and Dr J.B. Neilsen.

6 Hospital Services Commission of Ontario, annual statistical reports on public and private hospitals, 1956-60. At the same time, grants of roughly $2,000 provincial and $2,000 federal funds became available for new active-treatment beds, and lesser amounts for nurses' beds, bassinets, and interns' beds; also a grant per square foot by both governments for x-ray, laboratory, dispensary, physiotherapy, emergency, and outpatient departments.

7 See, for example, their calling to account a subcommittee member who was too frequently absent from meetings (October 1962). Amidst the proliferation of mysterious new technologies, the medical advisory board was cautious about what it would approve being done on an outpatient basis in day surgery – no blood transfusions and no D & C's (2 April 1962). It refused permission to give to the press a report of a surgeon's successful new techniques (January 1965); and it denied a chief permission to begin discussion with a prospective candidate for a staff appointment (4 November 1963).

8 For example, in 1963-64 the hospital acquired its first Jaeger fetal heart-monitoring device, a gastric hypothermia machine, an electronic volemetron, an echo-encephalography machine, and a new Mayo-Gibbon pump oxygenator. These devices represented approved requests from across the services: obstetrics, internal medicine, the laboratories, neurology/neurosurgery, and cardiovascular surgery.

9 The committee for investigating patients' stay in hospital, formed in November 1957, reported regularly 125 to 130 patients in hospital for more than thirty days. The admissions and discharge committee later took over this duty. See ASMH, Board Minutes, 23 April and 25 November 1959.

10 ASMH, U-1, no. 297, and U-2.

11 Ibid., 23 April 1959 and 25 November 1959.

12 ASMH, MAB Minutes, 7 January 1957 and 9 December 1963.

13 ASMH, GM-13, no. 067. The author is indebted to Inna Wester, MCPA, who, at the request of Grace Murphy, prepared a record of the development of the department while she served as a supervisor there for several years, beginning in 1962.

14 ASMH, MAB Minutes, 9 July 1962.

15 For these details, the author has drawn from a history of the department of urology (ASMH, M-ll, no. 180), prepared by Sister St Matthew, nursing supervisor in urology at the time.

16 ASMH, R-2, no. 514 *Research Society Abstracts*, 1967, no. 22. The author has drawn as well from a history of the development of the clinical investigation unit and metabolic service at St Michael's Hospital, prepared by Dr A Little (ASMH, GM-19, no. 067).

17 ASMH, GM-7, no. 067, Radioisotope Laboratory Report, circa 1974.

18 *Research Society Abstracts*, 1967, no. 4, J.K. Wilson and C.B. Baker, "Heart Surgery at St. Michael's Hospital: A Detailed Clinical Study of Patients Undergoing Valve Replacement."

19 These details, and those that follow, are taken from "A Report on the Development of the Cardiovascular Laboratory," prepared by Dr P. Forbath about 1974 (ASMH, GM-5, no. 067).

20 Author's interview with Jean Watson, O.R. theatre supervisor, 10 December 1991; Watson was present at the procedure. Also, author's interview with Dr Peter Forbath in the summer of 1992.

21 ASMH, brochure, *Course for Laboratory Technologists, St Michael's Hospital, 1952*. The course was approved by the Canadian Medical Association and led to registration in the Canadian Society of Laboratory Technologists.

22 *Research Society Abstracts*, 1967, no. 4. Here Drs Baker and J.K. Wilson reported on their study of seventy patients who had received the new artificial heart valves, a major breakthrough in prostheses, in 1963.

23 ASMH, MAB Minutes, 7 October 1963.

24 ASMH, R.T., no. 1303.

25 ASMH, GM-8, no. 067; also, taped interview of Dr Ross by Anita Wong and Marina Engelsakis.

26 The use of Betadine as a skin disinfectant interfered with the radioactive iodine uptake tests; the antidepressant wonder-drugs were found to be inappropriate for certain types of psychiatric patients; patient sensitivities to certain drugs needed to be documented, and alternatives found. Red arm-bands for patients with known drug sensitivities were introduced in 1964.

27 ASMH, A-10.

28 ASMH, Board Minutes, 28 February 1964 and 30 April 1965.

29 ASMH, MAB Minutes, January 1965.

30 ASMH, R-5, no. 651, Curriculum Vitae, James Alexander (J. Alick) Little.

31 ASMH, R-5, nos. 900 and 893, articles from *Medical Post*, 24 January 1984, and *Ontario Medicine*, 6 February 1984.

Notes

32 ASMH, GM 19, no. 067, Dr Little's letter to Grace Murphy, 3 September 1969, tracing the development of the clinical investigation unit and metabolic service.

33 See, for example, sociologist Aileen D. Ross's *Becoming a Nurse* (Macmillan, 1961).

34 Nettie D. Fidler, "The Preparation of Professional Nursing," address to the biennial meeting of the Canadian Nurses' Association held in Toronto, July 1946. Quoted in Katherine MacLaggan, *Portrait of Nursing* (Fredericton: New Brunswick Association of Registered Nurses, 1965).

35 Helen K. Mussallem, *A Path to Quality: A Plan for the Development of Nursing Education Programs within the General Education System of Canada*, PhD thesis, Columbia University (published by Canadian Nurses' Association, Ottawa, 1964), 179.

36 *Perspectives in Nursing Education: Educational Patterns – Their Evolution and Characteristics*, Sister Charles Marie Franck and Loretta E. Heidgerken, eds. (Washington, D.C.: Catholic University of America Press, 1963).

37 At Sister de Sales's graduation, her classmates wrote of her: "She mixed reason with pleasure, and wisdom with mirth" (ASMH, *Probe*, 1932 – the school of nursing's first yearbook).

38 The Howell sisters had held the record: Ann (1955), Kathleen (1957), Mary (1963), and Susan (1964); however, they were finally outnumbered by the McLeans: Lenore (1961), Sharron (1963), Denise (1965), Florene (1968), and Susan (1971).

39 In 1965, one eighty-bed teaching ward was reduced to a staff of one supervisor, two head nurses, one assistant head nurse, six registered nurses, and nine nursing assistants, with twelve first-year students two days a week, two second-year students, and four third-year students – for the three tours of duty.

40 The author of the team-nursing concept (Thora Kron, *Nursing Team Leadership*, [Philadelphia: W.C. Saunders, 1961]) was engaged to give a workshop to the nursing staff.

41 These were Drs Bruce Bird, Grant Bird, John Kempff, John Shea, and Joseph Sungaila (ASMH I, Board Minutes, 10 December 1957).

42 Ibid., 25 November 1959 and 20 April 1961.

43 AMSH, MAB Minutes, 11 September and 2 October 1961. The central planning committee was chaired by Dr W.E. Hall, with Sister Janet and Drs Day, Baker, P. O'Sullivan, Horsey, and Solmes as members. The architects were Govan, Ferguson, Lindsay, Kaminker, Langley, and Keenleyside.

44 ASMH, Board Minutes, 21 February and 29 April 1963.

45 One of the first items that Sister Mary Zimmerman, as the new administrator, had to bring to the board was the question of installing TV in the amphitheatre, the conduit for which would have to be provided for in the plans (ibid., 18 September 1963).

46 In seeking approval from Rome for permission to borrow the $4,000,000, Sister Maura McGuire, superior general, wrote: "It is essential that we provide our young Catholic doctors with the most up-to-date facilities ... at present there is no debt at all on the hospital" (ARCAT, Sisters of St Joseph Papers: General Correspondence, St Michael's Hospital, Sister Maura to Cardinal Valeri of the Sacred Congregation for Religious, Vatican City, 11 July 1962).

47 ASMH, M-11. In 1965 Dr Russell was granted a patent for the Russell ileostomy and colostomy appliance, developed for use after these procedures.

48 ASMH, Board Minutes, 23 January, 1962.

49 Ibid., 28 February 1964.

50 ASMH, MAB Minutes, 5 April 1965. The announcement was not a complete surprise: four years earlier the dean had outlined the proposed change and expressed "the hope that the three university hospitals would form three separate schools, taking care of a certain quota of medical students during the last two years .... [each school] would enjoy a certain autonomy .... St Michael's may be responsible for 50-60 students in each of the last two years" (ASMH, A-2-2-3, Dean MacFarlane, Minutes of Joint Hospital Relations Committee, 2 May 1961).

51 ARCAT, Sisters of St Joseph Papers: St Michael's Hospital, General Correspondence, Dr John Hamilton (dean) to Sister Mary, 26 April 1965.

52 Ibid. The pool of medicare fees accruing under the province's medicare plan for treatment of patients on the teaching units would be returned to participating teaching staff on an agreed-upon basis.

53 The hospital had earlier established a disaster plan, the need for which was probably triggered by the devastation and death resulting from Hurricane Hazel in 1956. See ASMH, MAB Minutes, 7 October and 2 December 1957; 6 January and 4 February 1958. The update referred to here was done in the fall of 1964.

54 ASMH, MAB Minutes, 27 April and 4 May 1964.

Chapter 8

1 By 1972, with a very substantial portion of health care for Ontario's residents covered under OHIP, the cost to the province had risen 263 percent over the 1960 costs. (See report of Health Planning Task Force [the Mustard report], 1974).

2 Sunnybrook purchase (1966), Donwood Institute (1967), North York General (1968), York-Finch (1970), Addiction Research Foundation/Clinical Institute (1971), Etobicoke General (1972). See *Canadian Hospital Directory*, vol. 26, August 1978.

3 ASMH, The Third Lecture in the Edward F. Brooks Memorial Lectureship at St Michael's Hospital, June 4, 1979, by Dr C.H. Hollenberg, Professor and Chairman of the Department of Medicine, University of Toronto.

4 Several members continued from the previous decade, among them, Hon. Wallace McCutcheon, Metro Chairman William R. Allen, Senator Joseph Sullivan, Hon. Frank Hughes, and Mr Justice H.G. Steen. Preston Gilbride was appointed in 1966. Then, as members retired, others were appointed: W.V. Moore, president of IBM in 1970; Hartland MacDougall, executive vice-president, Bank of Montreal, and Latham Burns, president of Burns Bros and Denton Ltd, in 1972; David Kinnear, vice-chairman of Bank of Montreal, in 1973; Frank Udall, vice-president of the Canadian Imperial Bank of Commerce, and Mr Justice C.L. Dubin in 1975. The president of the Women's (later Hospital) Auxiliary became an ex-officio member, beginning in 1973.

5 ASMH, Board Minutes, 28 April 1967; see also 10 April 1970.

6 ASMH, MAB Minutes, 2 December 1968.

7 Davies, quoted in interview with *Globe and Mail*, 23 October 1969.

8 ASMH, Board Minutes, February 1969.

9 Approximately $6 million in campaign funds was required for the purpose of establishing an application for statutory grants on a 2\3:1\3 basis.

10 ASMH, Board Minutes, 10 April 1970.

11 The architects were asked to prepare "not only a functional structure, but a building with imagination, and an exciting appearance" (ibid., 15 May 1970).

12 ASMH, J.A. Hamilton, *Report Concerning Health Sciences, Education, Research and Service* (University of Toronto, September 1970).

13 ASMH, MAB Minutes, 2 November 1970.

14 ASMH, Board Minutes, 25 August and 23 November 1971.

15 ASMH, A-6, no. 896, Letter from S. Martin, chairman of OHSC, 23 November 1971.

16 Kates, Peat, Marwick, "Health Services, Teaching and Research in Toronto Teaching Hospitals," 28 February 1972.

17 ASMH, MAB Minutes, 10 July 1972.

18 ASMH, Board Minutes, 6 September 1972.

19 Ibid., 6 September 1972.

20 ASMH, A-16, Davies's notes on meeting of 27 August 1973.

21 ASMH, A-16, Ministry of Health to John Law, president of UTHA, 24 September 1973.

22 ASMH, A-16, B.A. Monaghan, hospital solicitor, to deputy city clerk, 23 August 1974. The city council, in fact, first officially discussed the matter on 19 April 1974 – the day after expiry of the thirty-day period.

23 ASMH, A-16, J.J. Carthy, counsel to the Sisters of St Joseph, to the board of governors, St Michael's Hospital, 29 August 1974.

24 At only thirty-seven years of age, Davies co-authored the book *Canadian Corporation Precedents* (1962). He followed this with three years' service on the government-appointed Kimber Commission, which rewrote the Securities Act of Ontario; the revised act became a model for similar legislation in all the other provinces. He then became senior legal counsel to the select committee on company law, a body whose recommendations also led to significant statutory changes.

25 ASMH, Box A-3-4.

26 The particulars contained in this section are all from ASMH, NS-16.

27 At that time the congregation operated facilities containing more than 4000 beds – at St Michael's Hospital, St Joseph's Hospital, Providence Villa, Our Lady of Mercy Hospital, and Sacred Heart Child and Family Centre, all in Toronto.

28 Government of Ontario, "Guidelines for the Development of Health Technology Programmes within the Colleges of Applied Arts and Technology and Health Sciences Complexes in Ontario" (November 1970).

29 Discussions were held with representatives of the University of St Michael's College, York University, and Ryerson Polytechnical Institute; in addition, there was considerable discussion with the Toronto

Institute of Medical Technology.

30 In the final paragraph of her doctoral dissertation Sister Marion had written, "It is difficult to see how the system of diploma nursing education could be improved by moving totally within the larger system of the Colleges of Applied Arts and Technology until these unresolved questions (identified above) have been answered." Sister Marion then went on to recommend experimentation with an autonomous institute of nursing education–which would "relate to the general system of education ... and with the health field ...." See Sister Marion Barron, CSJ, MEd, "Possible Consequences for Diploma Nursing Education in Ontario as a sub-System of the System of the Colleges of Applied Arts and Technology," PhD thesis, the Catholic University of America, 1971.

31 ASMH, N-5-16, meeting of Sister Marion with Stan Martin of OHSC, 27 January 1972. The Ontario Hospital Association, with which Martin had long been associated, worried about the quality of the graduate and about losing the identity and character of each school, had campaigned for an affiliation with the colleges rather than integration. Many schools supported this position. The Registered Nurses Association of Ontario, which in 1967 had asked for the transfer into general education, was now anxious about the speed with which it was being made. Some students protested vigorously (see letters from two Toronto General students to the *Toronto Star*, 24 January 1973). Almost 10,000 nursing students from fifty-six Ontario schools of nursing moved into twenty-two community colleges beginning September 1973.

32 ASMH, NS-16, Sister Marion's notes on meeting with Milton Orris, curriculum coordinator of CAATS, (Colleges of Applied Arts and Technology) of the Ministry of Colleges and Universities, 5 June 1972.

33 The sisters were not the only ones to feel the loss. In submitting his resignation as chairman of the school's board, Mr Justice Steen confessed "a great deal of sadness in watching the school pass from the hands of the Sisters into the formal control of the Community College .... I have always been firmly convinced that the background of the school, together with the devotion of the Sisters and staff, was the best possible combination to produce nurses of real excellence" (ASMH, NS-16, his letter of 3 December 1973).

34 The five schools of nursing that formed the nursing division of George Brown College were those of the four hospitals – St Michael's, St Joseph's, Toronto General, and Toronto Western, as well as the Nightingale School of Nursing, connected with Mount Sinai Hospital.

35 ASMH, School of Nursing yearbooks, 1972 and 1974. Sister Marion's messages to graduating classes.

36 Some of the doctors who resigned were: Dr L. Swales and Dr S. Sims in 1965, to become chief of obstetrics and gynaecology at St Joseph's Hospital and Humber Memorial Hospital respectively; Dr James Lanskail, to become surgeon-in-chief at York-Finch Hospital in 1968; Dr W.E. Hall, to become physician-in-chief, Scarborough General, in 1969; Dr H.T. Van Patter, to be chief of laboratories at North York General in 1970; Dr P. Bailey, to be chief of anaesthesia at York-Finch Hospital, 1970-73; Dr H.P. Higgins, to be physician-in-chief of St Joseph's Hospital in 1976; and Dr A. Katz, to be pathologist-in-chief of Toronto Western Hospital in 1976.

37 See ASMH taped interview with Dr R. Ross, pathologist-in-chief. Dr A. Gottlieb of his staff worked closely with the cardiologists and CV surgeons. Others of his staff collaborated in different areas: Dr J. Bilbao, with the neurologists and neurosurgeons; Dr A. Lang, with the nephrologists; and Dr A. Chalvardjian, with the gynaecologists. Radiologists Dr N.L. Patt and Dr P. Samu did the large share of radiologist studies connected with the cardiac teams' laboratory. (ASMH, GM-5, notes by Dr Peter Forbath.)

38 In 1974 Dr Woolever and Dr P.F. Beirne organized, under the sponsorship of the Archdiocese of Toronto and St Michael's and St Joseph's hospitals, a two-day family planning symposium; all the choices available to Catholic couples were explored in depth. Dr J.J. Billings, author of "The Ovulation Method," was brought from Australia for the symposium.

39 ASMH, Board Minutes, 23 January 1970.

40 ASMH, MAB Minutes, 4 December 1972; 6 January 1975; and 3 March 1975.

41 ASMH, Board Minutes, 23 January 1970.

42 The Canadian Medical Association, the Canadian International Development Agency, the Trinidad Ministry of Health, and the British West Indian Airways (*Toronto Star*, February 1973).

43 The author has drawn from an overview of the department of anaesthesia prepared by Dr Dunn for the hospital archives (ASMH, An-1 no. 030).

44 ASMH, Board Minutes, 17 December 1965.

45 ASMH, M-11 no. 509. Sister St Matthew, nursing supervisor of urology at the time, recorded that Dr Colapinto in 1964 was one of the first urologists in Toronto to transplant a kidney in a dog, and have the dog survive. Sister Elaine Stockdale, RN, who had undertaken special studies at the University of Toronto in the care of research animals, was nursing administrator of St Michael's animal-research lab-

oratory from 1966 to 1981; she observed that animals "seem to have a sense of pain quite different from ours – they might have a kidney removed in the morning, and by evening would have taken a meal and be up walking around" (Author's interview with Sister Elaine, November 1989).

46 ASMH, MAB Minutes, 10 September 1973.

47 Ibid., 5 June 1972; 4 June and 9 July 1973.

48 See, for example, the *Reader's Digest* article of November 1977 where the story is told of a Trinidad policeman receiving at St Michael's the kidney of an eighteen-year old Burlington boy fatally injured in a car accident.

49 With Dr Ronald McCallum of St Michael's department of radiology, Dr Colapinto co-authored an authoritative text, *The Urological Radiology of the Adult Male Lower Urinary Tract* (Springfield, Ill.: Charles C. Thomas, 1973).

50 In an important document entitled "Criteria for the Determination of Neurological Death," Dr Horsey enunciated principles for the guidance of all involved in organ transplantation at St Michael's; published in the proceedings of Continuing Educational Course for Coroners, Dr Horsey's paper was entitled "Brain Death" and was delivered in Toronto, 24 October 1974 (ASMH, S-4).

51 The author recalls receiving a letter from a former patient in which he charged that "the rattling windows, the sputtering steam radiators, and the dripping bathroom tap made the place a Chinese torture chamber." In recognition of Yvonne Erwin's contribution to the work of the neurosurgical unit and the growth of the staff there, the Yvonne Erwin Memorial Scholarship for Neurosurgical Nurses was established in 1990.

52 ASMH, MAB Minutes, 7 July and 8 September 1969.

53 Dr Hudson became president of the World Federation of Neurosurgical Societies in 1985; in 1988 he was awarded an honorary doctorate in medical science from Tokushiwa University, Japan, for "enormous devotion in teaching young Japanese neurosurgeons over the last ten years" (ASMH, S-4).

54 ASMH, S-4, no. 1650. Dr Susan MacKinnon, a plastic surgeon and head of the hand service at Sunnybrook Hospital, worked with Dr Hudson on the transplantation.

55 See his paper "Are Doctors Obsolete?," the first in the Edward F. Brooks Lecture series, 1977 (ASMH, M-25, no. 222); his "Report on the Department of Medicine" to the board of directors, 1978 (ASMH, M 340); and the sentiments expressed by staff members (*Bond Issue*, June 1978) when Dr Marotta left St Michael's to become chief of neurology at Wellesley Hospital and to set up a clinic for epileptics there.

56 ASMH, X-2, *Bond Issue*, February/March 1976.

57 ASMH, O-1, no. 009, Dr Kelly to Sister Camilla Young, SMH archivist, 9 January 1974.

58 ASMH, 0-1, no. 929, Dr Michael Shea to L. Thalheimer, coordinator of hospital development fund-raising, 10 May 1984.

59 ASMH, 0-1, no. 009: letter from Dr Kelly to Sister Camilla Young, archivist, 9 January 1974.

60 Described in *Research Society Abstracts*, 1967 (ASMH, R-2, no. 514).

61 The chapter is entitled "Thermoelectric Cryosurgery," in *New and Controversial Aspects of Retinal Detachment*, Alice McPherson, ed. (New York: Hoeber Medical Division of Harper and Row, 1968).

62 See, for example, ASMH, MAB Minutes, December 1969 and 2 October 1972.

63 Ibid., Dr Alan Hudson to chairman of medical advisory board, 1 September 1977.

64 ASMH, S, no. 761, A. Smialowski and D.J. Currie, *Photography in Medicine*, and D.J. Currie and A. Smialowski, *Photographic Illustrations for Medical Writing* (Springfield, Ill.: Charles C. Thomas, 1960 and 1962 respectively). In 1978 Dr Currie authored *Abdominal Pain*, published by Hemisphere Publishing Corporation/McGraw Hill Book Company.

65 M. Barkin, C.R. Cowan, John A. MacDonald, and L.J. Mahoney, "A Portable Pump (Conjector) for Regional Perfusion Chemotherapy," *Canadian Medical Association Journal*, 19 November 1966, vol. 95, 1087-9.

66 See, for example, "Face to Face with Cancer," by Lillian Newbury, *Toronto Star*, 19 December 1978.

67 ASMH, S, no. 761. A *Globe and Mail* article of January 1967 carried a picture of Shamess "taking a stroll" with a patient who had had his arm completely severed in an industrial accident, and successfully replanted by a team of surgeons, which included Dr Leo Mahoney. Twenty years later the *Toronto Star* (21 October 1987) carried the story of a man transported by helicopter for reattachment of a severed arm, this time by Dr Mahoney's son, James – chief of plastic surgery at St Michael's.

68 ASMH, W-4, no. 98, Dr K. Kovacs to Sister Camilla, archivist, 12 February 1985. See also ASMH, H-15, Dr Higgins's address to board of directors of Ontario Hospital Association, and MAB Minutes, 2 February 1976.

69 See Dr McCulloch's seven reports to the medical advisory board between 7 June 1971 and 10 September 1973 (ASMH). The CHAP was the Certified Hospital Admission Program, a method whereby each admission was surveyed by computer and norms were established for patient turnover in various dis-

ease categories. In his clinical practice Dr McCulloch pioneered at St Michael's the administration of the chymo-papin enzyme for spinal pain, a treatment that attracted to his service a large number of Americans, who did not have access to the treatment in their own country.

70 A quick review of ASMH's MAB Minutes shows a modest $75,000 approved for twenty researchers in the years 1967-72.

71 Ibid., 3 April 1976 and 13 September 1976.

72 ASMH, E-7, no. 670. The straight internship was offered in either medicine or surgery and was forty-eight weeks in length. The rotating internship consisted of eight weeks in each of medicine, surgery, paediatrics, obstetrics and gynaecology, psychiatry, and emergency, plus four weeks of an elective posting. In the family practice internship, time was divided equally among medicine, emergency, paediatrics, and obstetrics and gynaecology; it qualified the doctor for licensing as a family practitioner. The mixed internship called for eight weeks in each of emergency, obstetrics and gynaecology, and paediatrics as well as twenty-eight weeks divided betwen medicine and surgery (twelve and sixteen or sixteen and twelve).

73 MAB, 3 April 1972; not all departments were remiss, but major offenders were cited, in the presence of the chiefs of those departments.

74 Ibid., 5 February and 5 March 1973.

75 See, for example, ibid., 3 September 1968 and 7 April 1970.

76 Ibid., 1 November 1976.

Chapter 9

1 In November 1991 the University of St Michael's College conferred on Sister Mary the degree of doctor of sacred letters, *honoris causa*.

2 Peter C. Newman, *The Acquisitors: The Canadian Establishment* (Toronto: McClelland and Stewart, 1981), 17. In 1981 the Canadian Council of Christians and Jews presented Griffen with their Human Relations Award, an honour they reserve for outstanding Canadians and humanitarians.

3 The *Bond Issue* was inaugurated in 1977, edited by Jean Matthews and a small staff. The well-researched articles in this publication have been a valuable resource and are gratefully acknowledged by the author. Jean Matthews was, as well, director of public relations for many years, a position to which she brought an unmistakeable flair, combined with good judgment and a strong sense of the hospital's mission and philosophy.

4 Hynes was a partner in the law firm of Fraser and Beatty; Barr was chairman, Moore Corporation; Mr Justice Dubin was a judge on the Supreme Court of Ontario; Braide was vice-president of Canadian Industries; Dilworth was an executive with Touche Ross and Partners; O'Donoghue was an executive with Marsh and McLennan; Dr Hollenberg was vice-provost, health sciences, University of Toronto.

5 In October 1980 twenty-five hundred interns and residents in the twenty-three teaching hospitals of Ontario engaged in a six-day strike to support their collective bargaining demands.

6 See, for example, ASMH, Dr C.H. Hollenberg's paper delivered at the Edward F. Brooks Memorial Lectureship, 4 June 1979. See also MAB Minutes, 3 March 1980, and Board Minutes, 27 March 1980, regarding extra-billing (beyond OHIP rates) by physicians. With regard to OMA job action, see Board Minutes, 10 April 1982, and the telegram from the minister of health calling on the board and the medical advisory committee to discharge their responsibilities under the Public Hospitals Act.

7 ASMH, MAB Minutes, 5 March 1979 – arrangements had been made for medical residents to have special training in gerontology, and the chief resident in psychiatry was moving into geriatric psychiatry.

8 An addressograph card designed to record patient information at this time made provision for twenty-nine different nationalities.

9 In January 1983 St Michael's banned the sale of tobacco products on its premises and restricted smoking to certain designated areas.

10 *Report of the Health Planning Task Force* (the Mustard report), ix-xii and 32, 33.

11 *Report of the Special Program Review*, 20 November 1975 (the Henderson report), recommendations 8.9, 8.10, 8.11.

12 ASMH, Board Minutes, 20 October 1975. Letter to John Law, chairman of UTHA, from Donald L. Gordon, chairman of a three-member committee set up to express views on the future of UTHA, 10 October 1975. See also ASMH, MAB Minutes, 2 February 1976.

13 ASMH, Board Minutes, 4 February 1976.

14 ASMH, *Globe and Mail*, 15 December 1978.

15 The hospital's unexpended portion of OHRDP funds in 1973 dollars, adjusted for inflation, had grown by 1977 to $25,754,747.

16 ASMH, Board Minutes, 22 September 1977. This would be changed in 1984, when the decision was

made to complete the operating room floor, as well as the ICU/ACU floor and the supply-processing-and-dispatch floor.

17 Ibid., 7 December 1982.

18 At the time of writing, St Michael's hopes to begin construction on a new building within two years (*Toronto Star*, 13 February 1992).

19 ASMH, MAC Minutes, 1 November 1982 and 7 March 1983.

20 Author's interview with Al O'Brien, director of plant and engineering, October 1991.

21 ASMH, Board Minutes, 18 May 1984. Renovation costs were projected as $1,400,000; equipment and furnishings, $1,093,000; and additional operating costs of more than $900,000 annually. The roof of the E-wing had earlier been enclosed to provide a community room for the sisters; a part of this space was renovated in 1984 to provide a dining-room for the sisters and, as well, they retained their eighth floor sleeping quarters.

22 ARCAT, *Archdiocesan Directories*.

23 ASMH, MAB Minutes, November 1977, March 1978, November 1979.

24 The x-ray equipment for this laboratory was the first of its kind to be installed in North America, and St Michael's cardiac team was the first in the world to experiment with this equipment to do biplane (capable of filming from two angles simultaneously) coronary angiography. Although the x-ray equipment was designed and built in France, and the computer components in the United States and Canada, St Michael's own planning and engineering department was heavily involved in the design and construction of the new facilities.

25 ASMH, MAB Minutes, 27 October 1977 and 8 September 1980.

26 ASMH, Dr P. Forbath to Dr P. Higgins, 16 March 1981. Forbath estimated that the cost of the new angiography equipment would be between $500,000 and $2 million, and the new physiological recorder $150,000.

27 The source of much of the data on the various surgical divisions has been the documents submitted by their chiefs to the future directions committee of the university's department of surgery, chaired by Dr N. Colapinto (ASMH, S-761).

28 In 1980 Dr Hudson rerouted nerves to restore movement in a patient's arm – a first-in-Canada operation, which involved removing nerves from the lower leg and joining them to the nerves between the ribs and in the arm. Much of the material here is taken from an overview of the division of neurosurgery prepared by Dr Hudson in 1982 (ASMH, S-4).

29 ASMH, M-629. Dr Higgins published more than twenty-five articles, alone or with others, during the years 1959-78.

30 ASMH, MAC Minutes, Dr Higgins's report, 5 April 1982. The calendar for the University of Toronto faculty of medicine for 1981-82 lists the eleven hospitals that were being used for teaching: Toronto General; Hospital for Sick Children; St Michael's; Toronto Western; Clarke Institute of Psychiatry; Sunnybrook; Women's College; Wellesley; Princess Margaret (The Ontario Cancer Institute); Mount Sinai; Clinical Institute of ADR Foundation; and Lyndhurst Hospital. Of the eleven, the first four were commonly referred to as the "major" teaching hospitals.

31 ASMH, H-15, address of Dr Higgins to the board of OHA, 1984.

32 ASMH, M-6, no. 1195, 1986 report of the division of nephrology.

33 Ibid. In 1982 St Michael's became the first hospital in Toronto to introduce self-care dialysis in a hospital setting, a procedure that required a highly motivated patient but that put less stress on the patient and family than did home dialysis (*Bond Issue*, December 1982).

34 ASMH, MAB Minutes, 3 December 1979.

35 Ibid., 3 November 1980; also, Dr Higgins's address to Board of OHA 1984.

36 ASMH, Board Minutes, Dr Marotta's report to the board on the department of medicine, 16 May 1978.

37 Ibid., 17 February 1983.

38 ASMH, G-2-2, Patrick Beirne, "A Specialist Looks at Natural Childbirth" (only pages 40-6 are on file). The name of the journal is not cited.

39 Dr Beirne's letter to the editor, *Catholic Register*, 25 April 1981. While strongly pro-life, Dr Beirne disassociated himself from the methods of some factions of the movement (see his letter).

40 See also ASMH, Board Minutes, 30 September 1980, Dr Beirne's report to the board on the department of obstetrics and gynaecology. In 1981 Dr Beirne's contributions were recognized by the pope, who conferred on him the papal honour of Knight of St Sylvester.

41 Ibid., 28 June 1978. The somewhat embarrassed chairman of the board told his fellow members that the department of nursing, however, had received a very favourable appraisal.

42 ASMH, MAB Minutes, 3 April, 1 May, and 5 June 1978.

43 The criterion audit is a method whereby the medical staff selects a diagnosis or condition, develops cri-

Notes

teria that reflect the essential aspects of medical care for the patient with that diagnosis, then reviews medical charts, noting variations from the criteria, develops and implements solutions, and reaudits to ensure effectiveness of the solutions (*Bond Issue*, December 1978).

44 ASMH, MAB Minutes, 4 June 1979.

45 Ibid., 5 January 1981: an electrolyte survey had turned up twelve sets of electrolytes ordered on the day of the survey for no medically justifiable reason.

46 ASMH, Board Minutes, 3 October 1979. The observation was made at the meeting that 50 percent of hospitals at that time had a two-year accreditation standing.

47 ASMH, Press release by Hon. R. Elgie, minister of labour, 27 April 1981.

48 The St Lawrence neighbourhood stretched from Yonge Street to Parliament Street, ten city blocks, and south from Front Street and the Esplanade to the embankment.

49 According to a published interview in the *Globe and Mail*, 21 January 1981, the centre was financed by a $150,000 capital grant from the Ministry of Health, which also would contribute $40,000 a year in operating costs and doctors' fees. Nursing services of about $80,000 were to be shared 2/3:1/3 between the hospital and the city's public health department.

50 This was Dr E. Stuart Macdonald, in a letter to the *Globe and Mail*, published following the newspaper's report of the issue, 21 January 1981. On the office wall of the centre's physician, Dr Howard Seiden, there hung a mezuzah – a piece of parchment inscribed with Old Testament passages sacred to the Jews; so the councillor's charge of insensitivity towards those not of the sisters' faith was not quite accurate.

51 ASMH, *Annual Report*, 1984-85.

52 L.M. Cathcart and P. Berger, "Medical Examination of Torture Victims Applying for Refugee Status," *Canadian Medical Association Journal*, vol. 121, July 1979.

53 ASMH, MAB Minutes, 12 September 1977, Dr Horsey's comments on the Agnew, Peckham study of emergency departments, commissioned by UTHA in 1977.

54 One of the shortcomings of these rapid developments was in the estimation of expenses and receipts; the hospital guaranteed a level of income to emergency physicians, and in return depended on them to bill, collect, and render receipts to the hospital. In 1983-84 payments to the emergency physicians exceeded receipts to the hospital by $389,000 (ASMH, audit committee of board of directors, 29 May 1984).

55 ASMH, MAB Minutes, 1 September 1977.

56 Ibid., 1 May 1978.

57 See, for example, ibid., 4 June, 10 September, and 1 October 1979, and 4 February 1980. The university was attempting to introduce a requirement for clinical teachers to spend a certain amount of their time on university activities; hence, a ceiling on their income was set, which was not fully accepted by the teachers, nor was the university's suggestion as to the use of what the full-time teacher earned over his/her ceiling (ASMH, Board Minutes, 3 October 1979).

58 ASMH, MAB Minutes. See his letter of 17 September 1979 to the chairman of surgery, faculty of medicine.

59 Ibid., 2 June 1980. This was sparked by correspondence to Dr Horsey, chairman of the medical advisory committee of UTHA, from the university vice-provost, health sciences, following an incident at one of the teaching hospitals.

60 Ibid., 2 February 1981, and Ministry of Health to Council of Ontario Faculties of Medicine, 7 December 1981.

61 Ibid., 2 February 1981, and Board Minutes, 24 September 1981.

62 ASMH, MAC Minutes, 19 October 1981. It appears that the CV surgical staff were concentrating on their service demands at the expense of their academic responsibility for research and publication. At the same time the three St Michael's medical residents assigned to St Joseph's Hospital were cut, and the division of neurosurgery was cautioned that unless it improved its academic output, it was next in line for reductions. Later pathology lost a resident. (Board Minutes, 24 June 1982.)

63 ASMH, MAC Minutes, 30 August 1982, regarding a Ministry of Health news release on reassignment of post-graduate training posts, 14 July 1982, and discussion at the committee.

64 ASMH, Board Minutes, 29 June 1981. Dr Higgins's memorandum to the board.

65 ASMH, MAC Minutes, 11 April and 6 June 1983; Board Minutes, 12 April 1983.

66 Ibid., 10 October 1981.

67 Ibid., 17 February and 27 June 1983.

68 Ibid., 10 June 1983, Dean Lowy to chairman of the Hospital Council of Metropolitan Toronto.

69 "Treatment of Trauma Patients in Metropolitan Toronto," A Report of the Trauma Centre Task Force of D.H.C., January 1984. In his original proposal Dr Waddell had advised the board that the trauma unit

371

was important as insurance against erosion of its teaching programs through resident cut-backs (see ASMH, MAC Minutes, 2 November 1981); probably the Toronto General had a similar tactic in mind.

70 ASMH, Board Minutes, correspondence of Griffin with Ministry of Health, 17 April 1984. In June 1984 the hospital began to equip a trauma room in emergency, using funds from an anonymous donor, to accommodate the referred trauma cases (ibid., 25 June 1984).

71 Ibid., notes from a meeting with Ministry of Health officials on 28 February, when the ministry announced an addition of $4 million to the base budget.

72 ASMH, *Report of the Investigation by Edward Lane, Ralph Coombs and Donald Holmes of St. Michael's Hospital, August 30, 1991.* See also Statement of the Minister of Health [Hon. Elinor Caplan] to the Legislature, December 22, 1987, where she stated "my officials will be discussing the need for additional funding at St. Michael's as its caseloads increase over the next two to three years."

73 See *Bond Issue*, July 1982; also, SMH, MAC Minutes, 31 January 1984; 23 May 1984; and 21 November 1984.

74 Author's interview with Sister Raphael Kane, secretary-treasurer in the early 1950s when that office handled the employment of, and simple personnel records for, most of the paid staff except for nursing. The hospital supplied white striped pants to the orderlies to distinguish them from the cleaners who, until Sister Janet's term (1956-63), did not have a distinctive uniform.

75 See *Bond Issue*, July 1981. St Michael's had at this time students from the University of Toronto (dentistry, dietetics, medicine, pharmacy, psychology, rehabilitation medicine); from the Toronto Institute of Medical Technology (medical-laboratory technology, radiology); from George Brown College (nursing, respiratory technology); as well as from its own school of health record administration. Of particular interest is the large number of PhD psychology interns (four) in a department of only four staff psychologists and one consulting psychologist (*Bond Issue*, July 1982).

76 Since the late 1960s St Michael's had availed itself of the computer at the Hospital for Sick Children sponsored by the Teaching Hospitals' Regional Computer User Groups, which by 1971 was extending its services beyond payroll to include programming for haematology, clinical chemistry, and similar applications.

77 See *Bond Issue*, July 1977, and ASMH, MAB Minutes, 12 September 1977.

78 ASMH, Q-1, A-14-2. Some small installations had, however, been put in place – for example, a computerized billing and accounting system for emergency physicians' billing (ASMH, Board Minutes, 17 February 1983) and the medical records department had been equipped with Wang word processors in its central dictating pool.

79 ASMH, MAC Minutes, 3 May 1982, report of joint university-hospital relations committee.

80 Ibid., 10 January and 7 February 1983, and Board Minutes, 17 February 1983 and 12 April 1983, St Michael's had 600 staff who fell within the Ministry of Health's recommended guidelines, mainly in the renal-dialysis, intensive care, and acute care units, and the operating room, blood bank, and emergency. The hospital chose to administer the vaccine, but the total number receiving it is not recorded.

81 See *Bond Issue*, June 1984.

82 Following several infant deaths at the Hospital for Sick Children in 1982 the minister of health commissioned Mr Justice Charles Dubin to head a review committee into the matter. Among the ninety-eight recommendations of the Dubin report – which the Ministry of Health asked each hospital board to review for possible application to its own situation – were twenty-seven that had relevance for St Michael's; the cost for implementing same was estimated at $2.5 million. Apart from the recommendations mentioned in this chapter, the Dubin report recommended that staff nurses should hold baccalaureate degrees; to implement this would have added $480,000 annually to St Michael's nursing budget (ASMH, Board Minutes, 17 February and 31 March 1985).

83 There are numerous references in minutes of the pharmacy and therapeutics committee of Andrasko's concern in this regard. For example, in a small 1983 study she found that in one-third of the cases where intravenous metronidazole was ordered the indications for its use were not supported by the literature (ASMH, MAC Minutes, 3 October 1983).

84 ASMH, MAB Minutes, 5 April 1971. St Michael's had several pieces of expensive ophthalmology equipment and was about to purchase an Argon Laser, all of which it offered for the use of patients from other hospitals, subject to the approval of Dr Kelly.

85 Ibid., 3 April 1978. Dr Bird chaired a small committee of Drs Briant and Kopplin and Director of Finance Larry Thalheimer to put this system in place.

86 Ibid., 7 May 1979. In April 1979 the medical budget committee had approved a cardioangiographic diagnostic unit and monitoring equipment for the 9-F laboratory at a cost of $650,000 in response to the CV committee's "deep concern about the desperate state of its equipment" (Ibid., 2 October 1978).

87 Ibid., 3 November 1980. Also, in October 1979 Dr Tim Murray had proposed that the Research Society

buy word processors for its scientists and investigators.

88 See, for example, ibid., 4 May 1981; 2 May 1983 and 20 April 1984.

89 ASMH, Board Minutes, budget and finance committee, 13 September 1984.

90 ASMH, MAC Minutes, 21 September 1984.

91 ASMH, Board Minutes, 4 February 1976.

92 ASMH, MAB Minutes, proposal from Dr Platt, 1 May 1978.

93 Ibid., 7 November 1977.

94 ASMH, Board Minutes, 22 September and 23 November 1977.

95 ASMH, MAB Minutes, 2 October 1978.

96 ASMH, Board Minutes, 14 November 1979 and 10 January 1980.

97 Ibid., and MAB Minutes, both 3 November 1980.

98 ASMH, MAC Minutes, 1 March 1982.

99 ASMH, Board Minutes, 26 February 1982.

100 Ibid., budget and finance committee, 2 June and 19 October 1982.

101 ASMH, Board Minutes, 24 June 1982. Of all the board members, former Metro chairman William Allen stands out as ceaselessly pressing for cost containment. See also Board Minutes for 10 November 1981 and 7 December 1982.

102 Ibid., 7 December 1982.

103 ASMH, MAC Minutes, June 1983.

104 ASMH, Board Minutes, 5 April 1984. It is not clear what the board had in mind as "draconian"; but it suggested that such measures as the cost-effective use of drugs by medical staff only "chip away at" the problem. It put "medical manpower quotas" in this latter category, although there is no real evidence that there had been such a quota.

105 The consultants made other significant recommendations: for example, more effective planning for major capital projects which affected operational costs (such as cardiovascular programs) and an effective medical-manpower-planning system.

106 ASMH, MAC Minutes, 3 December 1984.

107 The nursing cuts were made in December 1984, but it was soon apparent that additional staff was needed for unplanned needs – trauma, suicidal patients, and so on – and the director of nursing, new to St Michael's and little over a year in the position, found herself confronted with grievances over workload. The author estimates that nursing hours in excess of budgeted hours for the months April and May 1985, if continued, would have amounted to $2 million by year's end – the very figure the nursing department had been challenged to save. (See ASMH, Board Minutes, budget and finance committee, 14 June 1985.)

108 ASMH, Board Minutes, 5 February 1985.

109 Ibid., budget and finance committee, 31 March 1985.

110 ASMH, Ontario Hospital Association's circular, F.Y.I., 2 July 1976.

111 ASMH, Board Minutes, 17 June 1985.

112 ASMH, MAC Minutes, 1 June 1981.

113 Ibid., 14 September 1981.

114 ASMH, MAB Minutes, February 1979.

115 ASMH, MAC Minutes, 2 May 1983.

116 ASMH, MAB Minutes, 3 April 1978.

117 Ibid., letter from Dr Dunn, 13 March 1979, and MAC Minutes, 7 December 1981.

118 The *Toronto Star* carried an article on 6 May 1989 that referred to the Interlink service established by Foy and Gay Evans; the latter had served first as volunteer and then as instructor on St Michael's palliative-care team. The *Star* article reported that a $1-million grant had just been received by Interlink for support of its work.

119 Author's interview with Alice McNamara, former acting operating-room supervisor and theatre supervisor, a few days before her death in April 1989.

120 ASMH, Board Minutes, 4 June 1984, Mrs Louis Wilson's report to the board.

121 St Michael's and St Joseph's Hospitals, Providence Villa and Hospital, Our Lady of Mercy Hospital, Sacred Heart Child and Family Centre, and St Joseph's Infirmary (for sick sisters) were the original six member institutions of the Health Services Planning Committee. This was reduced to four when St Joseph's Hospital and Our Lady Mercy merged in 1979 to become St Joseph's Health Centre, and Sacred Heart Child and Family Centre withdrew. In 1980 Sister Janet was appointed on a full-time basis to chair the health services planning committee; she was assisted by a full-time planner (Neville Chenoy) and a part-time financial analyst, an indication of the serious efforts being made by the sisters at this time to coordinate the activities of their institutions.

122 *Bond Issue*, December 1979, and Sister Janet's address at symposium held at St Michael's and reported in *Bond Issue*, December 1980.

123 ASMH, MAC Minutes, 19 October, 2 November, and 7 December 1981. The Quo Vadis committee developed into the long-range planning subcommittee of the medical advisory committee; its members were Dr M. Shea (chairman) and Drs Platt, Bird, Higgins, Horsey, Murray, Nethercott, and Waddell.

124 Ibid., 10 January 1983.

125 ASMH, Board Minutes, 29 November 1982, and MAC Minutes, 7 February 1983.

126 ASMH, Board Minutes, 2 May 1983. Members of the strategic planning committee were: Lawrence Hynes (chairman); William Allen, Mrs Kristine Thompson, Graham Constantine, Sister Catherine McDonough, Drs J. Waddell, P. Higgins, and D. Murray, and Mrs Jeanne Foxwell. Departments and divisions were ranked: first priority – those that should be strengthened in all aspects (fifteen); second priority – those that should be strengthened only in specific aspects (two); and third priority – those that should maintain the current level of service activity (twelve). (*Bond Issue*, December 1984.)

127 Ibid., 10 March, 10 April, and 24 June 1982; 22 June and 26 October 1983; and 8 February 1984. At the February meeting it was announced that Dilworth would serve as chairman of an interim management committee "until such time as Mr Conrad Black should bring together his own team"; in the meantime, Black had secured the commitment of three deputy chairmen. However, by April 1984 Black, who had consistently expressed doubts about the possibility of reaching such a high campaign target, had stepped down to be one of three co-chairmen.

128 By 31 March 1989 more than $23 million had been raised ibid., 28 March 1989).

Chapter 10

1 Faced with a steep rise in liability-insurance premiums, the OHA established a group-liability plan, Hospital Insurance Reciprocal of Ontario, in 1987. St Michael's elected to stay with its own carriers; although St Michael's had paid out only $212,000 in liability claims in the previous twelve years, its insurance premiums increased from $116,000 to $584,000 in 1985-86, and the board considered a proposal to increase the liability coverage from $5 million to $10 million per incident. (ASMH, Board Minutes 30 July 1985; 18 November 1986; 23 June 1987.)

2 *Globe and Mail*, 6 April 1991, quoting Statistics Canada's news release of 5 April 1991. By June 1991, 13.9 percent of Ontario's under-sixty population were on social assistance (*Globe and Mail*, 3 April 1992, quoting Ministry of Community and Social Services).

3 *Toronto Star*, 5 February 1991, quoting Metro Toronto's Community Services Department; also, *Globe and Mail*, 29 March 1991, quoting commissioner of same department.

4 *Toronto Star*, 26 March 1991 and 9 February 1992. The best-known of the food banks was the Daily Bread Food Bank, established through the initiative of Sister Marie Tremblay, CSJ.

5 *Toronto Star*, 26 March 1991.

6 On 29 October 1986 royal assent was given to the Toronto Hospital Act, which approved merger of the 1000-bed Toronto General Hospital and the 660-bed Toronto Western Hospital (*Globe and Mail*, 7 November 1986).

7 ASMH, F.Y.I., 12 August 1987.

8 See, for example, ASMH, Board Minutes, 16 September and 18 November 1986, and Dilworth's memorandum to board members, 9 September 1986.

9 For the flavour of these years, as reflected in the health-care field, the reader is referred to *Hospital News*, a monthly paper published in Toronto, its nineteen-member editorial board made up of representatives from Toronto hospitals and the OHA.

10 ASMH, AX-1619.

11 *Toward a Shared Direction for Health in Ontario* (Report of the Ontario Health Review Panel, June 1987, chaired by John R. Evans, MD). This panel endorsed many of the recommendations from previous task forces: John Hastings, *The Community Health Centre in Canada*, 1972; Edward Pickering, *Report of the Special Study Regarding the Medical Profession in Ontario*, 1973; Fraser Mustard, *Report of the Health Planning Task Force* (1974); Fraser Mustard, *Final Report of the Task Force to Review Primary Health Care* (1982); Ontario Council of Health and Ministry of Health, *Health Care: the 80s and Beyond* (1983).

12 ASMH, F.Y.I., 15 July 1987, and MAC Minutes, 5 October 1987.

13 Liberal Minister of Health Elinor Caplan was replaced by NDP Health Minister Evelyn Gigantes in November 1990; she resigned in April 1991, and was replaced by Frances Lankin.

14 *Hospital News*, October 1990. Later, in an interview published in the *Toronto Star* on 29 October 1991, the minister of health said, "The Province is serious about shifting funding from large institutions to community clinics, day surgery, and home care."

Notes

15 *Toward a Shared Direction*, 62.

16 President of OHA, quoted in *Toronto Star*, 16 November 1991 (2,900 out of 15,000 acute-care beds had been taken out of service).

17 See ASMH, Board Minutes, president's report, 23 January 1990. Over 800 job descriptions, excluding those of unionized nursing staff, were reviewed and analyzed. See also *Hospital News*, April 1991, announcing the creation by the provincial government of a $150-million fund to assist hospitals in covering the cost of pay equity. For the employer health tax levy, see ASMH, Board Minutes, 28 February 1990, "Operating Budget 1990-91."

18 Ibid., president's report, 23 January 1990; at that same meeting an interim board of the integrated St Michael's-St Joseph's facilities was announced, with Sister Marie Paradis as interim president of the merged institutions.

19 Within the year the Sister Christine Gaudet Scholarship was established to recognize Sister Christine's commitment to St Michael's during her term; the scholarship is for St Michael's staff or their children who wish to pursue studies in health-care-related fields.

20 ASMH, AX, Dilworth's memorandum, 9 September 1986, also, his memo to J. Lavoie, 18 November 1987 (ASMH, AX-1619). P.J. Keenan, Rudolph Bratty, and Sister Catherine McDonough were elected to the board in July 1985, as was Councillor Betty Disero from the city. W. Allen, D. Kinnear, and the Reverend A.J. MacDougall retired.

21 ASMH, Board Minutes, 16 November 1987. On that same date Dilworth addressed an inter-office communication to Lavoie expressing his concern that the board might not be receiving all of the information that it should, particularly relating to proper use of hospital resources. See also the minutes for 29 November 1988 and the Annual Report, 1988.

22 The four ministers of health were Murray Elston, Elinor Caplan, Evelyn Gigantes, and Frances Lankin. Dean Frederick Lowy of the faculty of medicine was replaced by Dean John Dirks. In 1985 L. Hynes was elected vice-chairman of the board, and P.J. Keenan, Rudolph P. Bratty, Sister Catherine McDonough, and Councillor Betty Disero became new directors. In 1986 Burke Doran, Timothy Price, Bernard Syron, and Sisters Janet Murray and Mechtilde O'Mara were elected; Anthony Griffin, L. Hynes, F. Udell, and Councillor J. Piccininni retired. Keenan was elected vice-chairman. In 1987 D.F. Sullivan and M.O. Sanderson were elected, and D. Barr retired. In 1988 J.F. O'Donnell, W. Deluce, Scott Griffin, W. James, and Sister June Dwyer were elected, and L.C. Burns, H. MacDougall, and Sanderson resigned, as did Sisters Catherine and Mechtilde. In September 1989 F. Anthony Comper was elected, and in January 1990 P.J. Keenan became acting chairman as Dilworth assumed the interim chairmanship of the board which was to govern the merged St Michael's-St Joseph's institutions. Medical chiefs who retired or resigned were Drs Horsey, Beirne, Cathcart, Bird, Stauble, Baker, Wilson, and Noble. In nursing, Mrs Louis Wilson, who had come in 1984, left in 1989; in pharmacy, Mrs Martha Andrasko was replaced after twenty-two years, and Mrs Bronwyn Morgan was replaced after several years as director of personnel.

23 In 1987 human resources and hospital services were reassigned to vice-presidents, and the new vice-president, finance (J. Lavoie), reported directly to the president. Sister Catherine became executive vice-president. In a further restructuring in November 1989 only three senior line staff (executive vice-president – J. Lavoie; vice-president, patient care – Ms Anita Fisher; and vice-president, medical affairs – Dr J. Platt) reported to the president, while five vice-presidents reported to Lavoie. In this structure, Lavoie chaired the major operations committee, while Sister Christine chaired the management executive committee responsible for policy matters and adherence to the strategic plan.

24 ASMH, Board Minutes, 4 November 1987 and 19 January 1988. A board committee chaired by David Braide, assisted by Graham Constantine, vice-president, planning and development, undertook implementation of the strategic plan. While areas of concentration were clearly stated, the actual ranking of programs in terms of priorities was less well enunciated; nothing was eliminated, and as a result the budget dollar was severely strained.

25 ASMH, M-1-1-3, no. 1272, reprint from *Medical Post*, 22 December 1987.

26 ASMH, M-1-1-3. Dr Chisholm teamed up with cardiovascular surgeon Dr Samuel Lichtenstein in what was believed to be the first procedure of its kind in Canada, where a blockage was removed from the main artery of the heart without surgery (*Globe and Mail*, 25 February 1989). Two years later Chisholm successfully used the technique on a pregnant woman to correct a heart valve narrowed as a result of rheumatic fever, saving the life of both mother and infant (*Toronto Star*, 14 March 1991).

27 ASMH, S-2, curriculum vitae, Tomas A. Salerno, MD.

28 ASMH, MAC Minutes, 2 February 1987.

29 ASMH, AX-1621, president's report, 24 January 1989.

30 ASMH, AX-1621. *Investigation of Cardiac Surgery at St. Michael's*, February 1989, by Vicki Kaminski,

William Sibbald, and Sister Elizabeth Davis.

31 Kaminski, Sibbald, and Davis, *Investigation*. Recommendations to St Michael's and to the Ministry of Health were for multi-disciplinary committees regarding goals, resource allocation, and planning; computerized data base; a patient-information officer; definition of resource needs; evaluation of the scheduling/booking system; a medical coordinator for the service; central triage; and public education. Still another recommendation was that "nursing and perfusion staff recruitment and retention efforts be coordinated in Metro Toronto with the intention of reducing inter-hospital competition, and enhancing inter-hospital cooperation – immediately."

32 Ibid., 30. (In the margin of the report filed in ASMH there is a handwritten insertion that St Michael's Joe Lavoie "is the leading expert in Hospital Cost Accounting in Canada. He has pioneered the use of Resource Intensity Weight and Case Mix Groupings. This will enable all hospitals to cost any procedure."

33 In an extensive interview with the *Toronto Star*, published 30 March 1990, Dr Garvey commented on the experience, early in her career, of proving herself in the man's world of medicine.

34 Between 1982 and mid-1987 there were 426 cases of AIDS reported in Ontario, the majority of whom lived in Toronto (*Ontario Hospitals Today*, vol. 2, no. 11, August 1987). In 1985 St Michael's admitted fifty-five AIDS patients, eleven of whom required ICU care; 128 tests per patient were performed (ASMH, MAC Minutes, 9 April 1986) – an indication of the research that accompanied patient care.

35 Sister Margaret McNamara and Dr Patrick Higgins served on the first board of Casey House. On 17 May 1988 eight physicians were appointed to the courtesy staff, St Michael's department of family and community medicine, for Casey House. (ASMH, MAC Minutes, 17 May 1988.)

36 Nurses were further recognized in 1990 when the Yvonne Erwin Memorial Scholarship for Neurosurgical Nurses was established, in honour of Yvonne Erwin, deceased, who had served as head nurse on neurosurgery.

37 When reporting on the proposal to St Michael's board on 16 September 1986 Sister Christine stated that the "financial impact is staggering: equipment $2.1 million, site preparation $2.3 million; annual operating cost $1.0 million."

38 ASMH, *Annual Reports*, 1986 and 1988; see also *Toronto Star*, 30 April 1989, for an account of a six-pound tumour removed by Dr Bell from a patient's thigh and pelvis.

39 ASMH, *Hospital News*, November 1987.

40 ASMH, *Pulse*, 10 March 1989.

41 ASMH, Board Minutes, 14 April 1987; 29 September 1987.

42 Ibid., 27 March 1990 and *Pulse*, 7 May 1990.

43 ASMH, *Annual Report*, 1985-86.

44 ASMH, MAC Mimutes, 4 May 1987 and *Pulse*, 21 July 1989.

45 ASMH, *Capsule News*, June 1987; and *Annual Reports*, 1985-86 and 1990. *The Endocrine Journal* pronounced St Michael's pituitary pathology laboratory "the best in the world" (*Annual Report*, 1990).

46 ASMH, MAC Minutes, 5 October 1987. This decision required an additional 3.2 full-time equivalent staff, and an additional $281,500 annually in supplies. In 1990 Dr K. Jeejeebhoy, who had earned international recognition for his studies in nutritional abnormalities associated with bowel disease, was appointed to staff with a view to developing an expanded home TPN (total parenteral nutrition) program (ibid., 2 April 1990).

47 *Pulse*, 10 February 1989. Dr Murray's work in diagnosis of osteoporosis by measuring the mineral content of bone was facilitated by the acquisition of a dual photon bone densitometer, donated by Mrs Clarice Chalmers, a generous benefactor of many of the hospital's and medical staff's efforts. Dr Murray's work received significant support, as well, from the group Women Against Osteoporosis, who in 1990-91 raised $120,000 to support the bone and mineral group (*Pulse*, January 1991 and 9 December 1991).

48 The unit was dedicated to the memory of Wallace B. Chalmers, in recognition of his and his family's support of St Michael's Hospital.

49 ASMH, Board Minutes, 29 September 1987; 19 January 1988; 29 March 1988; 27 September 1988; 16 May 1989; 27 March 1990.

50 For example, in February 1990 the ministry made additional funds available "to cover additional cardiovascular and trauma costs" (ibid., 27 March 1990).

51 See, for example, ASMH, MAC Minutes, 2 November 1987.

52 ASMH, Board Minutes, 23 June 1987. The members of the interim board of each corporation were Dilworth, Sister Christine, and J. Lavoie, who were also members of the executive committee of the board.

53 Scott Griffin, president of Meridian Technologies, was the son of former board chairman A.G.S. Griffin (see ASMH, Board Minutes, 8 March 1988). Later in the year he was elected to the board.

Notes

54 Ibid., 29 March 1988.

55 Ibid., 24 January 1989.

56 Ibid., 14 August 1989.

57 ASMH, Board Minutes, President's Report to the Sisters at St Michael's, November 1989.

58 ASMH, minutes of executive committee of the board, 12 November 1990, and Board Minutes, 6 December 1990.

59 ASMH, *F.Y.I.*, 12 August 1987.

60 ASMH, Board Minutes, 19 January 1988, and president's report to board, 29 March 1988: "Neurooncology and breast oncology appear to be the only two programmes with major academic foci that will be at St Michael's." See also minutes for 28 November 1989.

61 *Pulse*, 27 May 1991.

62 *Capsule News*, 30 April 1985 and *Pulse*, 15 March 1991.

63 ASMH, Board Minutes, 17 May 1988, and Sister Christine's address to the sisters at St Michael's, November 1989.

64 ASMH, Cardinal Carter to Webster, 16 September 1988, also, Board Minutes, report of ethics committee, 16 May 1989.

65 Report of ethics committee, 21 June 1988 and 16 May 1989. See also Dr Webster's work, and his collaboration with Dr Robert Byrick, director of ICU, as reported in *Macleans*, 1 May 1989, and *Toronto Star*, 2 April 1989.

66 ASMH, Board Minutes, president's report to the board of directors, 20 January 1987.

67 ASMH, MAC Minutes, 1 April 1985. Dr John Schuman, of Providence Villa and Hospital, had been given a cross-appointment at St Michael's in 1981.

68 See *Bond Issue*, December 1987.

69 ASMH, planning and programs committee report, dated 20 March 1989, prepared for presentation to board of directors meeting of 28 March 1989.

70 ASMH, Board Minutes, 2 May 1985.

71 Ibid., executive director's report to the board, 19 November 1985 and 16 September 1986.

72 Ibid., president's report to the board, 23 June 1987.

73 Ibid., 28 November 1989. In 1989-90 the Women's Health Care Centre treated 17,000 patients (ASMH, a document entitled "61 Queen Street East St Michael's Health Care Centre," showing services and volumes on each floor, dated 23 January 1990).

74 Author's interview with Mrs C. Shevlin, nursing coordinator, 5 May 1992; the research here mentioned was guided by Ellen Hodnett, BScN, PhD, faculty of nursing, University of Toronto.

75 For these figures, and other details on community health care, see *Annual Report*, 1988 and *Bond Issue*, December 1989.

76 Peggy Ann Walpole and her work have been the subject of more than one newspaper article. See, for example, *Toronto Star*, 23 March 1990.

77 ASMH, Board Minutes, 20 June 1989, and *Pulse*, 5 October 1990. Dr Jenkins held a cross-appointment from the department of nutrition, University of Toronto. A world-authority on the place of dietary fibre in health and disease, Dr Jenkins worked with Drs Josse, Wong, and Wolever, of St Michael's staff, in his research. (*Annual Report*, 1985-86). The Kellogg Company of Battle Creek, Michigan, also made a substantial donation towards the centre (ASMH, Board Minutes, 20 June 1989).

78 The term is used in the *Annual Report*, 1990.

79 ASMH, Board Minutes, 8 September 1987.

80 ASMH, AX-1623, report by the IBI group, 27 August 1987.

81 Special joint meeting of their two committees, 28 August 1987.

82 ASMH, MAC Minutes, 2 March 1987 and 6 April 1987.

83 ASMH, report to special meeting of board of directors, 8 September 1987. A statement of space requirements was presented: 11,250 sq. ft. was needed immediately, but only 1,600 available; it was estimated that forty-two of eighty-one physicians with on-site offices could be relocated to the new building, freeing up their current space for other needs.

84 On 5 October 1987 Lavoie told the medical advisory committee there was a potential of $2 million in growth funds.

85 ASMH, Board Minutes, 29 September 1987. A document contained with the board materials for the 24 November 1987 meeting indicates that the building was purchased by 738215 Ontario Ltd. A puzzling entry in the *Annual Report*, 1988, states that the purchase was "fully financed by a unique offering to the Hospital," which may explain some of the later revelations of confusion surrounding the purchase. See also audit committee, 19 January 1988, whose report is among the documents for the January board meeting. This report was listed on the agenda, but minutes do not indicate whether it was ever discussed.

377

86 ASMH, MAC Minutes, 2 November 1987 and 24 November 1987. Only three out of eighty-one of these were paying rent.

87 ASMH, Board Minutes, report of building and property committee, 24 November 1988. The original estimate of $1 million for renovations had grown to $2,246,000; the eventual renovation cost was $4.3 million, plus interest costs because of the time delay.

88 Report by the IBI group.

89 ASMH, Board Minutes, president's report to the board, 27 September 1988, and "Historical Review of 61 Queen Street East," presented to board on 22 October 1990.

90 President's report, 27 September 1988, and ASMH, Board Minutes, 22 May 1990.

91 "Innovative Fund Raising: The St Michael's Hospital Health Centre," by George H. Pink, Raisa B. Debar, Joe N. Lavoie, and Eric Aserlind (Project No. 6606-3989-Ht, National Health Research and Development Program, Health and Welfare Canada, November 1989). The 61 Queen Street East project is examined as a case study of a "recent example of innovative financing" (1-31).

92 ASMH, Board Minutes, 17 June 1985.

93 ASMH, Board Minutes, president's report, 29 September 1987. *F.Y.I.* reported on 6 May 1987 that there were 1283 vacant RN positions in Ontario, 59 percent of which were in Metro and 38 percent in teaching hospitals.

94 ASMH, Board Minutes, executive director's report, 18 November 1986.

95 Ibid., Board Minutes, 17 June 1985.

96 Ibid., president's report, 29 September 1987.

97 Ibid., president's report, 24 October 1988.

98 ASMH, MAC Minutes, 16 September 1986 and 3 April 1989; Board Minutes, president's report, 31 October 1987.

99 Two 1988 studies on the question (one by RNAO and one by the Hospital Council of Metropolitan Toronto) revealed common threads: the desire of nurses for greater flexibility of work scheduling, better recognition, more support by administration, increased educational opportunities, and pay adjustments (*F.Y.I.*, 16 November 1988).

100 ASMH, Board Minutes, president's report, 21 June 1988; also, an update on nursing, August 1988. The picture may have been even worse: in September 1988 the director of nursing told the board that the use of registry nurses had increased the hospital's cost of providing nursing service by $3.8 million annually, only $1.3 million of which was in the approved budget (ibid., 27 September 1988).

101 Ibid., 20 June 1989; also, report on nursing issues, by A. Fisher, to the president, 19 November 1989, and *Hospital News*, February 1990. The report of the investigation into scheduling of cardiovascular surgery at St Michael's (October 1988) had commended the hospital on the success of its recruitment efforts, and its subsequent preparation of these nurses for their critical-care responsibilities.

102 ASMH, Board Minutes, document entitled "Situation of Nursing Staff Since Beds Have Closed," dated 24 October 1988; and president's report, 28 March 1989 and 19 September 1989.

103 Ibid., president's report, 16 May 1989.

104 See ASMH, MAC Minutes, April 1987 and 8 May 1987, and Board Minutes, 12 May 1987. Also, in an article published in the magazine *Health Management Forum* (Spring 1987), 42-52, Sister Catherine McDonough and Andrew P. Vaz reported on their review of utilization of the hospital's facilities at this time; they speak of the "sensitivity of the project," which was viewed by some as an encroachment on the "power" and "autonomy" of the medical staff.

105 Vice-presidents of nursing were attempting to get separate bargaining for nurses staffing the downtown hospitals (ASMH, Board Minutes, 19 September 1989).

106 ASMH, MAC Minutes, 3 October 1988 and 24 January 1989; Board Minutes, 23 January and 27 March 1990.

107 *Annual Report*, 1990.

108 Board Minutes, 27 March and 17 April 1990.

109 Ibid., 23 October and 6 December 1990.

110 Ibid., Report by Ray Briggs to board of directors, May 1985. Moore, president of Network Data Systems, had resigned his directorship on St Michael's board to chair this important project.

111 ASMH, Board Minutes, report of meeting with Ministry of Health and Ministry of Community and Social Services, 4 May 1985; and Board Minutes, 11 September 1985.

112 Ibid., 23 June 1987 and *CHIPS TODAY*, November 1987.

113 ASMH, planning and development project budget, 1987-88, contained with Board Minutes, September 1987.

114 See article "Curing what Ails the System," by Bruce Little in the *Globe and Mail*, 18 January 1992.

115 The "parent Board" of the St Joseph's Health System was to be concerned with enhancement of Christ-

ian values in the various institutions, as well as with overall financing and planning, development of shared projects, and evaluation of quality of service (ASMH, Board Minutes, Sister Janet reporting to St Joseph Health System board of directors, 9 April 1986).

116 Among the achievements during the two years 1986-88 were the appointment of Sister Ann Delaney to develop a process for evaluating adherence to the sisters' values (ASMH, Board Minutes, 9 April 1986); initiation of a joint proposal for acquisition of an MRI (ibid., 29 September 1987); initiation of a shared hospital information system (ibid., 14 April 1987); initiation of shared security, biomedical engineering, and printing services; and geriatric assessment, both at the inter-institutional and regional levels (ibid., 29 September 1987).

117 Ibid., Sister Janet, speaking to board of directors, 24 November 1987.

118 ASMH, Touche Ross, "Report to The St Joseph Health System," June 1988, 18, 35.

119 ASMH, Board Minutes, address by Sister Imelda Cahill, general superior and chairperson of board of St Joseph's Health System, to the board, 22 November 1989. Sister Imelda said that Providence Villa, because of its unique character, did not fit within the council's vision of integration for the time being. For the doctors' response to the merger, see ASMH, MAC Minutes, 4 December 1989.

120 ASSJ, circular letter from Sister Imelda Cahill to the congregation, 16 January 1990.

121 The name "Fontbonne" has had a very significant place in the history of the Sisters of St Joseph. Mother St John Fontbonne re-established the Sisters of St Joseph in Lyons, France, after they had been dispersed during the French revolution; in 1836 she sent her two nieces, Mother Febronia and Mother Delphine Fontbonne, to establish at St Louis, Missouri, the first foundation of the Sisters of St Joseph in North America. From there in 1851, as explained in Chapter 1, Mother Delphine, at the request of the bishop of Toronto, came to establish the first foundation of the Sisters of St Joseph in Toronto; she died five years later, having contracted typhus during her ministrations to typhus victims in their homes.

122 ASMH, Appendix A to hospital/university agreement, 1988-89. Appendix D to the agreement stated the specifications for a University of Toronto nursing-clinical unit, to be associated with the faculty of nursing. Increased liaison with the latter had evolved, with a nurse faculty member serving on the search committee for a vice-president, nursing, for St Michael's in 1989-90.

123 *Annual Report*, 1985-86 and 1989; also ASMH, MAC Minutes, 6 October 1986, which details success in LMCC examinations, and Board Minutes, 20 January 1987 and 16 May 1989.

124 Ibid., Board Minutes, 24 January 1989 and *Annual Report*, 1990.

125 In May 1988 Henry Botchford assumed the position of vice-president, development and external relations; he resigned on 1 December 1989. Mrs Ingrid Perry Peacock, who had extensive experience in fund-raising, was appointed director of development in early 1990.

126 ASMH, see the foundation's newsletter, *The Column*, vol.1, no.1, Spring 1991. Chaired by Hartland M. MacDougall, the initial board consisted of Dr Hans Abromeit, Conrad M. Black, Latham C. Burns, Timothy K. Griffin, Sister Margaret McNamara, Mrs Wendy Cecil-Cockwell, Mrs Judy L. Cohen, Mrs H. Ingrid Perry Peacock, Dr H. Patrick Higgins, Roger S. Hunt, Alan J. Dilworth, Richard R. Kennedy, Jack H. Kenney, Donald J. Smith, John H. Tory, and G. Kingsley-Ward, Sr.

127 ASMH, vol. 5, Minutes of the Women's Auxiliary Meeting, May 1943 to 13 March 1963. See minutes of ten meetings between 25 February 1947 and 25 May 1948. The name was changed to Hospital Auxiliary in the 1970s.

128 *Pulse*, 12 March 1990.

129 See *St Michael's Hospital Medical Bulletin*, vol.1, no.1 (1922).

130 *The Column*, vol.1, no.2 (Spring 1991); *Pulse*, 7 June 1991.

131 ASMH, Board Minutes, budget and finance committee, 21 March 1985.

132 Ibid., 16 May 1989.

133 Ibid., Financial Highlights, 31 August 1989.

134 Ibid., 27 March 1990.

135 Ibid., 16 May 1989.

136 Ibid., J. Lavoie to assistant deputy minister of health, 4 September 1990.

137 The February 1988 financial report to the board states "after discussion with our auditors we have decided to take the full amount of our billings into revenue ($850), and appropriate a reserve from equity for the amount in dispute."

138 *Report of the Investigation by Edward Lane, Ralph Coombs and Donald Holmes of St. Michael's Hospital, 30 August 1991*, 52.

139 ASMH, Board Minutes, J. Lavoie to assistant deputy minister of health, 4 September 1990. Lavoie was aggressive in his pursuit of the increased funding; in a "Record of WCB patients for 12 months ending March 31, 1990" there is a request for the per diem rate to be raised to $1,161 and an additional emergency charge fee of $450 charged for those patients (82) admitted through emergency. With 327 WCB

patients totalling 2488 days of care and an emergency fee, St Michael's had been maintaining a $3 million accounts receivable on its books for more than a year.

140 ASMH, MAC Minutes, 2 March, 6 April, 14 September, and 2 November 1987; 2 May and 17 May 1988. At this latest meeting a chief explained that many verbal agreements made years ago between certain staff and the hospital, entered into in good faith, would be terminated by the proposed policy. See also ASMH, Board Minutes, 8 September 1987, where it was noted that of the eighty-one physicians with on-site office space only three were paying some sort of rent. See also ibid., 24 November 1987; 27 September 1988; 3 January and 20 June 1989; and minutes of executive committee 6 March 1990.

141 ASMH, Board Minutes, 19 January, 27 September, 31 October, and 29 November 1988. While the January records suggested that $40 million-worth of assets would be for sale, the 31 October notes record "Sale of Assets – $21,650,000."

142 Ibid., 8 September 1987; 22 May 1990.

143 See ibid., 29 November 1988; also, report of G. Constantine, vice-president, programmes and planning, to the medical advisory committee (MAC Minutes, 5 December 1988). See Board Minutes, 29 March 1988, for board request for report on programs that had been, or would be, eliminated, and Board Minutes, 22 May 1990, requesting information as to what savings had been realized as a result of bed closings.

144 ASMH, MAC Minutes, 2 March 1987 and 1 June 1987; Board Minutes, 12 May 1987.

145 *Annual Report*, 1988; *Pulse*, December 1988; and ASMH, Board Minutes, 28 March 1989.

146 A quick check of the MAC and Board Minutes shows twenty-six appointments to the medical staff between 6 June 1988 and 20 June 1989 even as beds had been drastically reduced for lack of nursing staff.

147 ASMH, Board Minutes, 28 March 1989.

148 Ibid., Financial Highlights, 28 February 1990.

149 Ibid., Auditors' notes to financial statements, year ending 31 March 1990.

150 ASSJ, circular letter to the congregation from Sister Mary Beth Montcalm, 15 February 1991; See, as well, *Report of the Investigation by Edward Lane, Ralph Coombs and Donald Holmes of St. Michael's Hospital, 30 August 1991*. Lane was past chairman of Ottawa Civic Hospital and a director of Canada Post Corporation; Coombs was past president of Foothills Hospital, Calgary; Holmes was an auditor with Ernst and Young, Toronto.

151 Lane, Coombs, and Holmes, *Report*, 16, 21, 22, 24, 25, 32.

152 Ibid., 21, 22, 29, 30.

153 Ibid., 6, 7, 8, 29, 30, 54, 55.

154 Ibid., 31, 32, 37, 38, 41, 44, 45, 55, 57.

155 Ibid., 56.

156 Ibid., 89-102.

157 Ibid., 89.

158 Ibid., 89.

159 *Pulse*, 27 February 1992. See also *Toronto Star*, 2 March 1992. Among The Friends of St Michael's are actor John Candy, singer Gordon Lightfoot, author Joan Callwood, broadcaster Jeremy Brown, Police Chief William McCormick, Dave Garrick of the Skydome, Jack Kenney, president of the Jockey Club, and Nick Yioladassis, owner of St Michael's long-time neighbour, the Silver Rail.

160 Jeffrey Lozon became chief operating officer in September 1991 and president in April 1992 upon the resignation of Roger Hunt.

161 *Hospital News*, March 1992.

162 Author's interview with Jeffrey Lozon, 12 August 1992.

Index